Patient-Centered E-Health

E. Vance Wilson
Arizona State University, USA

Medical Information Science Reference

MEDICAL INFORMATION SCIENCE REFERENCE

Hershey · New York

Director of Editorial Content: Kristin Klinger
Senior Managing Editor: Jennifer Neidig
Managing Editor: Jamie Snavely
Assistant Managing Editor: Carole Coulson
Copy Editor: Laura Kochanwoski
Typesetter: Carole Coulson
Cover Design: Lisa Tosheff
Printed at: Yurchak Printing Inc.

Published in the United States of America by
Information Science Reference (an imprint of IGI Global)
701 E. Chocolate Avenue, Suite 200
Hershey PA 17033
Tel: 717-533-8845
Fax: 717-533-8661
E-mail: cust@igi-global.com
Web site: http://www.igi-global.com

and in the United Kingdom by
Information Science Reference (an imprint of IGI Global)
3 Henrietta Street
Covent Garden
London WC2E 8LU
Tel: 44 20 7240 0856
Fax: 44 20 7379 0609
Web site: http://www.eurospanbookstore.com

Library of Congress Cataloging-in-Publication Data

Patient-centered e-health / E. Vance Wilson, editor.
p. ; cm.
Includes bibliographical references and index.
ISBN 978-1-60566-016-5 (hardcover : alk. paper)
1. Medical informatics. 2. Medical telematics. 3. Medical personnel and patient. I. Wilson, E. Vance (Ellis Vance)
[DNLM: 1. Medical Informatics--trends. 2. Internet. 3. Medical Records Systems, Computerized--trends. 4. Patient-Centered Care--trends. 5. Self Care--trends. W 26.5 P2983 2009]
R858.P384 2009
610.285--dc22

British Cataloguing in Publication Data
A Cataloguing in Publication record for this book is available from the British Library.

List of Reviewers

Paul Ambrose
University of Wisconsin-Whitewater, USA

Natalie Armstrong
University of Leicester, UK

Michael Bliemel
Dalhousie University, Canada

Gloria M. Boone
Suffolk University, USA

Jed Bopp
University of Colorado at Boulder, USA

Nathan Botts
Claremont Graduate University, USA

Richard Burkhard
San Jose State University, USA

Joseph A. Cazier
Appalachian State University, USA

Elizabeth Cummings
University of Tasmania, Australia

Juanita Dawson
Claremont Graduate University, USA

Liqiong Deng
University of West Georgia, USA

Brian E. Dixon
Regenstrief Institute, USA

Omar F. El-Gayar
Dakota State University, USA

Jesus Favela
CICESE, Mexico

Stefano Forti
Fondazione Bruno Kessler, Italy

Linda M. Gallant
Emerson College, USA

Nicole Garcia
Claremont Graduate University, USA

Biswadip Ghosh
University of Colorado at Denver, USA

Amy Hennington
Middle Tennessee State University, USA

Morten Hertzum
Roskilde University, Denmark

Neset Hikmet
University of South Florida, USA

Abhi Jain
Northern Michigan University, USA

Jan-Are Kolset Johnsen
Norwegian Centre for Telemedicine, Norway

Nelson King
American University of Beirut, Lebanon

Richard Klein
Clemson University, USA

Nancy Lankton
Michigan State University, USA

Table of Contents

Detailed Table of Contents

In Chapter III we look at some fundamental aspects of communicating about ourselves and our health through technology. In particular, we examine how the social psychological theories of self-presentation and self-regulation might be applied to online health-communication. It is argued that the specific qualities of text-based communication might have unique benefits for health-communication through the interplay between the writing process and the concerns posed by health-issues. An understanding of how psychological processes are connected with online health communication is believed to be fundamental in understanding trends within self-help and user-driven health communication, and to predict possible outcomes of such behavior. Also, this knowledge might inform the design and development of patient-centered solutions for health-communication and heath-service delivery.

An increasing focus on e-health and a governmental push to improve healthcare quality while giving patients more control of their health data have combined to promote the emergence of the personal health record (PHR). The PHR addresses timeliness, patient safety, and equity, goals that the Institute of Medicine has identified as integral to improving healthcare. The PHR is vital to the National Health Information Network (NHIN) that is being developed to give all Americans access to electronic health records by 2014. This chapter looks at how PHRs address the needs, desires, and expectations of patients, explores the data quality concerns regarding patient-generated information (data capture, sharing and integration with other systems), discusses social implications of adoption, and concludes with a discussion of the evolving role that PHRs play in the growth of patient-centered e-health.

Newly disabled workers are often unemployed, uninsured, and indigent. They are in desperate need of Social Security OASDI monthly benefits, and the Medicare health insurance that follows 24 months after benefits begin. Applicants must prove that their medical conditions (excluding drug and alcohol abuse) have resulted in severe functional limitations that prevent them from any gainful employment. Delays and denials of benefits result when applicants cannot find or retrieve medical records from providers familiar with their medical history, health status, and functional limitations. The disability application workflow is complex, particularly for applicants with cognitive and mental health impairments. Health information technology (HIT) has been used to automate care delivery workflow through provider-controlled, electronic health record systems (EHRs). Disability applicants' workflow could, just as well, be automated through consumer-controlled, unbound, and intelligent personal electronic health record systems (PHRs), which are not tethered to a health plan or employer network, and which automatically exchange information updates with authorized providers' EHRs. Applicants' PHRs may later prove helpful with self-management of chronic conditions prior to Medicare coverage and with periodic reevaluations of their medical status.

In Chapter VI we review key concepts, using the marketing mix framework, to identify the needs of healthcare consumers, and the tools and services that can fulfill these needs. Unlike traditional healthcare delivery, patient-centered e-health (PCEH) involves the consumer as a partner and has a number of marketing implications. A more informed understanding of PCEH will help practitioners and researchers to formulate marketing strategies that improve healthcare outcomes and are acceptable to patients.

This chapter introduces the privacy management framework as a means of studying patient-centered e-health. The chapter raises some important issues in regards to the privacy domain of e-health and offers a privacy framework to look at the issue that addresses some of the concerns people and industries have regarding privacy. The framework does not neglect the important distinction between the different interests affected by e-health. It acknowledges the voluntary nature of the way in which individuals have surrendered control over personal information in exchange for the benefits that information technology brings. Because the applications of information technology are logically malleable, there are sufficient strategic reasons to suggest that privacy management as a concept and practice will survive, and that to ignore privacy issues might be fatal for the success of PCEH.

Patient-centered e-health (PCEH) offerings see the emergence of divergent, new third parties, through initiatives, including (a) medical content aggregation, (b) health-based online communities, and (c) patient-physician Internet-based portals. Here, the product is digital and heterogeneous for medical content aggregators; virtual and heterogeneous for online communities; and digital, context-specific, and asynchronous for patient-physician portals. With patients expressing privacy and confidentiality concerns in communicating personal health information electronically, growing numbers of PCEH initiatives give rise to many unique issues with respect to patient trust. Existing electronic commerce research focuses on trust in online vendors, potentially providing an incomplete picture with respect to patient trust in PCEH. An accurate and holistic understanding of patient trust encompasses different combinations of cognitive processes, disposition to trust, and institution-based trust, all shaping trusting beliefs in these different PCEH initiatives.

Chapter IX deals with the principles and practice of patient and public involvement in e-health research, and discusses some of the issues raised. In the first part of this chapter, we discuss the problems of defining an "e-health consumer," and discuss why, how and when to involve consumers in e-health research. We also set out principles to guide effective consumer involvement, and the benefits that this can bring in the e-health arena. In the second part of this chapter, we describe how consumers were successfully involved, through a variety of methods, in the development and evaluation of an Internet-based intervention to aid diabetes self-management. Patient and public involvement in research is not the same as undertaking research on patients or the public. It is about understanding, incorporating and benefiting from the relevant consumer perspective, at various levels, throughout the stages of a project.

This chapter presents a case study of using interaction design methods for exploring and testing usability and user experience of a personal health record (PHR) user interface based on visual and graphical elements. To identify problems and improve the design of PHR user interface we conducted two task-oriented usability testing based on the think-aloud technique for observing users during their interaction with a high-fidelity PHR prototype, and questionnaires and semistructured interviews for measuring user satisfaction. Our study demonstrates that a user-centered approach to interaction design involving the final users in an iterative design-evaluation process is important for exploring innovative user interfaces and for identification of problems in the early stages of the development cycle of a PHR

This chapter explores the use of Web sites to provide patients with understandable information about the quality and price of healthcare (healthcare transparency). Our first objective is to discuss patients' perceptions of empowerment and need for quality and cost information when choosing medical providers and facilities for healthcare procedures. To meet this objective, we address issues of patient awareness of sources of healthcare quality and cost information, perceived responsibility for managing healthcare costs, and knowledge of appropriate actions to exercise choice of providers. Our second objective is to investigate the potential of Web-based tools, which provide healthcare quality and cost information, to facilitate patients' decision-making processes regarding choice of provider for healthcare services, particularly common outpatient procedures. To meet this second objective, we use insights from user-centered design procedures (e.g., focus groups and in-depth interviews) associated with the development of a healthcare transparency Web-based tool.

This chapter is drawn from a comprehensive study that examined the effect Human-computer interaction usability factors had on rural residents' perception of trust in e-health services. Written comments provided by participants were drawn upon to develop a qualitative assessment of dimensions that are important to rural residents' perceptions of e-health. Identification of these dimensions will aid e-health system designers and administrators in creating better e-health applications.

This chapter explores how in developing patient-centred e-health systems it is possible to accommodate heterogeneous characteristics of end-users and their diverse health and care contexts. It concurs with conventional sociotechnical design paradigms that argue systems must be easy to use, fulfill a perceived need, and present a clear value proposition to ensure successful adoption and utilisation by patients. The chapter also highlights the need for awareness of a number of key challenges relating to emerging discourses on 'empowering patients' and 'e-health'. The implications of these challenges for the development of a truly patient-centred e-health approach are explored in a detailed case study. This chapter contributes to research focused on supporting patients to become genuine co-participants in their own care, health and well-being. However, it also acknowledges that part of the challenge of achieving this goal requires a focus on assisting clinicians to learn to respond to this shift in the autonomy of decision-making.

Chapter XIV investigates asthmatics' reasons for not adopting an e-health system for asthma self-management. An understanding of these reasons is particularly relevant, because clinical evidence indicates that, if used, such systems lead to better asthma management. The investigated asthma system is, however,

Foreword

Growing interest in consumer health informatics on the one hand, and continuing advances in health information technology (HIT) on the other are setting the stage for the emergence of the Patient-Centered E-Health (PCEH) discipline. Expectedly, this specialization of e-health and emerging PCEH applications are directly benefiting patients and their caregivers. Indeed, given its appeal to both patients and their caregivers in recent years, PCEH promises to not only strengthen the patient-provider relationship, but also bridges their communication gaps in the twenty-first century and beyond. Herein lies the distinguishing contribution of this work to the broadening diversification found in the extant e-health literature. A major significance of this compendium, therefore, is in shaping the future and focus of e-health research in a domain that is aligned with a more informed patient population, a trend towards greater individual accountability for self-care, a cry for more public accessibility, improved availability and affordability of healthcare, and an effort to make delivery of e-health services on an increasingly global scale. In a nutshell, PCEH represents one of the paradigm shifts that I have noted in today's *e-Healthcare Information Systems Age* where not only is the role of healthcare providers being redefined, but where the expectation bar for consumers to participate actively in decisions leading to their own health, as well as the overall quality and acceptability of e-healthcare informatics and services are being raised.

How, then, should one go about accumulating and documenting the theories and methods underlying the structures and limitations, and the range of applications still waiting to be explored in the PCEH knowledge domain? In this light, Dr. Vance Wilson has provided us an excellent showpiece covering a wide range of PCEH-related topics generated from a multitude of disciplinary perspectives. An examination of how the chapters of this volume have been ordered, integrated, and presented showed that both foundational areas and applications are key to our understanding of the PCEH field. On the foundation side, the reader's interest is first perked with an opening chapter on how e-health technology redefines the relationship between the patient and the healthcare provider. This is followed by insights on new methods for PCEH system design and development, by illustrative thoughts on ways to improve health literacy and communications through e-technology, by emerging concepts of personal health records (PHR) to securely and robustly capture, store, and exchange sensitive health information, and finally, by detailed discussions on privacy, trust, and e-technology marketing ideas not only for the typical patient and the general public, but also for the needy, the disabled, and the underserved. On the application side, the contributed pieces focused on PCEH system acceptability and usability factors, and several other key PCEH-related technology adoption factors, and the use of Web-based tools to enhance healthcare transparency. A study on predicting PCEH system use as moderated by effects of facilitating conditions and patients' behavioral intention serves to close this part of the discussion.

What ingredients, specifically, are critical to ensure the success and significance of future PCEH research and development? Dr. Wilson noted a combination of three such ingredients in his *Preface*, namely, PCEH systems that are *patient-focused, patient-active,* and *patient-empowered.* In this regard, I concur with his view and would like to further emphasize why these ingredients are particularly important for future PCEH initiatives. First, a system that is *provider-focused* will not be appealing to the patient. Unfortunately, the majority of HIT applications developed have mostly been *provider-focused*, rather than personalized to the patients so that they could be connected to "their own physicians, clinics, and records" interactively. Second, to elicit the active participation of the patient, the system should have all of the necessary characteristics that enhance use and acceptance by the patient (user). Here, Wilson noted the example of personal health records (PHR) where implementation failure is probably a result of "poor usability [...] privacy issues (or) lack of health content integration." I find this true to many of my own research—for example, in designing the *eHealthSmart system*, a PCEH system to close the disparity gap for seniors in key specific areas of health promotion, such as smoking cessation and weight control, much of our software development effort has to be devoted to designing a user interface that meets the needs of the elderly person, whether it be to overcome their hearing problem, deteriorating eyesight, or their ability to maneuver the keyboard and the mouse. Finally, the use and design of *patient-empowered* systems such as the ability of the patient to schedule a doctor's visit online via a PCEH application puts PCEH in the forefront of health information sciences and consumer health informatics. After all, if many of the individual patient's concerns can be fixed through self-help with the aid of various PCEH applications, it would translate to a highly efficient, low cost, safe, and good quality e-healthcare service delivery system that would gradually transform and replace our aging traditional healthcare delivery system.

This volume challenges the next generation e-health researchers and practitioners to promote the awareness of PCEH concepts, methods, and applications and how they differ from other forms of e-health. Those who have been the early adopters of these concepts, methods and applications have now opened the doors of the PCEH knowledge domain to future innovation, research, and development.

Joseph Tan, PhD
Professor of Business and Healthcare Informatics,
Wayne State University
Editor-in-Chief, IJHISI

Preface

Patient-Centered E-Health (PCEH) encompasses a foundational set of perspectives and approaches toward using the Internet to deliver healthcare services to patients and their caregivers (for brevity, "patients" is used hereafter to indicate both groups). Thus, PCEH is not a type of information technology (IT), but instead represents a new way of thinking about how to apply IT for the betterment of patients. This preface describes the trends that motivate development of a PCEH discipline, and the attributes that are essential for PCEH initiatives to succeed.

Trends That Drive Patient-Centered E-Health

Motivation for PCEH derives from three transformative trends that cross healthcare industries and society at large. The first trend accompanies the ongoing diversification of e-health (i.e., "health services and information delivered or enhanced through the Internet" (Eysenbach, 2001)). E-health has grown to encompass purely clinical applications, such as physicians consulting on a diagnosis (Wiecha & Pollard, 2004), patient records (Anderson, 2007), emergency health communication applications (Fruhling & De Vreede, 2006; Rizo, Lupea, Baybourdy, Anderson, Closson, & Jadad, 2005), online procurement and claims management (Deluca & Enmark, 2000), disease-focused applications such as diabetes self-management support (McKay, Glasgow, Feil, Boles, & Barrera, 2002), electronic prescription refills and appointment scheduling (Wilson & Lankton, 2004), applications to support online communication between patients and physicians (Wilson, 2003), and commercial applications such as WebMD (Itagaki, Berlin, & Schatz, 2002). As e-health applications diversify into increasingly unrelated areas, this limits potential for the work of researchers or practitioners in one branch to be helpful to those in other branches. Developing a specialization toward e-health that is used by patient represents a natural response to the increasing diversification within the e-health universe (Wilson, 2008).

The second trend motivating PCEH results from the diffusion of Web applications into the business and personal activities of most adults in developed nations. As more of the population becomes familiar with the Web and relies upon the Web for services—such as information searches, banking, and shopping—consumer demand increases for Web access to other services. Although healthcare has lagged banking and other industries in providing online access to customers, demand is building among patients for such health services as online appointment scheduling, billing and payment services, and online health communication with physicians and clinical staff (Homan, 2000; Taylor & Leitman, 2002). The demand for online health services is complicated further by entrainment of Web users to expect interfaces that are easy to use and understand (Lankton & Wilson, 2007; Zeithaml, Parasuraman, & Malhotra, 2002). These factors imply that it is essential to build high-quality, user-centered applications in order for patients to accept and use e-health that is directed toward them.

The third trend motivating PCEH is an emerging consensus that IT can and should be used more effectively to improve healthcare. Much of this new interest in health IT was sparked by two Institute of Medicine reports recommending improvements in health IT as a remedy to preventable medical errors and other healthcare quality problems (IOM, 1999, 2001). Other studies show that health IT can reduce or contain healthcare costs (Devaraj & Kohli, 2000; PricewaterhouseCoopers, 2007). To date, new government pronouncements and programs have been developed toward improving health IT infrastructures (HHS, 2004), and investment in health IT has increased substantially (Carpenter, 2005). Although much of this attention centers on development of a standardized electronic medical record (EMR) and other IT improvements to organizational infrastructure, the importance of e-health is also becoming recognized. As Microsoft Corporation Chairman Bill Gates (2007, pp. A17) writes in a Wall Street Journal opinion titled "Healthcare Needs an Internet Revolution":

What we need is to place people at the very center of the health-care system and put them in control of all their health information. Developing the solutions to make this possible is an important priority for Microsoft. We envision a comprehensive, Internet-based system that enables health-care providers to automatically deliver personal health data to each patient in a form they can understand and use.

Individuals also understand the importance of e-health, and over half say their choice of physicians is influenced by quality of e-health services (Taylor & Leitman, 2002). Development of effective e-health for use by patients is buoyed by the emerging consensus that increased use of health IT is key to improving quality, increasing efficiency, and managing costs in healthcare.

PCEH can accommodate these trends by meeting objectives of (1) instantiating a specialized discipline around which research and practice can coalesce to address issues that are specific to e-health that is used primarily by patients and (2) promoting development of high-quality e-health applications that are desirable to patient-users and responsive to quality, efficiency, and cost objectives. To accomplish these objectives, three attributes are essential: PCEH must be patient-focused, patient-active, and patient-empowered (see Figure 1).

Figure 1. Essential attributes of patient-centered e-health

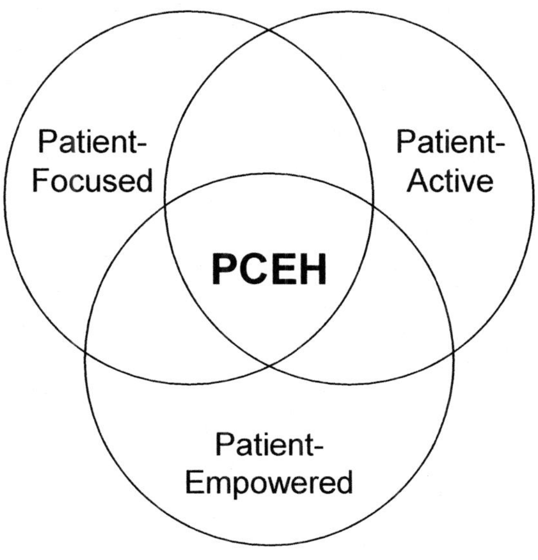

Patient-Focused E-Health

A patient focus refers to the condition where attention of e-health designers and administrators is primarily directed toward the patient-users. It may surprise readers, but much of the e-health that has been created to date for patients to use is not patient-focused. The first e-health applications were developed by commercial interests while healthcare organizations initially observed "from the sidelines," due to concerns over risk, liability, and start-up expense (Lazarus, 2001, pp. 33). The e-health applications produced by these early consumer-focused initiatives specialized in providing encyclopedic health content and promoting health products and services. Because healthcare providers are not involved, e-health designed with a pure consumer focus cannot deliver the personalized features and interactions with their own providers that patients desire (Homan, 2000; Taylor & Leitman, 2002).

As healthcare organizations began to offer e-health to patients, this created the opportunity to develop personalized, interactive services connecting patients to their own physicians, clinics, and records. Yet this opportunity has been obstructed in many cases by an excessive focus on organizational objectives. Despite lagging other industries in information technology (IT) investment, healthcare has grown to support a substantial IT industry, which for most of its existence has been oriented almost exclusively on developing clinical and transactional systems for use within the healthcare organization. Health IT designers have focused narrowly on organizational goals and, where user interactions are considered, it is the clinicians, technicians, and office staff who are targeted for study (Jamar, Mattison, Orland, Giatt, Karat, & Coble, 1998). Where e-health is developed within an organization-focused initiative, design decisions tend to be based upon organizational goals and assumptions that e-health developers and administrators make regarding patients and their e-health needs (Wilson, 2008). Although this approach may be practical in traditional healthcare settings, such as in-hospital procedures, it is not effective where system use is voluntary. Patients typically have alternatives to using an e-health service, and they will reject e-health that does not meet their actual needs—even if the designers' intentions were entirely directed toward the good of the patient (Payton & Brennan, 1999).

E-business application designers have come to understand that it is essential to create a high-quality "user experience" in order to build and retain Web traffic (Becker & Mottay, 2001; Molla & Licker, 2001) and avoid rejection by intended users. This can be accomplished only by focusing on users (Alpert, Karat, Darat, Brodie, & Vergo, 2003). E-health designers serve a population of patients who are increasingly dependent upon and proficient in using Web applications, and these patients expect their experience with e-health to be as satisfying as with other Web applications. Instead of treating patients as objects to be manipulated through e-health—such as consumers of pharmaceuticals, or receivers of medical instructions—it is necessary for designers of patient-focused e-health to understand and act upon patients' needs, preferences, and perspectives.

Healthcare is a profession of compassion and concern, yet the culture of healthcare is based to a large extent on a paternalistic model of physician-patient relationships (Emanuel & Emanuel, 1992) in which physicians control virtually all aspects of their interaction with patients (Eysenbach & Jadad, 2001). It is important that researchers and practitioners confront this situation explicitly in developing patient-focused e-health so as to avoid reprising the paradox Warren Winkelman (2004, pp. 1) describes in his review of a study assessing a patient-accessible electronic patient record system:

[The system] shares a common identity paradox with these other systems in that it portends to be patient-centered while employing physician-centered design and evaluation frameworks. It is therefore not surprising that, in their study, patient access has little measureable impact on patient-specific health outcomes.

In order to create patient-focused e-health, patients must be seen as the overriding reason for designing e-health services, the principle source of design requirements, and the key evaluators of e-health success. This is not to say that commercial and organization goals cannot be considered in design of patient-focused e-health, just that these considerations must be secondary.

Patient-Active E-Health

Patient-active means that patients are given meaningful abilities to provide information as well as consume it, a perspective that has numerous implications for potential uses of e-health and the types of services that e-health should offer. A number of patient-active e-health services are becoming common, including electronic prescription refills, online appointment scheduling, and e-mail-style communication that patients can initiate (Lazarus, 2001). However, support for patient activity can be nuanced, and in some cases, achieving highly patient-active e-health will require reconceptualization of healthcare processes and information flows.

Consider the example of the personal health record (PHR). The PHR is a comprehensive personal health information repository that is controlled by the patient and potentially covers the patient's entire lifespan (Lafky, Tulu, & Horan, 2006). E-health that offers a PHR with these characteristics provides a certain level of patient activity, in that patients are primarily responsible for making entries and maintaining these records. But there is a problem—although PHR software is offered by a number of vendors, including freely accessible versions, hardly anyone uses it (Taylor, 2004). A number of reasons have been offered for this situation, ranging from poor usability, to privacy issues and lack of health content integration (Wilson, 2006), yet numerous other software applications have overcome similar handicaps, especially where these are perceived by users as providing meaningful capabilities (Lee, Kozar, & Larsen, 2003). The PHR is typically conceptualized as being distinct from the legal medical records that institutions are required to maintain (AHIMA, 2005). In practice, this distinction has been implemented by creating a wall between the patient's PHR and the healthcare provider's EMR, which effectively obstructs much of the value that patients could gain from maintaining a PHR. The patient cannot enter any information into the EMR, and typically cannot incorporate information from the EMR into the PHR. This situation constrains the PHR to simply storing and organizing information that is provided by the patient, a process which requires substantial effort to achieve limited benefits. To build a PHR that is highly patient-active, linkage should be provided to the EMR as well as other data sources to which the patient has legitimate interests, including patient records held by employers, insurers, and governmental agencies.

The ultimate goal of patient-active e-health is to provide services that allow patients to initiate and conduct all actions that they desire to perform. This will require e-health designers to develop effective strategies for removing barriers to information exchange in an environment which is both policy-driven and highly regulated. While the challenge is difficult, similar user-activity barriers have been overcome in numerous online activities, including personal finance and investment, commercial sales and auctions, and social networking.

Patient-Empowered E-Health

Patient empowerment is achieved through providing powerful e-health tools that allow patients to control far-ranging aspects of their healthcare. Increasingly, patients expect to be empowered in their own healthcare decisions (IOM, 2001), and the expectation of personal control is especially strong for e-health applications (Lafky et al., 2006; Markle Foundation, 2004).

In the context of e-health, it should be recognized that empowerment has more than one dimension. First, patient empowerment implies that patients must have meaningful control of e-health services. However, this requires designers to overcome two important obstacles. As discussed previously, the paternalistic culture and attitudes which are common in healthcare can conflict with the very principle of patient control. Attitudinal biases against patient empowerment can take many forms, and these frequently are couched in concerns for the patient's well-being (Ross, Todd, Moore, Beaty, Wittevrongel, & Lin, 2005). Tension between paternalism and empowerment is a recurring phenomenon in healthcare (Yeo, 1993), but it is important to recognize that e-health per se does not create new conflicts. Patients principally expect e-health to support activities which they already can control—for example, by making a personal visit to their health clinic. Designers should be ready to argue for extending existing forms of patient empowerment into the e-health domain wherever this can be done.

Security and financial issues can also block patient empowerment, and these may be difficult to overcome (Wilson, 2008). Healthcare organizations have the legal responsibility to maintain security and privacy of patient and provider data, and providing patient access can increase exposure to security breaches. In addition, interconnecting e-health application to internal systems can increase development expenses, especially where the internal systems have limited interoperability. Because e-health holds the promise of increasing patient services and containing costs, designers should press for long-term commitment toward interconnecting e-health with other organizational IT, even if pragmatic constraints prevail in the short term.

A further aspect of patient empowerment is ensuring that e-health provides a high level of usability. In particular, patients must be able to understand and communicate effectively within the e-health environment. From the patient's perspective, e-health is an extension of the healthcare providers' other services, thus it is reasonable for patients to expect e-health to be generally understandable, and for the provider to offer better explanations if the need becomes apparent. In patient-empowered e-health, it is not acceptable for designers to insist that patients' health literacy must increase before they can use e-health services, as is suggested by Norman and Skinner (2006). Patients' need for healthcare services is not dependent upon their literacy level, and requiring patients to be highly literate in order to use e-health is no more defensible than requiring literacy in order to schedule medical examinations or other healthcare services (Wilson, 2008). The examples of online banking and financial services demonstrate that people who are only marginally literate can successfully interact with Web applications when they are provided with an effective interface. Usability of e-health applications can be increased by applying user-centered design (UCD) principles and related methods (Nielsen, 1993; Preece, Rogers, & Sharp, 2002). These methods have greatly improved usability of Web applications in general (Becker & Mottay, 2001) and in the healthcare contexts where they have been applied (Johnson, Johnson, & Zhang, 2005).

Patient-empowered e-health is not a call to give patients controversial new forms of control or to require patients to change how they interact with healthcare providers. Instead, the key objective is to bring as many aspects of patients' existing empowerment online as possible.

How PCEH Contributes to Research and Practice

This book introduces PCEH as a conceptual framework, but it must be recognized that study and development of e-health centered around patient needs is not new. Around the world, researchers and practitioners are engaged in creating e-health applications that intermingle patient focus, patient activity, and patient empowerment, the essential attributes of PCEH. Furthermore, this development is being undertaken across multiple fields—prominently including medical services, user-centered design (UCD), computer science, information systems (IS), and consumer health informatics. Advances are occurring, but they mostly arise within "development islands" which are isolated by geography and training. Recognition of PCEH as conceptually distinct from other forms of e-health is an important first step in bringing these islands together and increasing information exchange and mutual understanding. However, it is becoming clear that PCEH has important disciplinary characteristics, viewpoints, and methods beyond its conceptual impact which can be important to improving the productivity of research and design. Thus, the further purposes of this book are to organize and integrate PCEH activities that are occurring spontaneously, promoting research and development as a PCEH discipline forms and evolves.

Organization of the Book

The book is organized within two sections: Foundations and Applications. Nine chapters in the Foundations section address central topics of philosophy, structure, and research methodologies underlying PCEH. A brief description of each Foundations chapter follows:

Chapter I explores the role e-health plays in the broader context of patient-centered care. The authors conduct a historic review of the development of health IT and the patient-centered care movement. They then present a conceptual framework of the considerations and requirements that are essential for PCEH to bridge these two disparate fields.

Chapter II identifies techniques of user-centered design (UCD) that are particularly appropriate to PCEH. The authors describe the techniques and administration procedures in an understandable manner and in sufficient detail to be used as a guide by practitioners and researchers who do not have previous experience with UCD.

Chapter III presents a foundational discussion of the psychological issues inherent in applying computer-mediated communication (CMC) to the context of e-health. The authors' contention that certain aspects of CMC may actually benefit patient health motivates an important discussion of future research directions in PCEH.

Chapter IV introduces the personal health record (PHR) as a central component of PCEH. This chapter reviews historical development of the PHR, including objectives of governmental and regulatory agencies and challenges to success.

Chapter V explores the role of PCEH in the under-researched context of disabled workers. The author argues that health IT can profoundly change the application and maintenance processes for disabled workers to receive benefits, concluding with a set of recommendations for automating these processes.

Chapter VI confronts the issue of PCEH as a marketing venue. The authors present a clear and well-balanced overview of the marketing methods that are most applicable to PCEH. Their approach promotes the constructive benefits of marketing that is well targeted and sensitive to patients' interests.

Chapter VII introduces a privacy management framework for PCEH. In grounding this framework, the author rigorously reviews privacy and privacy management literatures, and explicitly addresses the diverse interests involved in patients' use of e-health services.

Chapter VIII addresses the issue of trust as a means of overcoming patients' concerns regarding privacy and confidentiality in PCEH. The authors review the trust literature and identify how trust relates to e-health developed by medical content aggregators, health-based online communities, and patient-physician portals.

Chapter IX comprehensively discusses ways to involve patients and the general public in e-health research. The authors propose key principles to guide researchers in designing and conducting e-health studies, and then describe how they used these principles to gain public involvement in an Internet-based intervention to aid diabetes self-management.

A further seven chapters present research findings from actual applications of PCEH. A brief description of each Applications chapter follows:

Chapter X presents a case study in which interaction design and usability evaluation methods were applied to improve the user interface of a personal health record (PHR). The authors applied the think-aloud technique for observing PHR users through two design iterations, finding that significant improvements could be made from a relatively small number of observations.

Chapter XI uses focus group research methods to explore patients' perceptions of empowerment and need for quality and cost information when choosing healthcare providers. The authors' study suggests that a previously-proposed theoretical compatibility model can have utility in predicting patients' healthcare decisions.

Chapter XII describes results of a survey conducted among rural Nebraska residents, which asked their perceptions regarding access to e-health. Special attention in this study is directed toward identifying key dimensions of rural residents' perceptions about e-health from a qualitative analysis of their open-ended responses.

Chapter XIII uses interview methods to study effects of an e-health application to aid self-management of chronic respiratory conditions. Qualitative analysis of interview data identified important ramifications regarding evidence-based medicine, the doctor-patient relationship, and the role of e-health in improving collaboration and communication with patients.

Chapter XIV investigates asthmatics' reasons for not adopting e-health for asthma self-management. The authors interviewed four asthmatic individuals to identify why a well-funded e-health application had failed to gain acceptance, finding that the designer's image of asthmatics as primarily striving to be symptom-free was incompatible with interviewees' actual objectives.

Chapter XV studies hospital e-health Web sites in a design based upon an extended version of the technology acceptance model (TAM). From interviews with 30 study participants, they find usefulness, ease of use, trust, privacy, and personalization are important elements in deciding whether to use hospital e-health.

Chapter XVI develops and tests a new rational-objective (R-O) model of e-health use that accounts for effects of facilitating conditions as well as patients' behavioral intentions. Results from a longitudinal survey design show that predictions of actual use were improved by more than 300% by considering effects of facilitating conditions.

REFERENCES

AHIMA. (2005). The role of the personal health record in the HER. *Journal of AHIMA, 76*(7), 64A-D.

Alpert, S.R., Karat, J., Karat, C-M., Brodie, C., & Vergo, J.G. (2003). User attitudes regarding a user-adaptive ecommerce Web site. *User Modeling and User-Adapted Interaction, 13*(4), 373-396.

Anderson, J.G. (2007). Social, ethical and legal barriers to e-health. *International Journal of Medical Informatics, 76* 480-483.

Becker, S.A., & Mottay, F.E. (2001). A global perspective on Web site usability. *IEEE Software, 18*(1), 54-61.

Carpenter, D. (2005). Spending spree. *Hospitals & Health Networks*. Retrieved May 28, 2008, from http://www.hhnmag.com/hhnmag_app/jsp/articledisplay.jsp?dcrpath=HHNMAG/PubsNewsArticle/data/0505HHN_FEA_Finance_Supplement_Story1&domain=HHNMAG

Deluca, J., & Enmark, R. (2000). E-health: The changing model of healthcare. *Frontiers of Health Services Management, 17*(1), 3-15.

Devaraj, S., & Kohli, R. (2000). Information technology payoff in the health-care industry: a longitudinal study. *Journal of Management Information Systems, 16*(4), 41-67.

Emanuel, E.J., & Emanuel, L.L. (1992). Four models of the physician-patient relationship. *JAMA, 267*(16), 2221-2226.

Eysenbach, G. (2001). What is e-health? *Journal of Medical Internet Research, 3*(2), e20.

Eysenbach, G., & Jadad, A.R. (2001). Evidence-based patient choice and consumer health informatics in the internet age. *Journal of Medical Internet Research, 3*(2): article e19.

Fruhling, A., & De Vreede, G.J. (2006). Field experiences with eXtreme Programming: Developing an emergency response system. *Journal of Management Information Systems, 22*(4), 39-68.

Gates, B. (2007). Healthcare needs an internet revolution. *Wall Street Journal*, October 3, 2007, A17.

Health and Human Services (HHS). (2004). Harnessing information technology to improve healthcare. *U.S. Department of Health & Human Services Fact Sheet.* Retrieved May 28, 2008, from http://www.hhs.gov/news/press/2004pres/20040427a.html

Homan, Q. (2000). Healthcare satisfaction study final report. *Harris Interactive/ARiA Marketing Report.* Retrieved May 28, 2008, from http://www.harrisinteractive.com/news/downloads/harrisariahcsatrpt.pdf

Institute of Medicine (IOM). (1999). *To err is human: Building a safer health system.* Washington, D.C.: Institute of Medicine, National Academies Press.

IOM. (2001). *Crossing the quality chasm: A new health system for the 21st century.* Washington, D.C.: Institute of Medicine, National Academies Press.

Itagaki, M.W., Berlin, R.B., & Schatz, B.R. (2002). The rise and fall of e-health: Lessons from the first generation of internet healthcare. *Medscape General Medicine, 4*(2). Retrieved May 28, 2008, from http://www.medscape.com/viewarticle/431144_Print

Jamar, P., Mattison, J., Orland, M., Giatt, J., Karat, J., & Coble, J. (1998). Human-computer interaction in healthcare: What works? What doesn't. In *Proceedings of the Conference on Human Factors in Computing Systems (CHI'98)* (pp. 80-81). Los Angeles, CA. Retrieved May 28, 2008, from http://delivery.acm.org/10.1145/290000/286539/p80-jamar.pdf?key1=286539&key2=0417346911&coll=GUIDE&dl=GUIDE&CFID=45207284&CFTOKEN=30559769

Johnson C.M., Johnson, T.R., & Zhang, J. (2005). A user-centered framework for redesigning healthcare interfaces. *Journal of Biomedical Informatics, 38*, 75-87.

Lafky, D. B., Tulu, B., & Horan, T. A. (2006). A user-driven approach to personal health records. *Communications of the Association for Information Systems, 17*, 1028-1041.

Lankton, N. K., & Wilson, E. V. (2007). Antecedents and dimensions of online service expectations. *IEEE Transactions on Engineering Management, 54*(4), 776-788.

Lazar, J. (2001). *User-centered web development.* Sudbury, MA: Jones & Bartlett.

Lazarus, I. R. (2001). Separating myth from reality in e-health initiatives. *Managed Healthcare Executive, June,* 33-36.

Lee, Y., Kozar, K. A., & Larsen, K. R. T. (2003). The technology acceptance model: Past, present, and future. *Communications of the Association for Information Systems, 12*(50), 752-780.

Markle Foundation (2004). Achieving electronic connectivity in healthcare. Markle Foundation. Accessed December 20, 2007 from http://www.connectingforhealth.org/resources/aech_exec_summary.pdf

McKay, H. G., Glasgow, R. E., Feil, E. G., Boles, S. M., & Barrera, M. (2002). Internet-based diabetes self-management and support: Initial outcomes from the Diabetes Network Project. *Rehabilitation Psychology, 47*(1), 31-48.

Molla, A., & Licker, P.S. (2001). E-commerce systems success: An attempt to extend and respecify the DeLone and McLean model of IS success. *Journal of Electronic Commerce Research, 2*(4), 131-141.

Nielsen, J. (1993). *Usability engineering.* San Diego, CA: Academic Press.

Norman, C. D., & Skinner, H. A. eHealth literacy: Essential skills for consumer health in a networked world. *Journal of Medical Internet Research, 8*(2), e9.

Pagliari, C., Sloan, D., Gregor, P., Sullivan, F., Detmer, D., Kahan, J. P., Oortwijn, W., & MacGillivray, S. (2005). What Is eHealth (4): A scoping exercise to map the field. *Journal of Medical Internet Research, 7*(1), e9.

Payton, F. C., & Brennan, P. F. (1999). How a community health information network is really used. *Communications of the ACM, 42*(12), 85-89.

Preece, J., Rogers, Y., & Sharp, H. (2002). *Interaction design: Beyond human-computer interaction.* New York: John Wiley & Sons, Inc.

PricewaterhouseCoopers (2007). *The economics of IT and hospital performance. PricewaterhouseCoopers Report.* Retrieved November 26, 2007 from http://www.pwc.com/techforecast/pdfs/HealthIndex_web-X.pdf

Rizo, C. A., Lupea, D., Baybourdy, H., Anderson, M., Closson, T., & Jadad, A. R. (2005). What internet services would patients like from hospitals during an epidemic? Lessons from the SARS outbreak in Toronto. *Journal of Medical Internet Research, 7*(4), e46.

Ross, S. E., Todd, J., Moore, L. A., Beaty, B. L., Wittevrongel, L., & Lin, C. (2005). Expectations of patients and physicians regarding patient-accessible medical records. *Journal of Medical Internet Research, 7*(2), e13.

Tan, J., Cheng, W., & Rogers, W. J. (2002). From telemedicine to e-health: Uncovering new frontiers of biomedical research, clinical applications & public health services delivery. *Journal of Computer Information Systems, 42*(5), 7-18.

Taylor, H. (2004). *Two in five adults keep personal or family health records and almost everybody thinks this is a good idea: Electronic health records likely to grow rapidly.* Health Care News, 4(10), Retrieved December 12, 2005 from http://www.harrisinteractive.com/news/newsletters_healthcare.asp

Taylor, H., & Leitman, R. (2002). *Patient/physician online communication: Many patients want it, would pay for it, and it would influence their choice of doctors and health plans.* Health Care News, 2(8). Retrieved December 13, 2005 from http://www.harrisinteractive.com/news/newsletters_healthcare.asp

Thompson, T. G., & Brailler, D. J. (2004). *The decade of health information technology: Delivering consumer-centric and information-rich health care.* Washington, DC: Department of Health and Human Services.

Wiecha, J., & Pollard, T. (2004). The interdisciplinary eHealth team: Chronic care for the future. *Journal of Internet Medical Research, 6*(3), e22.

Wilson, E. V. (2008). Creating patient-centered e-health. In N. Wickramasinghe and E. Geisler (Eds.), *Encyclopedia of Healthcare Information Systems,* (pp. 318-324). Hershey, PA: IGI Publishing.

Wilson, E. V. (2003). Asynchronous health care communication. *Communications of the ACM, 46*(6), 79-84.

Wilson, E. V., & Lankton, N. K. (2003). Strategic implications of asynchronous healthcare communication. *International Journal of Healthcare Technology and Management, 5*(3/4/5), 213-231.

Wilson, E. V., & Lankton, N. K. (2004). Modeling patients' acceptance of provider-delivered e-health. *Journal of the American Medical Informatics Association, 11*(4), 241-248.

Wilson, E. V. (2006). Building better e-health through a personal health informatics pedagogy. *International Journal of Healthcare Information Systems and Informatics, 1*(3), 69-76.

Winkelman, W. J. (2004). Reconciling the patient's role in the improvement of health outcomes: Medical informatics' newest frontier. *Journal of Medical Internet Research, 6*(2), e14.

Yeo, M. (1993). Toward an ethic of empowerment for health promotion. *Health Promotion International, 8*(3), 225-235.

Zeithaml, V.A., Parasuraman, A., & Malhotra, A. (2002). Service quality delivery through web sites: A critical review of extant knowledge. *Academy of Marketing Science Journal 30*(4), 362-375.

Acknowledgment

This book would not be complete without my acknowledgement of the extensive help and guidance provided by colleagues. First, I commend the editorial staff at IGI for providing a clear and complete plan for book development. While the production schedule was definitely not "relaxed," it turned out to be realistic and attainable. Frequent communication and reminders from IGI and quick responses to my questions were a great help in staying on schedule.

The second group I must acknowledge are the authors who contributed to *Patient-Centered E-Health*. I had thought that a major obstacle to recruiting chapters might be my inability to "sell" the idea that such a book is actually needed. Instead, I found a cadre of contributors who not only recognize the need, but are passionate about this emerging field.

A third group I am deeply grateful to are the 55 reviewers who gave up a significant part of their summer break to evaluate and improve book chapters. This group includes many of the chapter authors, as well as numerous topic specialists who graciously volunteered their efforts.

Fourth, I wish to acknowledge my fellow faculty members in the Information Operations and Technology Management (IOTM) Department at the University of Toledo who were exceptionally understanding about the time I spent focusing on book editing and production in lieu of departmental business. I especially thank our IOTM secretary, Chris Humbert, for her assistance with mailing and logistics.

Finally, I thank Betty Wilson for conducting final checks of citations, references, indexing, and formatting for all the chapters. Betty is not only a skilled graphic designer and copy production specialist, but is also my wife, so I am especially pleased that we are still on good terms following book production.

E. Vance Wilson, PhD
Toledo, Ohio, USA
June 2008

Section I
Foundations

Chapter I
Towards Patient-Centered Care:
The Role of E-Health in Enabling Patient Access to Health Information

Juanita Dawson
Claremont Graduate University, USA

Bengisu Tulu
Worcester Polytechnic Institute, USA

Thomas A. Horan
Claremont Graduate University, USA

ABSTRACT

This chapter provides a conceptual foundation by exploring the existing literature on traditional healthcare, patient-centered healthcare, and the progression of e-health in enabling the movement towards patient-centered care. This chapter also discusses enhancing the relationship between the patient and the healthcare provider through e-health. We conclude with a discussion of the future of patient-centered e-health and future research opportunities in this area.

INTRODUCTION

Access to information is important for enabling effective collaboration between patients and their healthcare providers. Use of information systems (IS) in patient-centered care renders an opportunity to provide individuals access to their own health information (Bailey, 1998) as well as other resources. Today, technological advances have changed how patients and healthcare providers regard health information.

- The concept of individual access anytime, anyplace, and anywhere is taking shape with the help of online applications that promise greater participation of patients in their own healthcare decisions (Wickramasinghe & Goldberg, 2005).

- Patients' access to information can be of benefit or detriment to health outcomes (Carrigan, 1993), and it is important to optimize information delivery and guidance to promote benefits.
- Individuals from all social and economic backgrounds need to better manage their health, so it is important that an information divide is not created as an unintended consequence of e-health (Currie & Guah, 2006; Luce, Phillips, Benjamin, & Wasson, 2006; Wasson, 2006).

It is important to make the distinction between patient-centered e-health (PCEH) and traditional health IS before we continue our discussion. Traditional health IS were designed to meet the needs of healthcare providers and were used by health workers to assist them in patient care. Many healthcare providers are now developing e-health for use by patients to support searches for health information as well as other interactions with the provider. Key distinctions between traditional health IS and these new forms of PCEH are presented in Table 1. The authors' vision is that patients' ability to access to information through PCEH can be used to economically empower them to better manage their health.

This chapter provides a conceptual foundation by exploring the literatures relating to traditional healthcare, patient-centered healthcare, and the role e-health has played in enabling the movement towards patient-centered care. The chapter concludes with a discussion of the role, status, and future of PCEH and future research opportunities. The authors hope to stimulate awareness of the progress PCEH is making in providing individuals with the capability to create and manage their own health information.

BACKGROUND

Healthcare Delivery Systems and Health IS

For centuries, hospitals have been a primary means for healthcare delivery (Carrigan, 2003). Services including patient care and record keeping were rendered at the physical location of the hospital building. The healthcare provider's access to patient information was also limited to the physical boundaries of the hospitals. These services were traditionally provided using paper and pen and other manual technologies such as photocopying and hand delivering documents to departments within the hospital (Koska, 1990) or to the patients. Responsibility for collecting and storing patient information was left to the

Table 1. Traditional health IS and PCEH

	Traditional Health IS	PCEH
Emphasis	Record-keeping	Access to patient information
Users	Provider personnel	Patient and provider
Interaction	Provider → Patient	Provider ← → Patient
Supports	Provider activities	Patient health management
Services available	At hospital location	Anywhere, anytime
System accessibility	Accessed locally	Accessed globally
Patient access	Patient has only indirect access to patient information	Patient has direct access to patient information

healthcare provider. This information typically was documented in paper files and stored in free-standing file cabinets. Some functions within the traditional healthcare delivery system focused on the operational areas such as laboratory and radiology examinations being sent out to specialized facilities for interpretation of results and then returned to the healthcare provider to share with the patient. Direct access by the patient to his/her health information was not a capability provided by the traditional healthcare delivery system.

The first health IS provided an electronic means for record keeping and billing information only. Information was stored on the computer and used to manage the healthcare facility or assist the physician and staff (Wickramasinghe & Mills, 2001). Health IS impacted the way the facility was operating and did not focus on patient-care information (Woodard, 2005). These health IS were mainly stand-alone systems that were not integrated among functions.

Although the healthcare industry has lagged in adoption of information technologies (Wang, Helian, & Jayaram, 2002), over time, hospitals have become more dependent on IS and have strengthened their infrastructure to accommodate new systems that were designed to support patient care. This new set of systems is focused on storing and providing patient information in electronic format—for example, as electronic medical records (EMR). These health IS enable the healthcare provider to access electronic laboratory and radiology results at the time the tests are entered into the system (Wickramasinghe & Goldberg, 2005). Moreover, the new systems enable information to flow among departments as needed for review and analysis. But even though advanced health IS, including EMRs, are now used by many providers to support the effective delivery of healthcare, these continue to be focused on the healthcare organization (Wasson, 2006) and do not facilitate patients' direct access to health information.

The Patient-Centered Care Initiative

The term *patient-centered care* was created in 1988 by researchers at the Picker Institute (http://www.pickerinstitute.org) to spearhead the concept that healthcare of a patient should be centered on the individual patient's needs and wants and based upon the patient's perspectives. The patient-centered care initiative focuses on the enhancement of knowledge, skills, or power with the objective of enabling individuals to become partners in their own healthcare (Goldberg, 1995).

From the authors' perspective, shown in Figure 1, patient-centered care is impacted by six factors relating to effective and efficient information exchange:

1. **Knowledge:** Enhancing the patient's knowledge about health concerns is valuable in understanding health issues that affect individual health maintenance and care. Knowledge of health information and the means to collaborate is associated with positive outcomes for the patient.
2. **Empowerment:** Empowering patients to take action is vital in keeping them involved in their own healthcare and maintenance process. A key aspect to empowering patients to take part in managing healthcare is for them to be informed regarding the control-points that exist in their individual care situations.
3. **Decisions:** Insofar as possible, patients should be helped to understand the decisions that healthcare providers make daily. Along with healthcare professionals' willingness to educate patients, a further necessary ingredient for patients to achieve understanding is the availability of credible health information.
4. **Collaboration:** Collaboration between the patient and healthcare provider is essential in managing immediate health concerns and in framing discussions regarding future

healthcare decisions. Information exchange is an essential element of collaboration.

5. **Quality:** Quality of healthcare is strongly impacted by the quality of information exchange. Quality issues in healthcare—including reducing medical errors, improving facilities scheduling, and enhancing the match between patient needs and healthcare providers' strengths—all can be addressed to a large degree by increasing the quality of information exchange.
6. **Participation:** The role of the patient is expanding, and patients are participating in managing their health even in areas where they do not expect to be in control. A key aspect of increased participation is the recognition that patients are important in providing and sharing health information as well as simply consuming it.

The patient-centered care initiative was supported by the introduction of the patient-centered clinical method as a framework (Beckman, Fernandez, & Coulter, 1996). This framework describes the clinical process that integrates the needs of both doctor and patient in order to facilitate positive outcomes. Within the framework, "disease-centered" or "doctor-centered" behaviors are no longer the primary focus in rendering a diagnosis or opinion (Beckman et al., 1996). Instead, understanding the patient's needs and shaping the services provided to the patient is the foundation to building the physician-patient relationship.

The movement toward patient-centered care creates new challenges in controlling and reducing the cost of healthcare (Tobias, 1996). The spending level of healthcare has increased, without any significant increase in the quality of care (Baucus, 2005). Therefore, there is an assumption that what we pay for healthcare and what we get are misaligned (Safavi, 2006; Sofaer, Crofton, Goldstein, Hoy, & Crabb, 2005). While there is general agreement that the healthcare system is in dire need of reform, an understated—but vital—aspect of this reform is actively engaging patients to manage their healthcare efficiently. By empowering patients, the patient-centered initiative holds out

Figure 1. Patient-centered care focus

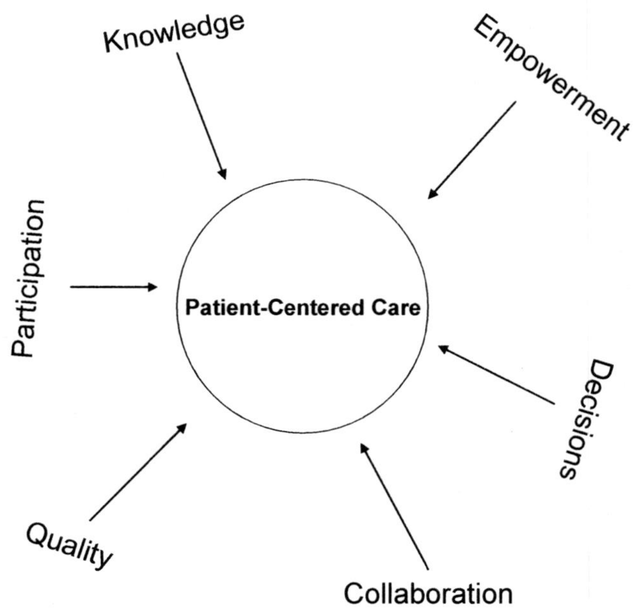

the possibility of system-wide improvements as well as individual benefits.

E-HEALTH

A common concern among healthcare organizations is the need to share information in a manner that facilitates health delivery, yet protects the interests of patients (Tang & Lansky, 2005; Wang et al., 2002). Application of e-health to support the patient-centered care initiative in the form of PCEH meets both needs. Leveraging the use of a common electronic information exchange facilitates an environment for improving healthcare delivery, and concerns about privacy, security, and information control are appropriately directed toward the patient's own needs.

Requirements for Patient-Centered E-Health

As we have discussed above, PCEH derives from the two disparate traditions of health IS and patient-centered care. Neither field supplies all the elements necessary for PCEH to succeed. Health IS has no tradition of direct patient accesses, and patient-centered care focuses on health treatments, rather than technology. We propose the following requirements are necessary to support effective PCEH (see Figure 2). These include: (1) developing an infrastructure that will support PCEH, (2) providing precautions that protect the privacy and security of patient health information, (3) developing a standard format to share patient information in an understandable manner, (4) aligning business goals and operations with the patient-centered approach, (5) enhancing the collaboration between patients and providers, and (6) providing ubiquitous access to the patient. We discuss each of these topics in the following sections.

Figure 2. Requirements to support effective PCEH

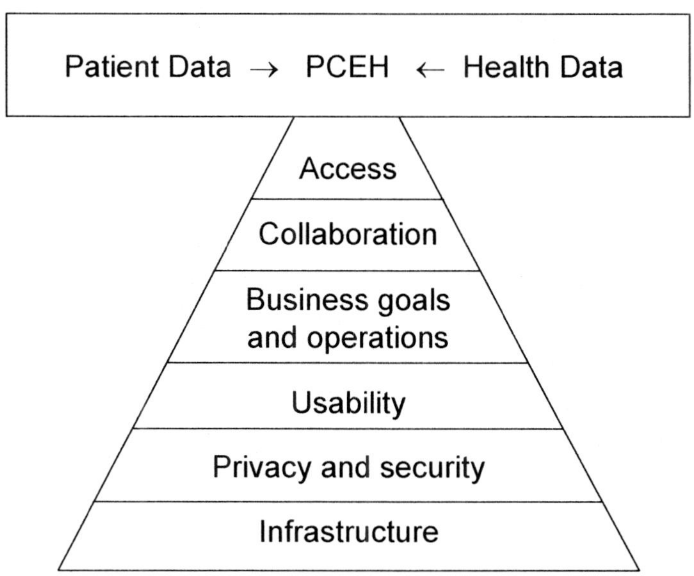

Infrastructure

Patient access to health information implies that a general, common, and collective information infrastructure must be created, which can eliminate inconsistencies in the use of patient information (Berry, Seiders, & Wilder, 2003). There is a need to define the infrastructure that will facilitate the needs of the healthcare industry in electronically exchanging health information in a secure environment (Siau, Southbard, & Hong, 2002; Tauzin, 2006). Potentially, this effort may be aided by the National Health Information Network (NHIN), which provides an overall architecture for implementing patient-centric health IS.

Privacy and Security

Protecting the privacy and security of patient health information is a concern for both patients and healthcare providers. The Health Information Portability and Accountability Act of 1996 (HIPAA) and other information privacy and security regulations have put a premium on designing secure health IS platforms (Christiansen, 1999; Tulu & Chatterjee, 2003). Yet, organizational trends such as common infrastructures and information sharing have raised challenges in implementing secure, shared environments. There is no single standard currently in place to ensure privacy and security of health information. However, efforts to develop integrated standards are underway, and policy makers, healthcare leaders, and healthcare providers support the need for standards (Stead, Kelly, & Kolodner, 2005).

Usability

Patients want healthcare information to be delivered in a format that is understandable. While the healthcare industry uses a great amount of specialized terminology and jargon, patients expect online health communication to be easy to use and readily accessible (Wilson, 2003). Developing easy-to-use formats to share patient information in an understandable manner will promote use of PCEH and increase cost effectiveness to the healthcare providers who fund it. It is particularly important to ensure usability across diverse populations, including those who may experience access or communication barriers.

Business Goals and Operations

In order to gain management support for PCEH in healthcare organizations, it is imperative to align business goals and operations with a patient-centered perspective. IS professionals are experienced in identifying user requirements in order to develop quality tools that facilitate healthcare as a business. The challenge is to integrate patient needs into the work processes and workflow of patient-health system interactions.

Collaboration

Where health information sharing and exchange initiatives have succeeded, this is largely due to effectively applying information technologies to support collaboration (Lorenzi, 2003). Patients look to e-health to provide health information that can enhance their knowledge, and thereby allow them to participate more effectively in their own care (Wickramasinghe & Mills, 2001). Enhancing collaboration between patients and healthcare providers is implicit in the principles of patient-centered health.

Access

In order to be effective, PCEH must be widely accessible and offer patients meaningful access not only to general information—such as encyclopedic health content—but to their own medical records, test results, appointment schedules, prescriptions, billing records, and other personal health information to which they rightfully have "ownership" (Pratt, Unruh, Civan, & Skeels,

2006). This means PCEH will need to be well-integrated into existing health IS, and not simply used as a public relations tool.

FUTURE TRENDS AND RESEARCH DIRECTIONS

PCEH faces substantial technological transformations in the form of electronic, mobile, and hand-held technologies and devices (Sneha & Varshney, 2005). The compact size of many new technologies will allow for increased range of access to health information by patients and will offer the opportunity to incorporate better information sharing with the healthcare provider, for example, to enable real-time monitoring of a patient's health condition. A number of new services are likely to enable advancements in future PCEH. For example, video and voice technologies will be integrated into PCEH to provide the patient with alternative modes of communication (Walters, Barnard, & Paris, 2006). It is unclear what applications and interface designs will be most adventitious for these new PCEH technologies, and we anticipate this to be a productive topic for new research.

As is the case with most new information technologies, PCEH will likely bring about social changes, and it is imperative that we understand the social impacts of this technology. In particular, there are consequences to increasing patients' responsibility for health management when they may have limited understanding as to what to do with the information. Many patients can effectively manage their own care when provided with the proper resources (Davis, Schoenbaum, & Audet, 2005; Moore & Wasson, 2006). Yet, an incorrect assumption or misinterpretation of health information can be costly and can defeat the intention of good health management (Korpman, 2001). More research is needed in ways of creating greater health literacy among PCEH users without making these systems hard for patients to use. In addition, the e-health literature has focused primarily on patients who were interested in playing a more significant role in their own health management. However, the population of patients that has traditionally been underserved by healthcare-the underprivileged, impoverished, uninsured, uninformed, and uninterested-has not been adequately studied. Future research is needed to better understand how PCEH can be utilized to promoted access to health information among diverse patient groups.

CONCLUSION

This chapter provided a brief review of literature underlying the development of a patient-centered initiative in the domain of e-health. PCEH can economically provide patients access to health information that can be delivered virtually anytime, anyplace, and anywhere (Wickramasinghe & Goldberg, 2005). Yet this information is not always beneficial to patients (Carrigan, 1993), so it is important to find ways of developing PCEH that promote benefits and reduce risks. Further, access to PCEH is limited, due to an unresolved information divide across social and economic dimensions (Currie & Guah, 2006; Luce et al., 2006; Wasson, 2006).

Although PCEH has technological roots in traditional health IS, its objectives have been formed largely from the perspective of patient-centered care. We have proposed that this situation requires a new approach that explicitly addresses infrastructure, privacy and security, usability, business goals and operations, collaboration, and access in PCEH development. Further research will be necessary, but we believe our vision is achievable—that giving patients the ability to access information through PCEH will provide an economical means of empowering them to better manage their health.

REFERENCES

Bailey, P.G. (1998). Best healthcare system in the world: Where healthcare should go in the 21st century. *Vital Speeches of the Day, 64*(8), 245.

Baucus, M. (2005). Looking at the U.S. healthcare system in the rear-view mirror. *Health Affairs, 24*, 544-545.

Beckman, J.F., Fernandez, C.E., & Coulter, I.D. (1996). A systems model of healthcare: A proposal. *Journal of Manipulative and Physiological Therapeutics, 19*(3), 208-215.

Berry, L.L., Seiders, K., & Wilder, S.S. (2003). Innovations in access to care: A patient-centered approach. *Annals of Internal Medicine, 139*(7), 568-575.

Carrigan, M. (1993). The future of healthcare information systems. *Hospital Material Management Quarterly, 15*(1), 1-13.

Christiansen, J.R. (1999). Health information technology and privacy: The legal perspective. *MDComputing: Computers in Medical Practice, 16*(4), 15-16.

Currie, W.L., & Guah, M.W. (2006). IT-enabled healthcare delivery: The U.K. National Health Service. *Information Management, 23*(2), 7-22.

Davis, K., Schoenbaum, S.C., & Audet, A. (2005). A 2020 vision of patient-centered care. *Journal of General Internal Medicine, 20*, 953-957.

Goldberg, M.C. (1995). If we're lucky, the patient will complain. *American Journal of Nursing, 95*(2), 52-53.

Inguanzo, J.M. (1992). Taking a serious look at patient expectations. *Hospitals, 66*(17), 68.

Korpman, R. (2001). Managed care and e-health. *Health Management Technology, 22*(2), 12-14.

Koska, M.T. (1990). Patient-centered care: Can your hospital afford not to have IT? *Hospitals, 64*(21), 48-54.

Lorenzi, N.M. (2003, December 16). Strategies for creating successful local health information infrastructure initiatives. *Local Health Information Infrastructure Success/Failure Report.*

Luce, P., Phillips, J., Benjamin, R., & Wasson, J.H. (2006). Technology to support community health alliances. *Journal of Ambulatory Care Management, 27*(3), 399-407.

MacStravic, S. (1988). The patient as a partner: A competitive strategy in healthcare marketing. *Hospital & Health Services Administration, 33*(1), 15-24.

Moore, L.G., & Wasson, J.H. (2006). An introduction to technology for patient-centered, collaborative care. *Journal of Ambulatory Care Management, 29*(3), 195-198.

Pratt, W., Unruh, K., Civan, A., & Skeels, M. (2006). Personal health information management. *Communications of the ACM, 49*(1), 51-55.

Safavi, K. (2006). Patient-centered pay for performance: Are we missing the target? *Journal of Healthcare Management, 51*(4), 215-218.

Siau, K., Southbard, P., & Hong, S. (2002). E-healthcare strategies and implementation. *International Journal of Healthcare Technology and Management, 4*(1-2), 118-131.

Sneha, S., & Varshney, U. (2005, August 11-14). A wireless ECG monitoring system for healthcare. In *Proceedings of the Eleventh Americas Conference on Information Systems* (pp. 2539-2549). Omaha, NE.

Sofaer, S., Crofton, C., Goldstein, E., Hoy, E., & Crabb, J. (2005). What do consumers want to know about the quality of care in hospitals? *Health Services Research, 40*(6), 2030.

Stead, W.W., Kelly, B.J., & Kolodner, R.M. (2005). Achievable steps toward building a national health information infrastructure in the United States. *JAMIA, 12*(2), 113-120.

Tang, P.C., & Lansky, D. (2005). The missing link: Bridging the patient-provider health information gap. *Health Affairs, 24*(5), 1290-1295.

Tauzin, B. (2006). Building a healthcare system. *Vital Speeches of the Day, April 1, 2006, 72*(12), 378-381.

Tobias, R. L. (1996). Healthcare in the information age: An integrated system wide approach. *Vital Speeches of the Day, April 15, 1996, 13*, 411.

Tulu, B., & Chatterjee, S. (2003, August 4-6). A new security framework for HIPAA-compliant health information systems. In *Proceedings of Americas Conference on Information Systems (AMCIS)* (pp. 929-938). Tampa, FL.

Walters, B., Barnard, D., & Paris, S. (2006). Patient portals and e-visits. *Journal of Ambulatory Care Management, 29*(3), 222-224.

Wang, F., Helian, N., & Jayaram, N. (2002, June 6-8). A management information system for public health. *European Conference on Information Systems 2002* (pp. 1454-1464). Gdansk, Poland.

Wasson, J.H. (2006). When all things are not equal. *Journal of Ambulatory Care Management, 29*(3), 235-237.

Wickramasinghe, N., & Goldberg, S. (2005, June 6-8). A framework for delivering M-health excellence. In *Proceedings of the 18th Bled eConference eIntegration in Action* (pp. 1-21). Bled, Slovenia.

Wickramasinghe, N., & Mills, G.L. (2001, June 27-29). Knowledge management systems: A healthcare initiative with lessons for us all. In *Proceedings of the 9th European Conference on Information Systems* (pp. 763-774). Bled, Slovenia.

Wilson, E.V. (2003). Asynchronous healthcare communication. *Communications of the ACM, 46*(6), 79-84.

Woodard, T.D. (2005). Addressing variation in hospital quality: Is six sigma the answer? *Journal of Healthcare Management, 50*(4), 226-236.

Chapter II
Patient-Centered E-Health Design

Alejandro Mauro
Hospital Italiano de Buenos Aires, Argentina

Fernán González Bernaldo de Quirós
Hospital Italiano de Buenos Aires, Argentina

ABSTRACT

This chapter introduces a series of techniques and tools useful for developing patient-centered e-health. As information technology (IT) is revolutionizing health care delivery, a wide range of personal health information management tools have become available to the patients. The variety and quality of information delivered by these tools will determine how useful consumers find them. Equally important is how the information is delivered. To create quality e-health, designers must attend to the needs and wants of users by engaging them in the design and testing processes. User-centered design (UCD) is a formal approach to ensuring that new products address the needs, wants, skills, and preferences of the user throughout the tool's development. UCD is a design and evaluation process which pays special attention to the intended users, what they will do with the product, where they will use it, and what features they consider essential. This iterative approach ensures that users' needs and wants are met and ultimately increases the likelihood users will accept the final product. This chapter focuses on UCD methods and techniques, giving examples of how to use them and when.

INTRODUCTION

E-health use by patients is steadily increasing, perhaps due to the patients being empowered by physicians and the health system itself (Andreassen, Trondsen, Kummervold, Gammon, & Hjortdahl, 2006; Baker, Wagner, Singer, & Bundorf, 2003; Coulter, 1997; Eysenbach & Kohler, 2003; Street, 2003). Personal health records, patient portals, and pathology-oriented information are just a few areas of growth in patients' use of e-health. However, to be useful these applications must be easy to use and meet patients' real needs and capabilities. This is a major challenge for the development of new interfaces and systems.

Designing usable systems is difficult, and designers need effective and accurately-tested tools. Nowadays there are multiple user-centered design (UCD) methods which make system design more efficient and effective. Inquiring, inspection and testing methods are essential when planning a UCD, and although there is plenty of information about the importance of UCD in software development, many development programs fail to comply with key principles. When failing to comply, the software can be difficult to use, and this paves the way to failure. This failure can be observed both in software which is not completely put into use or is rejected due to user dissatisfaction.

When developing interfaces and designing software for medical patients to use, developers must thoroughly understand patients' needs and capabilities. Sometimes patient's needs are difficult to assess. Patients can become seriously frightened or anxious when diagnosed with a disease and they may hide important information. Lack of health literacy is another factor that makes it difficult to assess patients' needs. In any case, patients are known to have *unrecognized needs and capabilities* which are important to be considered when developing e-health. The concept of patient-centered design is intended to identify patients' needs and capabilities through tailored application of UCD principles to the context of e-health.

UCD is a highly structured, comprehensive software development methodology that is driven by clearly specified, task-oriented business objectives, and recognition of user needs, limitations and preferences (Mauro, 2000). Information collected using UCD analysis is scientifically applied in the design, testing, and implementation of products and services. When rigorously applied, a UCD approach meets both user needs and the business objectives of the sponsoring organization, such as managing risks (Siegel, 2003). UCD can make the difference between success and failure of software applications and can contribute to innovation by revealing unsuspected opportunities for innovative design, including aspects that would not emerge in other forms of idea generation.

APPLYING UCD TO DESIGN OF PATIENT-CENTERED E-HEALTH

UCD is a design philosophy and a process where the user is the design cornerstone, and his/her limitations, hopes and objectives are given extensive attention at each stage of the design process. UCD seeks to answer questions about users and their tasks and goals, and then uses those findings to drive development and design (Katz-Haas, 1998). The chief difference from other interface design philosophies is that user-centered design tries to optimize the user interface around what people may need and what their capabilities are in order to fulfill a task, rather than force them to adapt to designers' preferences.

There are countless methods, tools and techniques intended to help designers evaluate a target product or service (for brevity these are referred to hereafter simply as *products*) from the point of view of the user. By choosing an appropriate method, it is possible to learn in just a few hours

Table 1. User-Centered Design Principles (UsabilityNet, 2006)

Designing for the users and their tasks
Being consistent
Using simple and natural dialogue
Reducing unnecessary mental effort by the user
Providing adequate feedback
Providing adequate navigation mechanisms
Letting the user drive
Presenting information clearly
Being helpful
Reducing errors

how to improve usability of a product (Mauro, 2000). In this chapter we profile several useful tools and methods which will help an e-health design project to comply with the key principles of UCD. An exemplar set of UCD principles (UsabilityNet, 2006) is shown in Table 1.

Inquiring Research Methods: Understanding What Users Want

The proper identification of what users need and what the product should offer are essential at an early stage. Inquiring methods generally gather data in an open-ended way through interviews or observation, and these data are then progressively interpreted by the investigators.

Several types of methods are typically used in combination. A general classification of these methods can be summarized as follows (Friedman & Wyatt, 2006).

- ***Observation methods***: When using these methods investigators immerse themselves in the domain under study. The investigator may act purely as a detached observer and rely on multiple "informants" as a source of information, or he/she can be a participant-observer by becoming to some degree a member of the work team, empowering him/her with a more vivid impression of the living or working environment under study.
- ***Interviewing methods***: These are conducted as *formal interviews*, where both the investigator and the interviewee are aware that the answers to questions are being recorded, or *informal interviews*, occurring as spontaneous discussions between the investigators and the observational subjects. Formal interviews vary in their degree of structure. At one extreme is the unstructured interview where there are no predetermined questions, and between the extremes is the semi-structured interview where the investigator specifies in advance a set of topics he/she would like to address, but is flexible to the order in the pre-specified list (field interview). At the other extreme is the structured interview with a set of questions which are presented to each participant using the same words and in the same order (questionnaires).
- ***Document analysis /artifact analysis***: This activity consists of analyzing documents and other artifacts produced by the organized human activity in a given place. These can include written notes and forms given to patients by their physicians or administrative personnel and accesses to the patient's

Personal health record (PHR). Automatically-generated user log files are key artifacts in this analysis. Data from these records are often quantifiable, and can be important for subsequent analysis.

Specific inquiring methods are describe below.

Contextual Inquiry

The *contextual inquiry* is conducted through interviews and observation in the field and is based upon three fundamental principles: understanding the context in which the study object is used, knowing that the user is one of the most important parts of the design process, and having a precise focus or study object (Hom, 1996). Goals for the contextual inquiry should be established in advance, and include development of interview questions and observation tasks to achieve each goal. The overriding goal of contextual inquiry is to understand how and why something is done or why something is not done (Beyer & Holtzblatt, 1998). During interviews, the interviewer must create a bond with the interviewee and ask questions aimed toward creating a dialogue where the interviewee can express not only experiences or opinions, but also describe his/her involvement in the problem. When the interview is over, a careful analysis of the interview transcript should be conducted to assess if the goals have been achieved and to determine if there are further questions that need to be asked in subsequent visits.

Contextual inquiry is one of the best methods to understand issues from the patient's perspective. Many times the environment in which people use a system influences their use of a product. For example, if patients ordinarily access the Internet from a cybercafé they may prefer to have their PHR display health related information displayed in a more discreet form than if they are working at their home. Contextual inquiry is also very useful when researchers do not have a clear understanding of the domain being studied, such as in the early stages of development. Because much of the information obtained through contextual inquiry is subjective, it is important to confirm the results using other methods which are more objective in nature.

Method in practice: Let's consider that you are planning to change the procedure in which patients confirm their arrival at a large ambulatory patient practice. Contextual inquiry can be applied to initially assess the needs of people involved in the process. The patients can be requested to think about what would make their waiting time easier; and what design changes would help their waiting and would avoid the queuing. In this way they become partners in the design process and their opinion will be carefully analyzed. The researcher should stay focused on one thing at the time: in this specific case, the focus would be only on reception and waiting times. It was possible for the Hospital Italiano de Buenos Aires to improve on this process by developing a system for the patients to confirm their arrival at a kiosk, therefore avoiding the need for a hospital employee to be present and increasing the rate at which patients are checked in (Plazzotta, Otero, Campos, Pedernera, Navas, Martínez, Plazzotta, et al., 2005).

Ethnographic Study / Field Observation

Ethnography (from the Greek ethnos (εθνος), "people", and grapho (γραφω), "I write") is a method of anthropological investigation in which data is gathered in the field with the members of a given community acting as informants. Analysis of this data is used to provide a compact and detailed description of their customs, beliefs, myths, genealogies and history. Similar to the contextual inquiry, ethnographic study identifies how a product is personally experienced and used by each individual within his/her cultural and organizational contexts. Observing people in the field is often one of the best ways to determine their needs and capabilities, as observation can illuminate the concepts and premises of what people understand unconsciously but may not be able to articulate. Another aspect of field observation is informally interviewing people about the way they perform tasks and the way they use the product.

Ethnographic study of patients in a hospital has been used to evaluate the various hospital domains, including waiting rooms, blood laboratory rooms, information boards, patient's wards and consulting rooms (Schultz, Bottorff, & Johnson, 2006). As an alternative, Kaufman and colleagues have applied ethnographic study methods remotely, by video-recording patients using a diabetes management software from their homes (Kaufman, Patel, Hilliman, Morin, Pevzner, Weinstock, et al., 2003).

The idea behind ethnographic study methods is to understand how tasks are done and how products are used within actual contexts of use, including aspects which the people under study may not be aware of. It is advisable to apply this method in the early stages of development, when it is most important to understand the aspects related to the use of a product rather than other characteristics of the product.

Method in practice: Continuing with the scenario begun in the initial assessment, investigators should consider the conditions in which patients arrival is checked, whether there is a receptionist, if there is a long waiting queue to confirm their arrival, if patients have to repeat their name or last name more than once in spite of having shown their identity card, or if the queues are the result of receptionists doing other things apart from checking on patient's arrival. Every detail of the place where the patients are asked to confirm their arrival should be evaluated. It is essential not only to study the desk to which the patients come to and the number of patients standing in the queues, but also the practice room itself. Every detail should be carefully assessed, including the room's tidiness, the colors of the room and the noise levels.

Focus Groups

Focus groups are carefully planned group discussions conducted by trained moderators. A small number of questions, developed in advance, are used to generate in-depth consideration of a narrowly defined topic. By using this method a direct interaction with participants is established as they are asked to express their opinions about the topic, for example, relating to interface functionality or design (Pope & Mays, 2006).

This method involves identifying questions through which it will be possible to gather relevant information about a topic or a product. It is important to frame questions as widely as possible in order to facilitate discussion in which subsequent interaction among the participants can bring out varied and thoughtful ideas, such as identifying problems which might arise when using the product.

This method can be used at any stage of system development, as long as questions are appropriate to the context. This can begin at very early stages of development, when the product requirements are still being designed, and continue through the time following product release, where the objective may be to test customer satisfaction (Kinzie, Cohn, Julian, & Knaus, 2002).

Method in practice: Let's imagine that the manager of a medical practice notices that the patients are becoming annoyed by the delays they have encountered while waiting for an appointment. He therefore decides to interview some of the patients in the waiting room to tackle this problem. He then analyzes what steps the patients take before seeing the physician in order to understand what drawbacks there are in the system. Next he organizes a focus group that includes participants who represent those involved in the situation (patients, receptionists, physicians among others) and moderates a discussion on delays in order to assess whether his observations were correct and complete and to identify potential solutions to the problem.

Questionnaire Surveys

The two terms *questionnaire* and *survey* are often confused, and some people consider surveys as a synonym for questionnaires. However this is not so. The survey is a process of investigation across a substantial population, whereas the questionnaires is a specific tool that can be used to implement the survey. Thus, the term *questionnaire survey* indicates a survey investigation conducted through the use of a questionnaire, versus other methods, such as an interview survey.

The questionnaire survey is exceptionally useful to efficiently obtain information from large numbers of individuals. This method consists of a set of questions on the subject of study which can be administered on paper or electronically.

Surveys are inherently interactive. The function of a surveyor is to lead the respondent in such a way to bring light to all the topics or ideas the surveyor wants to learn about. Design of the questions is the most important step of the survey development process. The questions should be as open and clear as possible, but this can be difficult for novices to achieve. It is helpful to consult a focused guide to creating and evaluating survey questions, such as (Rea & Parker, 2005).

It is possible to make a quantitative analysis with the results from the questionnaire survey through interpretation of charts and graphs or use of statistical analysis software. The last part of survey analysis is interpretation of the patterns and trends that arise in the results.

Method in practice: Having improved the standards by which patients confirm their arrival through a kiosk, it might be necessary afterwards to use a questionnaire to assess level of satisfaction among a larger sample of the people involved in this process. Questionnaires are a very efficient mechanism for administering this type of assessment. One example is the QUIS, a validated questionnaire for assessing users' satisfaction with interfaces that was designed at the University of Maryland at College Park. The QUIS has been widely used and can help developers to estimate the impact the new product will have (Chin, Diehl, & Norman, 1988).

Other Inquiring Methods

Other methods of inquiry may be useful at various stages of the process. Among these are *screen snapshots,* where a prototype of a product is tested (usually at mid-stage of development) and screen snapshots are taken to document users' actions at specific points, and *journaled sessions,* where journaling software is used to record user's actions, including cursor movements, mouse clicks, and other interface interactions. Journaling software can also provide dialogue boxes in which the user types in comments or observations while performing the tasks. Both approaches can provide valuable information about the usability of the software and are relatively inexpensive to implement. Internet development offers the opportunity to expand the reach of journaling software, lowering costs further and allowing large-scale product tests.

Inspection Design Methods: What the Analyst Can See

Usability inspection is the generic name for a set of methods that are based on having analysts inspect a user interface. A *usability analyst* is a trained professional specialized in applying usability methods (including UCD) to ensure the ease-of-use and positive user-experience of products. Typically, usability inspection is aimed at finding usability problems in the design, with some methods also addressing specific issues such as the severity of the usability problems and the overall usability of an entire system. Inspection methods are based on the concept of task analysis, where the evaluation takes place within information processing tasks. However, inspection methods also lend themselves to the review of user interface specifications that have not necessarily been implemented yet, meaning that inspection can be performed early in the usability engineering lifecycle (Nielsen & Mack, 1994).

There are several methods of inspection, but for practical reasons this chapter focuses on two that are particularly well-suited for evaluating interfaces for patients. These are the heuristic evaluation and cognitive walkthrough methods.

Heuristic Evaluation

Heuristic evaluation is an informal method of inspection involving usability experts who judge whether each dialogue element or task follows established usability and design heuristics, i.e., rules that are intended to be applied flexibly rather than followed rigidly (Nielsen & Mack, 1994). The analyst inspects the user interface system, often by carrying out a specific task while using the system, and notes any violations of a predefined set of heuristics. It is essential, therefore, that analysts are well trained. They must clearly understand the heuristics and also be experienced in applying them across a range of situations. Nielsen and Landauer (1993) observe that most usability problems can be identified if there are between three to five analysts working on the project.

Each analyst should check the interface at least twice, observing the function of each of its elements carefully and evaluating its design, location and implementation according to the heuristic list. Analysts independently evaluate the user interface and generate a list of heuristic violations. These are then combined into a joint list of all violations reported by all the analysts. The results of the heuristic evaluation can be summarized and presented to the design team along with recommendations for improvement.

Nielsen & Mack (1994) provide the following ten heuristics as guidelines for user interface design.

1. **Visibility of system status.** Keep users informed about what is going on, through appropriate feedback in a timely fashion.
2. **Match between system and the real world.** Speak the users' language, using words, phrases and concepts familiar to the user, rather than system-oriented terms. Follow real-world conventions.
3. **User control and freedom.** Users need a clearly marked "emergency exit" to escape from any unwanted state. Support undo and redo. A goal is for the user to feel he/she is in control of the system.
4. **Consistency and standards.** Use standard conventions for all aspects of the interaction, including navigation and carrying out basic operations. Adopt all conventions of the operating system or platform.
5. **Error prevention.** Where possible, avoid problems before they can occur. Eliminate error-prone conditions or check for them and present users with a confirmation option before they commit to the action.
6. **Recognition rather than recall.** Minimize the user's memory load by making objects, actions, and options visible. Make all information that is not visible easy to find and retrieve..
7. **Flexibility and efficiency of use.** Provide mechanisms to increase efficiency by experienced users, such as control key functions and shortcuts, and to support novice users in using the product and learning use processes.
8. **Aesthetic and minimalist design:** Remove all extraneous information from dialogs with users. Avoid distractions.

9. **Help users recognize, diagnose, and recover from errors**: Error messages should be expressed in plain language that clearly indicates what the problem is and suggests solutions where this is practical.
10. **Help and documentation**: Sources for help should be indicated clearly. Where documentation is included, it should be easy to search, be focused on the user's task, list concrete steps to be carried out, and not be excessively large.

The heuristic evaluation can be used at any stage of development, but it is especially practical at the early stages, when the product is not yet ready to be shown to non-expert users. It is also possible to provide paper models or even design details to the trained analysts and to thereby detect many usability problems before software development begins.

Method in practice: Carroll and his collaborators used heuristic evaluation to inspect a clinical decision support system (CDSS). They were able to make changes in the interfaces and develop a visual thermometer in an Electronic Health Record which allowed both patients and clinicians to readily identify absolute cardiovascular risk factors (Carroll, Marsden, Soden, Naylor, New, & Dornan, 2002).

Cognitive Walkthrough

The cognitive walkthrough is a method used to identify usability issues in software or web sites by focusing on how easy it is for new users to accomplish tasks within the system. This method is based on the fact that users typically prefer to learn a system by using it rather than studying a manual. Analysts construct task scenarios and then role-play the part of a user engaged in "walking through" the interface and note which user actions are needed to carry out the steps, what goals/subgoals the users would have and what potential problems might be encountered at each step. The objective of the cognitive walkthrough is to uncover possible errors in design that would interfere with user's ability to learn how to use the system and carry out tasks. Analysts complete a series of representative tasks from which an encompassing report of potential issues is compiled and used to guide improvements to the interface.

Cognitive walkthrough has been applied to the study of usability and learnability of several distinct medical information technologies (Carroll et al., 2002; Kushniruk, Kaufman, Patel, Levesque, & Lottin, 1996; Patel & Kaufman, 1998). For example, Kaufman and collaborators used this method to improve a home-based telemedicine system for a diabetic population (Kaufman et al., 2003). Cognitive walkthroughs identified aspects of the interface that were suboptimal or impeded the performance of certain tasks and patient-related factors that constituted barriers to productive use, such as numeracy and psychomotor skills.

The cognitive walkthrough can be effective in identifying potential problems which then can be evaluated via usability testing methods, which involve testing with representative users in real situational contexts. These are described in a subsequent section of the chapter.

Method in practice: Cognitive walkthroughs help to identify whether a product meets the user's goals and can be used efficiently to accomplish the purpose of each task. This can be seen in a system of geographical location for patients at a hospital kiosk, where a patient can ascertain, for example, the location of the laboratory where she has to get her blood tested. The patient's goal will be to find, among other tasks, where exactly the laboratory is located, what part of the building or on which floor it is and which lift she needs to take to get there. The various tasks the patient should perform will be first to identify the correct key she must press to start looking for the place she wants to reach, and then to find the laboratory in an interactive map. When analysts "walk through" the interface, it is important to identify if the patient will have difficulties in performing the tasks, for example, because the keys are not easily seen or the labels are not clear or she is distracted by other options.

Other Inspection Methods

Other helpful inspection methods include *formal usability inspections*, developed by IBM and used, among others, to identify bugs in programming, *standard inspections* which ensure compliance with industry standards and *guideline checklists* which can help ensure that usability principles will be considered in a design.

Usability Testing Methods

Usability testing refers to the evaluation of information systems by testing with representatives of the target user population as they perform representative tasks using the product in a particular context, such as patients using an e-health application to schedule an appointment. Usability testing is a means for measuring how well people can use a product for its intended purpose(s). The aim is to observe people using the product in an as realistic a setting as possible, in order to discover errors and identify areas that need improvement. Researchers report that 80% of the usability problems can be detected through these usability testing of as few as eight to ten representative subjects (Nielsen, 1993; Rubin & Hudson, 1994).

Kushniruk & Patel (2004) have defined nine phases for applying usability testing to the evaluation of clinical information systems that must be followed in order to ensure that the intended users of a clinical system, including patients, physicians, and nurses, can carry out the tasks efficiently and effectively. These phases are summarized as follows.

The **first phase** is the identification of the evaluation objectives, which may vary considerably according to the product being tested and the target users. The **second phase** is the sample selection; the subjects should be *representative* of end users of the system under study, for example, chronic disease patients in the case of a Pathology portal. It also is important to apply criteria for classifying subjects in terms of their prior computer experience. **Phase three** is the selection of representative tasks and contexts for analysis to adequately represent real scenarios. The tasks for analysis should be carefully chosen if the testing is in a usability laboratory; use of a real life scenario (naturalistic study) increases the ecological validity of the test. For example, Kaufman used a video-analytic approach to study how patients used home-care software in their own homes (Kaufman et al., 2003). The **fourth phase** is the selection of background questionnaires that can be administered either before or after the usability testing. These questionnaires are used to obtain historical information about the participants that will help evaluators to understand their behavior and performance during the test. The **fifth phase** is the selection of the evaluation environment, which can be either a usability laboratory with controlled experimental conditions, or the place where the user works or lives or uses the system, for example, selections addressed by Kushniruk and collaborators include the waiting room for testing a scheduling kiosk system for patients, automated interviewing and automated triggering questionnaires in a web-based system (Kushniruk, Patel, Patel, & Cimino, 2001). The **sixth phase** is data collection from video and audio recording, VCR recordings of the video screens or people faces were commonly used, but now screen recording tends to be software based. There are several software systems that allow recording the screens, mouse movements and clicks, as well as audio. Video recording provides a remarkably rich and vivid reproduction of an encounter. It also provides a permanent record of an event and supports multiple viewings and re-analysis of data (Jordan & Henderson, 1995). The **seventh phase** is the analysis of the video and audio files. The transformation of data into recommendations involves qualitative and quantitative analysis of the video-based usability data. The **eighth phase** is the interpretation of the findings, where the collected data are compiled and summarized in a number of aspects of a system (task accuracy, user preference data, time to completion of task, frequency and classes of problems encountered). The **ninth phase** is the iterative input into design, where the system is improved on the basis of the problems that usability testing identifies and is then re-tested to determine how the changes affect the system's usability.

Think-Aloud Protocol

The think-aloud protocol is one of the most useful and simple evaluation methods to emerge from the study of cognitive science. Subjects are instructed to "think aloud" (i.e., verbalize their thoughts) as they perform a set of specified tasks. They are asked to verbalize whatever they are looking at, thinking, doing, and feeling, as they go about their task (Lewis & Rieman, 1994). It is useful to record user actions during this process to support detailed analysis of actions, such as mouse clicks and menu selections in conjunction with audio recording of subjects verbalizations (Kushniruk, Patel, Cimino, & Barrows, 1996).

The think-aloud protocol allows the researcher to identify how the user approaches and performs tasks using the interface (Kaplan, 2003). Analyzing this information, it is possible for the researcher to better understand the user's mental model of his/her interaction with the product. There are other benefits as well, such as the ability to repeat tasks that are problematic or to introduce changes into the terminology used, as the user typically will express clearly what exact instructions he/she would have needed to have at hand when performing the task. (Johnson, Johnson, & Zhang, 2000). The think-aloud protocol is effective at all stages of development once a prototype is available for use, however, repeated testing with this method requires availability of new users in order to be effective.

Method in practice: Let's take the case of a researcher developing an application for patients to see laboratory results from their homes. He should keep in mind that laboratory reports are often difficult for patients to understand. Performing a think-aloud protocol would be a useful tool for identifying interface problems, such as visual display of laboratory numbers and test history results, the order in which buttons are displayed, or the terminology that is used.

Question-Asking Protocol

The *question asking protocol* goes beyond the think-aloud protocol by posing questions to users (Lindgaard, 1994). As with the think-aloud protocol, in the question asking protocol the user is shown a prototype or a final version of an interface and is requested to perform certain tasks while verbalizing his/her thoughts. The observer will shadow (stay behind the user watching the user's movements) and ask direct questions at specific stages to obtain more information on a given item or action. Both the readiness (ease-of-use) or drawbacks (difficulty-of-use) the user reports can be used to identify which parts of the interface are clear and which parts need to be improved.

Method in practice: While developing a health information web page, the researcher may wish to test whether an item of information is easily found. He will ask a patient to look for information about a flu vaccine. The patient will reply according to what she can see or according to what she believes should be the right place to find this information. The patient may also answer according to her experience of other interfaces and these responses will provide insights into her mental model of the product in addition to her ongoing verbalization.

Prototyping Methods

Prototyping is the process of quickly putting together a working model (a prototype) in order to test various aspects of a design, illustrate ideas or features and gather early user feedback. It allows testing to begin early in the design process. When the prototype is sufficiently refined and meets design goals relating, for example, to functionality, robustness, and manufacturability, the product is ready for production.

There are various methods in prototyping, ranging from working with a sheet of paper and a pencil (paper prototyping), to developing working but not fully capable computer applications (high-fidelity prototyping). Prototyping can be used at any time in during product development. At the early stages it can be useful to study the needs and desires of users, at a midstage it will provide information about the development of the product and how usable it is, and at later stages it will provide the necessary information to make alterations in areas which need to be refined.

Paper Prototypes

Paper prototyping is a method that lets the designer of a project mock up, test, and refine a design on paper before writing program code. It allows informal usability tests with real users to be undertaken at early stages of product development. Users can also participate in developing paper prototypes, as is detailed in a case study presented subsequently in the chapter.

A number of benefits have been identified in using paper prototypes to develop health care applications (Marill, Miller, & Kitendaugh, 2006; Plovnick & Zeng, 2004). This include the following:

1. **Paper prototypes make the researcher focus on keeping the interface simple**. Various approaches to the design of an interface can be tested with several users to see which one is the preferred.
2. **They are time savers**. Creating paper prototypes requires relatively less effort than coding, so paper prototypes can be easily abandoned if they are not working.
3. **They allow the researcher to start at an unsure stage**. Because paper prototypes have no code, they free the designer from the necessity of building a working platform for the interface. The designer can start with the parts he/she has the most questions about, rather than those that are most stable.
4. **They allow the testing of new terminology at early stages of development**. This is an important feature of paper prototypes in health related designs as many health systems and web pages face problems in presenting terminology that patients can understand.

The aim of this section is to show how it is possible to start with a simple method such as paper prototyping and produce useful improvements in usability. The following case study reports an example of using paper prototyping in the context of designing e-health software applications from a patient-centered perspective.

Case Study: Paper Prototyping in Developing a Personal Health Record (PHR)

The Hospital Italiano de Buenos Aires Experience

Since 1998, The Hospital Italiano de Buenos Aires has gradually implemented a full scale Health Information System (HIS), including ambulatory Electronic Medical Record (EMR), inpatient discharge summaries, administrative systems, scheduling systems, inpatient tracking systems, pharmacy systems and complementary studies report and visualization. It is currently working on the development of a Personal health record (PHR) to support patients' access to various functionalities and services from HIS. For this purpose, patients of the HMO were invited to participate in the activity "Internet Use: can it improve your health care?" by means of a notice published on the hospital's website and in a newsletter sent monthly by post.

Two activities were carried out in two hours. In a brief introduction it was explained to the participants what a PHR is. Then they were divided into 4 groups so that over the next 25 minutes they could discuss and write down what services or information they thought a PHR should offer. Table 2 shows participants' characteristics, based on a survey they answered at the end of the activities.

Even though the study participants were patients and potential users of the system being developed, during the session they were not in a real context of use. For this reason, the first activity used a focus group technique rather than an inquiring method, such as ethnographic study. However, their discussion included experiences and impressions of the context and their personal relationships, which offered relevant information and generated ideas. Each focus group wrote down notes about what they believed were the most important aspects a PHR should offer. At the end of the activity each of the groups shared its results with the other groups, while one investigator wrote down the information on a whiteboard.

To carry out the second activity, each group was given a photocopied sheet of paper in the form of a monitor screen and design materials (scissors, markers, papers, cardboard, and stickers). Participants were instructed to create a paper prototype of a web portal which would provide the services and information listed in the previous activity. When they finished, each group presented its prototype, explaining each of the components chosen and the function and/or information which each component should offer. An example is shown in Figure 1.

During both activities one investigator acted as moderator while another took down notes. To ensure the quality of the record, the two hours were filmed and recorded. At the end of the activities, each patient completed an anonymous questionnaire survey for us to get to know details of gender, age, educational level, access to Internet, and the perceived usefulness of the patient portal components. The information gathered through the activities was useful in:

- **Identifying users' needs and desires for a personal health record.** Focus groups, questionnaires and video-recording analy-

Table 2. Characteristics of study respondents

	All (n=17)
Age in years (range)	59.88 (34-81)
Female gender	11 (64.7%)
University level of study	11 (64.7%)
Internet access	15 (88.2%)
Broadband connection	13 (86.6%)
Internet health information*	12 (70.6%)
* Used Internet in the past to access health related information	

Figure 1. Example Paper Prototype

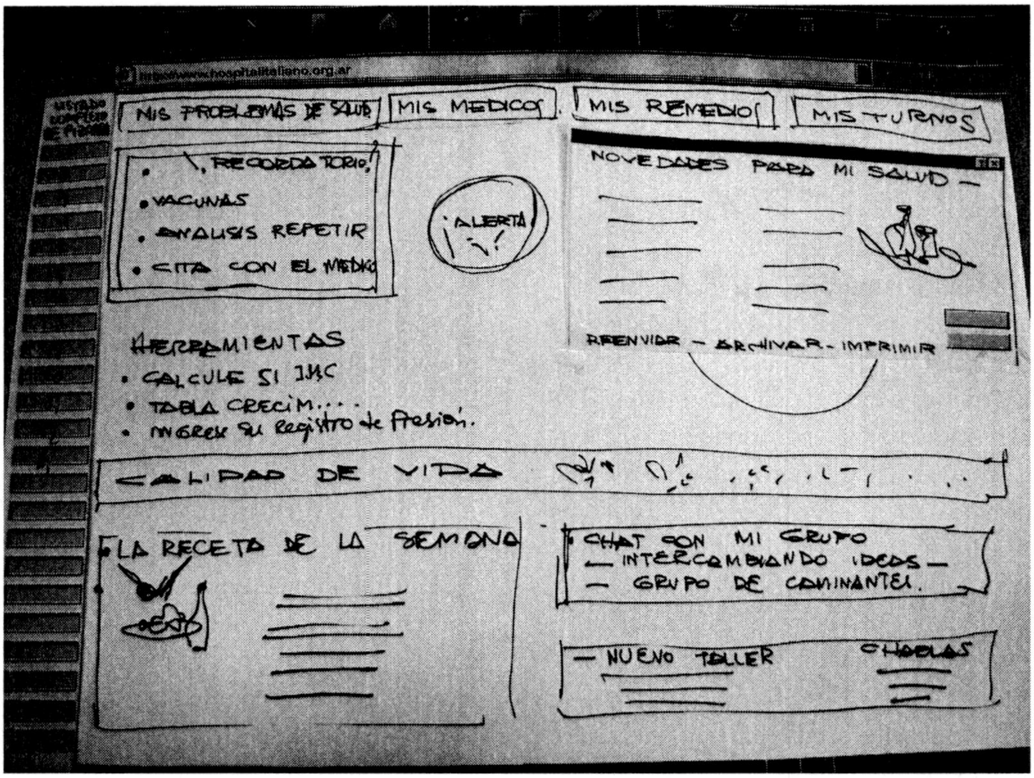

sis were useful methods for gathering this information. These are some examples of participants' needs and desires that were identified:

"...we give priority to basic pathology" "we would like all the information about diabetes to be together" "in reality, what we want is that the information should be integrated" [Problem-oriented information need]

"I don't want just to know what my clinical physician thinks; I want to know what the neurologist says, the opinion of the pharmacist, the nurse's recommendations." [Integrated information]

- **Identifying user's motivations and fears.** Focus group discussion revealed several motivations and fears on the part of participants which may not be observable otherwise.

"I am afraid that with so much technology we'll lose contact with the doctor... It would be important to have access to the e-mails of the different doctors who are concerned with my health" [New ways of communication]

"I would also like to be have access to a Chat room which allowed me a more spontaneous consultation in case some drug made me feel unwell" [New ways of communication]

"We need a patients' forum, a network where we feel represented, a space where we don't feel unprotected" [New ways of communication]

"I would like to be able to access my clinical history, and that the doctors should have access to my portal, but on condition that I should be able to decide which doctor sees what, because there are things I talk about with one doctor while with another I feel embarrassed" [Access to Clinical Histories, and Data Privacy]

- **Identifying user's ideal visual display of the interface**. Paper prototyping allowed participants to contribute to PHR design.

"We would like certain criteria to be complied with for the navigation of the portal, for example that it should be easy to change the size of the letters for those who have sight difficulties" [Interface Flexibility]

"We would like a section of favorites links" "that every illness should have links to pages with information that could be useful, associations, or that would put us in contact with groups of patients who suffer from the same pathology" [Access to Information Sources]

"I would like the system to warn me in case of my forgetting to vaccinate my children by giving me an alert in red" [Warnings in red]

- Identifying user's wish and desired terminology to be seen on the screen.

"I would like to be able to understand the medical terms used. I would expect the PHR to use every day language" "Seeing my medical record from my physician's monitor screen I had to ask him what Leiomyoma was. He told me that it were the uterine fibroids I had been complaining about for a long time" [Terminology issue]

By using UCD methods the developers were able to obtain sound information about patient's needs and desires and at the same time learn about the patient's preferred methods of information display. The use of prototyping methods are highly relevant to e-health developers, as these will provide information early in design stages when it is inexpensive and quick to initiate product changes.

CONCLUSION

UCD methods can be applied effectively with patients, even to the point of allowing patients the opportunity to contribute to product design. The resulting *patient centered design* is an essential step when undertaking development of e-health that is intended to meet patients' needs and address their capabilities. However it is necessary to keep in mind that there are motives, fears, and challenges which will influence results of interaction with patients. The methods described in this chapter can be very useful in overcoming these challenges, especially when used in combination as in the case study we presented.

REFERENCES

Andreassen, H. K., Trondsen, M., Kummervold, P. E., Gammon, D., & Hjortdahl, P. (2006). Patients who use e-mediated communication with their doctor: New constructions of trust in the patient-doctor relationship. *Qualitative Health Research, 16*(2), 238-248.

Baker, L., Wagner, T. H., Singer, S., & Bundorf, M. K. (2003). Use of the Internet and e-mail for health care information: Results from a national survey. *JAMA, 289*(18), 2400-2406.

Beyer, H., & Holtzblatt, K. (1998). *Contextual design: Defining customer-centered systems*. San Francisco: Morgan Kaufmann.

Carroll, C., Marsden, P., Soden, P., Naylor, E., New, J., & Dornan, T. (2002). Involving users in the design and usability evaluation of a clinical decision support system. *Computer Methods and Programs in Biomedicine, 69*(2), 123-135.

Coulter, A. (1997). Partnerships with patients: the pros and cons of shared clinical decision-making. *Journal of Health Services Research & Policy, 2*(2), 112-121.

Chin, J. P., Diehl, V. A., & Norman, L. K. (1988). *Development of an instrument measuring user satisfaction of the human-computer interface.* New York: ACM Press

Eysenbach, G., & Kohler, C. (2003). What is the prevalence of health-related searches on the world wide web? Qualitative and quantitative analysis of search engine queries on the internet. *2003 AMIA Annual Symposium Proceedings,* 225-229.

Friedman, C. P., & Wyatt, J. (2006). *Evaluation methods in medical informatics* (Second edition). New York: Springer.

Hom, J. (1996). *The usability methods toolbox.* from http://jthom.best.vwh.net/usability

Johnson, C. M., Johnson, T., & Zhang, J. (2000). Increasing productivity and reducing errors through usability analysis: A case study and recommendations. *2001 AMIA Symposium Proceedings*, 394-398.

Jordan, B., & Henderson, A. (1995). Interaction analysis: Foundations and practice. *Journal of the Learning Sciences, 4*(1), 39-103.

Kaplan, B. (2003). Deriving design recommendations through discount usability engineering: Ethnographic observation and thinking-aloud protocol in usability testing for computer-based teaching cases. *2003 AMIA Annual Symposium Proceedings,* 346-350.

Katz-Haas, R. (1998). Ten guidelines for user-centered web design. *Usability Interface, 5*(1).

Kaufman, D. R., Patel, V. L., Hilliman, C., Morin, P. C., Pevzner, J., Weinstock, R. S., et al. (2003). Usability in the real world: Assessing medical information technologies in patients' homes. *Journal of Biomedical Informatics, 36*(1-2), 45-60.

Kinzie, M. B., Cohn, W. F., Julian, M. F., & Knaus, W. A. (2002). A user-centered model for web site design: Needs assessment, user interface design, and rapid prototyping. *Journal of the American Medical Informatics Association, 9*(4), 320-330.

Kushniruk, A., Patel, V., Cimino, J. J., & Barrows, R. A. (1996). Cognitive evaluation of the user interface and vocabulary of an outpatient information system. *1996 AMIA Annual Symposium Proceedings*, 22-26.

Kushniruk, A. W., Kaufman, D. R., Patel, V. L., Levesque, Y., & Lottin, P. (1996). Assessment of a computerized patient record system: A cognitive approach to evaluating medical technology. *MD Computing, 13*(5), 406-415.

Kushniruk, A. W. & Patel, V. L. (2004). Cognitive and usability engineering methods for the evaluation of clinical information systems. *Journal of Biomedical Informatics, 37*(1), 56-76.

Kushniruk, A. W., Patel, C., Patel, V. L., & Cimino, J. J. (2001). 'Televaluation' of clinical information systems: An integrative approach to assessing Web-based systems. *International Journal of Medical Informatics, 61*(1), 45-70.

Lewis, C., & Rieman, J. (1994). *Task-centered user interface design: A practical introduction.* Retrieved December 13,2007 from http://www.hcibib.org/tcuid/

Lindgaard, G. (1994). *Usability testing and system evaluation: A guide for designing useful computer systems.* London: Chapman & Hall.

Marill, J. L., Miller, N., & Kitendaugh, P. (2006). The MedlinePlus public user interface: Studies of design challenges and opportunities. *Journal of the Medical Library Association, 94*(1), 30-40.

Mauro, C. L. (2000). Formal definition of user-centered design (UCD). Retrieved May, 2007, from http://www.taskz.com/definitions.php

Nielsen, J., & Landauer, T. K. 1993. A mathematical model of the finding of usability problems. *Proceedings ACM/IFIP INTERCHI'93 Conference* (Amsterdam, The Netherlands, April 24-29), 206-213.

Nielsen, J. (1993). *Usability engineering.* Boston: Academic Press.

Nielsen, J., & Mack, R. L. (1994). *Usability inspection methods.* New York: Wiley.

Patel, V. L., & Kaufman, D. R. (1998). Medical informatics and the science of cognition. *Journal of the American Medical Informatics Association, 5*(6), 493-502.

Plazzotta, F., Otero, P., Campos, F., Pedernera, F., Navas, H., Martínez, M., et al. (2005). *Estrategias para agilizar la atención ambulatoria: integración de los sistemas de información.* Paper presented at the 8mo Simposio de Informática en Salud - 34 JAIIO, Santa Fé, Argentina.

Plovnick, R. M., & Zeng, Q. T. (2004). Reformulation of consumer health queries with professional terminology: a pilot study. *J Med Internet Res, 6*(3), e27.

Pope, C., & Mays, N. (2006). *Qualitative research in health care* (Third edition). Malden, MA: Blackwell Pub./BMJ Books.

Rea, M & Parker, R. A. (2005). *Designing and conducting survey research: A comprehensive guide* (Third edition). San Francisco: Jossey-Bass.

Rubin, J., & Hudson, T. (1994). *Handbook of usability testing: How to plan, design, and conduct effective tests.* New York: John Wiley & Sons, Inc.

Schultz, A. S. H., Bottorff, J. L., & Johnson, J. L. (2006). An ethnographic study of tobacco control in hospital settings. *Tobacco Control, 15*(4), 317-322.

Siegel, D. A. (2003). The business case for user-centered design: Increasing your power of persuasion. *Interactions, 10*(3), 30-36.

Street, R. L., Jr. (2003). Mediated consumer-provider communication in cancer care: The empowering potential of new technologies. *Patient Education Counseling, 50*(1), 99-104.

UsabilityNet (2006). Key principles of user-centred design. Retrieved June 2006, from http://www.usabilitynet.org/management/b_design.htm

Chapter III
Connecting with Ourselves and Others Online:
Psychological Aspects of Online Health Communication

Jan-Are K. Johnsen
Norwegian Centre for Telemedicine, University Hospital of North Norway, Norway

Deede Gammon
Norwegian Centre for Telemedicine, University Hospital of North Norway, Norway

ABSTRACT

In this chapter, we look at some fundamental aspects of communicating about ourselves and our health through technology. In particular, we examine how the social psychological theories of self-presentation and self-regulation might be applied to online health-communication. It is argued that the specific qualities of text-based communication might have unique benefits for health-communication through the interplay between the writing process and the concerns posed by health-issues. An understanding of how psychological processes are connected with online health communication is believed to be fundamental in understanding trends within self-help and user-driven health communication, and to predict possible outcomes of such behavior. Also, this knowledge might inform the design and development of patient-centered solutions for health-communication and heath-service delivery.

INTRODUCTION

The degree to which we are able to express our health concerns and needs can be decisive for the appropriateness of the help we receive. In fact, patients' stories are found to be the most significant source of diagnostic findings, while clinical examinations and/or laboratory tests determine less than one third of diagnostic conclusions (Peterson, Holbrook, Von Hales, Smith, & Staker, 1992).

Nevertheless, communicating about personal health can be a challenge for many reasons. We may, for example, be confused and anxious about what is wrong with us, embarrassed, and/or just unable to put into words our thoughts and feelings. Such challenges may also differ depending on our relationship with those we are communicating with, whether they would be our peers, our family, persons of authority (such as doctors), or even anonymous strangers.

This chapter examines some fundamental aspects of communicating about ourselves and our health through technology. Throughout our discussion, it is useful to keep in mind that research on electronically mediated health communication (more widely known as e-health) is still in its infancy. Thus, much of the research we refer to is conducted outside the realm of healthcare under general headings such as such as computer-mediated communication (CMC) and Internet psychology (Joinson, McKenna, Postmes, & Reips, 2007). We believe that efforts to incorporate this research into the more applied endeavours of designing evidence based e-health hold promise.

The chapter starts by offering a brief overview of the classical theories of CMC as an introduction to the perspectives developed in this chapter. Based on these theories and related psychological research, some specific aspects of CMC that we believe are particularly relevant to health communication are outlined. This includes fundamental processes involved in communicating to others and ourselves about our health. The discussion is concluded by presenting research on some of the failures of traditional face-to-face healthcare settings in achieving patient-centeredness. We confront traditional assumptions about the superiority of face-to-face communication in healthcare—that e-health is invariably a second best alternative forced on us by resource constraints. Accepting the essence of patient-centeredness as systems *"(...) designed around the patient with respect for a person's preferences, values and/or needs—and to formulate tools and targets to achieve this"* (Harkness, 2005, pp. 4), we argue that understanding people's current uses of CMC for health purposes is crucial if we are to exploit it for enhancing patient-centeredness in healthcare.

THEORIES OF COMPUTER-MEDIATED COMMUNICATION

Quite simply, CMC can be defined as communication between two or more individuals using computers. This includes use of e-mail, instant messaging, chat, as well as similar functionalities offered through mobile phones such as the Short Messaging System (SMS).

Much of the research within the multidisciplinary field of CMC is based on the idea that different communication media affect the communication process and its outcomes based on the way information can be transmitted in a particular medium. A basic assumption is that media differ in terms of "richness," defined as a medium's ability to change understanding within a time interval, for instance measured by performance on persuasion tasks (e.g., how well are we able to get our view across to another person). This term was introduced through the media richness theory (MRT) (Daft & Lengel, 1986), which claimed that the richness of a medium could be judged by looking at four criteria: feedback, multiple cues, language variety, and personal focus. Accordingly, face-to-face communication was viewed as the richest medium, followed by telephone, e-mail and letters. Later, the emergence of real-time, interactive video would be viewed as somewhere between face-to-face and telephone with regards to richness (e.g., Isaacs, Whittaker, Frohlich, & O'Conaill, 1994). Developed for research on use of communication technology in organizations, MRT specifically claimed that rich media would be best suited to equivocal tasks, while written media (lower degrees of richness) would be suited for unequivocal tasks. Despite the fact that MRT was hardly meant to explain the informal social phenomena that have unfolded on the Internet during the past 10 years, it has nevertheless dominated research on online social interactions.

Indeed, MRT is consistent both with our common sense notions about communication, in particular social communication, and the preferences of people when asked about communication. Users almost invariably say they would prefer "richer" modes of communication (e.g., video over text), but these preferences cannot predict actual use and task performance (Schliemann, Asting, Følstad, & Heim, 2002). Also, the research literature on CMC is filled with surprising findings and apparent paradoxes not easily reconcilable with MRT. Asynchronous lightweight text messaging—like SMS and IM—are excessively popular and clearly foster informal interpersonal communication (Nardi, Whittaker, & Bradner, 2000), while classic theories (e.g., MRT) predict that they should not.

Modern CMC theories hold that relationships via media that lack nonverbal cues develop just as well as face-to-face, it just takes a longer time (Lea & Spears, 1995; Walther & Burgoon, 1992). Studies have also shown that relationship formation varies depending upon system features for instance, synchronous vs. asynchronous communication (Parks & Floyd, 1996; Parks & Roberts, 1998). While these results do not fit a neat and unified theory, they nevertheless give relatively clear indications of some critical factors in online interaction. In the next sections, we explore some of these critical factors in more depth.

SELF-DISCLOSURE

The act of revealing personal information about oneself to others is commonly referred to as self-disclosure (Archer, 1980, as cited in Joinson, 1999), and is crucial to the development of personal relationships, (e.g., Laurenceau, Barrett, & Pietromonaco, 1998). Both experimental and anecdotal evidence suggest that general CMC can be characterized as containing high levels of self-disclosure (Joinson, 1999, 2004), and research shows that people often reveal more about themselves via a computer than face-to-face (Joinson, 2001a; Joinson, 2001b). Few would have predicted the popularity of clumsy user-interfaces such as SMS (mobile phones), chat or instant messaging for highly emotional and intimate communication for better and worse (e.g., flirting, bullying). These examples of increased self-disclosure, along with a related concept—disinhibition—are often attributed to the lack of social restraints that accompany CMC compared to face-to-face communication. The Reduced Social Cues Model (Spears, Lea, & Postmes, 2001) offers an interesting explanation for this. This model emphasizes the role of reduced nonverbal cues and contextual information online compared to face-to-face communication. Although the model has mostly been applied to "deindividuation"[1] and corresponding "antinormative behaviour," it is equally interesting in light of more positive social behaviour. For example, several claim that new, meaningful relationships can be formed online *because of*, not despite, its known limitations (e.g., lack of nonverbal cues) (McKenna & Bargh, 1998; McKenna, Green, & Gleason, 2002; Tidwell & Walther, 2002).

Health-Related Self-Disclosure

The above findings from more traditional research on CMC appear equally relevant for communication about health-issues. Joinson (1999) outlined some of the studies illustrating these issues. For example, medical patients tend to report more symptoms and undesirable behaviours when interviewed by computer than face-to-face (Greist, Klein, & VanCura, 1973). Clients at a sexual disease clinic report more sexual partners, more previous visits, and more symptoms to a computer than to a doctor (Robinson & West, 1992). Ferriter (1993) found that pre-clinical psychiatric interviews conducted using CMC compared to face-to-face yielded more honest, candid answers. In the U.K., the Samaritans report that although only 20% of telephone callers report suicidal feelings, this number increases to around 50% of e-mail contacts (The Scotsman, 24, Feb., 1999, cited in Joinson, 1999). Also, a study of Norwegian online mental health forums found that 45% of those who participated (N=492) claimed they had never discussed the same issues with anyone outside the Internet (Kummervold, Gammon, Bergvik, Johnsen, Hasvold, & Rosenvinge, 2002). Since the quality of healthcare depends on the quality of information provided by patients, these examples are worth understanding in more depth.

Several factors might play a role in facilitating health-related self-disclosure. First of all, a patient communicating through text-based CMC might feel more able to control and set the agenda for the interaction. As an example, the self-disclosure model proposed by Kam and Chismar (2003) includes the concept of perceived control in terms of eliciting personal health information from respondent. Here the ability to backtrack in a Web-based questionnaire reduced tendencies to respond in socially desirable ways. As a result, the information gathered by these means might be more correct than information gathered from less controllable applications. Also, through the adaptation of uncertainty reduction theory to CMC (Berger & Calabrese, 1975, cited in Tidwell & Walther, 2002) we might argue that self-disclosure is one of the few communication strategies available in mediated-contexts where self-relevant information is exchanged. Further, nonverbal cues are unavailable as a source of social information in most forms of CMC. Thus, participants have to obtain such information by asking specific questions along with disclosing information about themselves (direct strategies for uncertainty reduction). The resulting self-disclosure "effects" are valid for many situations in CMC where self-presentation concerns are central.

These "side effects" of the use of mediated communication technology could be used advantageously for designing health-services that help patients respond candidly to diagnostic and therapeutic processes that otherwise may be difficult for various reasons (confusion, embarrassment). However, a better understanding of why people use technology to communicate about health issues is needed. Indeed, online health-related communication is largely user-initiated, and grasping the reasons for this use is crucial in efforts to improve patient-centred healthcare by means of technology.

Writing and Health

When people use communication technologies to communicate about their health-needs outside of official health-channels, they turn to low-tech, text-based media, typically discussion forums and e-mail lists (for instance, King & Moreggi, 1998). Self-disclosure is an important element in keeping a diary or writing about oneself, even though one may never end up sharing this information with others. Interestingly, the process of writing is associated with health effects. In particular, studies within the "writing cure" tradition of Pennebaker and colleagues (Pennebaker, 1997; Pennebaker & Beall, 1986; Pennebaker & Francis, 1996) found that the act of writing about emotional experiences has positive effects for those with and without health complaints. "Emotional writing" typically consists of structured writing tasks, where participants are asked to write about emotional upheavals or traumatic experiences over three–five days for about 15–20 minutes each time. Outcomes are compared to that of a control group (non-emotional writing). Emotional writing has been shown to positively influence frequency of physician visits, immune function, stress hormones, blood pressure, and a host of social, academic, and cognitive variables

(Campbell & Pennebaker, 2003). These findings appear to be reliable (e.g., Smyth, 1998), although conflicting views of the results have been voiced (Littrell, 1998).

It is argued that no single theory or perspective will convincingly explain the health effects of emotional writing (Pennebaker, 2004; Smyth, 1998). Writing about emotions affects people on multiple levels. Consequently, a number of different explanations have been put forward. These range from Freudian notions of catharsis and insight to behavioural concepts of habituation and extinction, cognitive oriented ideas related to perception, memory, self-regulation, and constructivist notions of meaning.

While elements of all these ideas may be at play in conjunction with self-disclosure, evidence suggests that the introduction of structured tasks to assist self-regulation is important (Cameron & Nicholls, 1998). These include focused emotional disclosure (about a specific problem), as well as formulating intentions or plans for addressing or solving the problem. Interestingly, a study by Guastella and Dadds (2006) further shows that writing tasks might be structured to lead to differential emotional processing. That is, by providing research participants with specific instructions about how they should write about their traumatic experiences, meaningful changes in emotional responses are detected. Also, Pennebaker and Francis (1996) investigated the language of emotional writing, and found that health-effects appeared related to the degree of structure and cohesiveness of the language used. This suggests a more complete understanding of the problems described, including that of causality (Pennebaker, Mayne, & Francis, 1997). Health-effects observed from writing about purely imaginary trauma suggest that the task itself might make people more resilient to coping with real-life trauma through establishment of mental coping mechanisms (Greenberg, Wortman, & Stone, 1996). Thus, rather than being only cathartic, emotional writing appears to affect the ways people think about their emotions and themselves.

SELF-PERCEPTION: HOW WE VIEW OURSELVES

Understanding the positive health-effects of writing would seem uniquely relevant for predicting possible implications of online health communication. Exploring this in more depth requires a more detailed understanding of how the process of self-perception unfolds—how people actually look at and think about themselves, also as "sick," "healthy," "patient," and so on.

Theories of self-perception are most often defined relative to the work of Daryl Bem (1972). His theory states that the way we make inferences about our own attitudes and emotions is not very different from the process by which we infer about others' attitudes and emotions. This means that we identify and label our attitudes and emotions—also related to our health—in part through observation of our behaviours and the setting in which these behaviours occur. Such inferences are quite fundamental to a child's development of self-perception, and adults' (especially parents') role in its development. For instance, responding to a child's temper tantrum by saying "You are a hot-headed kid" contributes to the child's sense of self as hot-headed. Interestingly, adults also use similar strategies when trying to identify their own reasons for behaving in certain ways. For example, when asked a question you have never really thought about such as; "What type of films do you like?" one may have to review ones own behaviour to find the answer: "Well, since the last films I've seen are drama, I must like drama." Making inferences about ourselves by observing our own behaviour is particularly employed when the attitudes and feelings are uncertain or ambiguous.

The self-perceptions we form by observing our own behaviour in this fashion serve important motivational functions. A good example of this is the "discounting phenomenon." This can arise when an external cause of behaviour, for instance a reward, makes us totally disregard other (internal) reasons for our behaviour—for example, that we enjoy what we are doing. Correspondingly, people can end up losing intrinsic interest in activities where there is a clear external cause (e.g., payment, coercion). This is often referred to as the "overjustification effect" (Deci & Ryan, 1985). Oppositely, when we engage in an activity without external factors or explanations, this will often lead us to conclude that we are genuinely interested in this activity. In sum, the thoughts and ideas we hold concerning our behaviour are very relevant in terms of motivating us to perform these actions.

Understanding what motivates people plays an important part in many areas of health research, perhaps no more so than research focusing on adherence to treatment. Research shows that having negative or erroneous self-perceptions related to health decreases adherence to health-care regimens (Wichowski & Kubsch, 1997). Such "incorrect" or ambivalent self-perceptions might reflect what Parsons (1951) called a "sick-role conflict." He poses that in order to adhere to treatment, patients need to internalize, or identify, with certain behaviours and attitudes consistent with "being sick," including allowing others to care for them and seeking medical advice.

However, in modern, "empowered" conceptualizations of the patient-role, these internalizations might also include greater sense of personal control over the illness through, for example, receiving sufficient information to cope with the illness. Also, many new medical concepts, such as "lifestyle diseases," might contribute to ambiguous attitudes from the patient's perspective. This might be particularly true if these health-issues are viewed as resulting from either neglectful or harmful behaviours on part of the patient. In such cases, construction of a positive self-perception in relation to the problem is highly important, as changes in life-style (i.e., the patient's own behaviour) is often the best way to resolve the problem. Acquiring the motivation to undertake these changes is a core challenge for interventions targeting lifestyle diseases.

Given the evidence suggesting that the writing cure health-outcomes can be attributed to cognitive processing of emotional issues, the question might be asked: Can text-based CMC function as a tool for revising potentially ambiguous health-related self-perceptions? Indeed, cognitive behavioural therapies (CBT), which are based on similar principles, have shown success and are being incorporated into self-help programs (Christensen, Griffiths, & Jorm, 2004; Griffiths, Christensen, Jorm, Evans, & Groves, 2004). Here, counteracting dysfunctional thought-patterns and attitudes, including perceptions of stigma related to depression and/or the treatment process, is crucial.

Also, the choice people make simply by visiting a given health-site might be relevant to self-perceptions. For example, choosing to join a particular discussion forum and contributing to the discourse, might "tell ourselves" something about our attitudes and goals that may in turn influence our health behaviour. Because such activities are often initiated voluntarily by the user, this undertaking might very well play a central role in consolidating a health-related self-image that includes taking an interest in ones own health and exercising personal control over treatment. This kind of health-related self-perception can increase the possibility that people engage in health-promoting activities. An example of this might be found in the results from a European e-health trend survey, where 33% of the sampled populations say they have increased willingness to change their diet and/or lifestyle after visiting a e-health Web site (Andreassen, Bujnowska-Fedak, Chronaki, Dumitru, Pudule, Santana, Voss, & Wynn, 2007).

SELF-REGULATION THROUGH TEXT: REHEARSING AND REPROCESSING

While the popularity of text-based communication channels for health-communication may arguably be linked to a lack of equally cheap and practical alternatives, we believe such arenas are uniquely suited for the needs of those who use them. This belief is also based on the findings associated with the writing cure and how self-perceptions might be revised through text. The possibilities afforded by the text-medium, that people are allowed to reflect on their problems and reprocess information relevant to them, might be very similar to the term "zone for reflection" coined by Suler (2000). This concept is defined simply as the time that exists between exchanges to think and compose a reply. The theoretical foundations for the intuitive correctness of this notion might be found with the media synchronicity theory (MST) (Dennis & Valacich, 1999). This theory is an extension of the MRT (Daft & Lengel, 1986) and proposes that communication through ICT might be best understood from an information processing perspective.

Whereas the concept of "richness" was closely tied to increased social presence, MST focuses on how information can be processed and handled by the individual during communication. MST proposes a number of traits that describe the information processing in different media, and rates communication technologies from low to high on these traits. These five traits are immediacy of feedback, symbol variety, parallelism, rehearseability, and reprocessability. Ratings based on these traits yield quite different results when compared to ratings of richness from MRT. For instance, face-to-face communication, which is commonly identified as the richest form of communication (according to MRT), is rated "low" on three of five dimensions in MST. From this perspective face-to-face communication is only unique with regards to its ability to support rapid feedback during communication (high rating for "immediacy of feedback"). In contrast, text-based communication (specifically "asynchronous groupware"), one of the "least rich" media according to MRT, receives "high" ratings for three of five dimensions. Such media would enable multiple conversations to exist simultaneously (high rating for "parallelism"), and give the user the opportunity to fine tune the message before sending it (high rating for "rehearseability"), as well as the ability to reexamine the message at a later stage during communication (high rating for "reprocessability"). Thus, MST challenges a conceptualization of richness mainly based on social factors.

For this reason the view proposed by MST is useful for analysing health-related CMC. Instead of focusing on how traditional social goals can be achieved or approximated through text, we might ask how text helps individuals manage information differently from the face-to-face setting (or other rich settings), and how this helps them achieve their goals. Interestingly, the prototypical "online health" communication arenas (discussion forums, e-mail) consistently score high on the reprocessability and rehearseability traits proposed by MST. As outlined above, reprocessability refers to the extent to which a message can be re-examined or processed again, while rehearseability refers to whether the medium allows the sender to rehearse or fine tune a message (Dennis & Valacich, 1999). We argue that these traits are central to health-related use of the Internet.

Indeed, the possibilities of revision and storage of information might serve as important facets with regards to the psychotherapeutic process, and the concept "zone for reflection" (Suler, 2000) is originally proposed in this context. Using text or diaries in therapeutic work is not uncommon (Stensland & Malterud, 1997), but relinquishing control over this process might be viewed as threatening from the therapist's perspective (Wangberg, Gammon, & Spitznogle, 2007).

However, we believe this process might enable people to build self-perceptions of themselves as competent and potent actors with regards to their own health. Viewed from the perspective of "normal", paternalistic health-behaviour and the traditional patient-role, such activities are probably unique to the electronically mediated setting. It is important to note that this positive outcome is not automatic. Evidence suggests that certain health problems can be more sensitive than others with regards to the construction of negative self-perceptions, an example being eating disorders (for instance, the "pro-ana movement," see also Johnsen, Rosenvinge, & Gammon, 2002). However, such outcomes reflect an interplay processes within the individual and the contexts within which social interactions are played out. Some of these aspects are examined in the following section.

HEALTH-RELATED SELF-PRESENTATION: TURNING TEXT INTO A SOCIAL ACT

Many can probably relate to the situation of having written something with a vague intention of sharing it with others. The decision whether to press "send" or not, can entail a whole range of considerations, including "is this really how I feel?" and "how will others view me when they read this?" Indeed, these considerations might very well prohibit us from sharing our stories or points-of-view. If such hesitations can lead us to abstain from communicating with others, then reassurances that we will not be misunderstood and misinterpreted might sway us in the opposite direction. As we have seen, computers and the text-based user-interface allow individuals to process information about their health and illnesses in more thorough and controlled ways than in "richer" modalities. We have argued that this enhanced processing has special significance for health-issues, for example through the interplay between health-related self-perceptions and health-behaviours. However, people do not write (or rather type) about their health-issues in a vacuum or solitarily. Many of the health-related activities online involve communication, and as we have seen self-disclosure is profoundly tied to CMC.

In efforts to make sense of these findings, it is natural to view anonymity as playing a central role. But experiences or behaviours of users are not simply reducible to questions of anonymity or no anonymity. As made apparent by the discussion of MRT and MST, social factors are not able to fully explain the observed phenomena, even when the contents of communication are highly social in nature. Indeed, from basic research on human-computer interaction we have seen that the design of user-interfaces is capable of changing patterns of communication. For instance, the varying the size of message windows have been shown to change how much people write, although the contents would easily fit within either window (Cech & Condon, 1998). Also, how we think about ourselves might be influenced by interface design (how much a person is allowed to type) even when anonymity is constant (Johnsen, 2007).

These results suggest that anonymity[2] cannot be used as a singular explanation of people's behaviour online. In addition to our theoretical objections to the anonymity concept, there is the issue of practicality: Because anonymity is not an option when communicating in a clinical health-care context (e.g., patient records, health legislation), an understanding based on this concept is not useful as a foundation for designing healthcare services. We believe the process of self-presentation is a more relevant approach to analysing both general online health-communication and, more specifically, (potential) online diagnostic and therapeutic work. Furthermore, self-presentation theory, more so than anonymity, offers a less "reductionistic" understanding of how public health-services should view CMC in addressing the needs and preferences of patients.

Self-Presentation

The process by which we manipulate, monitor and control the information conveyed to others about ourselves is referred to as *self-presentation*[3]. An important premise of self-presentation theory is that people are motivated to present themselves in a desirable way to others, and to maintain a desirable impression (Fiske & Taylor, 1991). Indeed, the role attributed to anonymity in terms of facilitating self-disclosure might be closely related to the *importance of making a positive impression.*

However, this motivation regrettably often interacts negatively with health, since behaviours that are deemed self-promoting, or at least are viewed as such, are often detrimental to health (Leary, Tchividjian, & Kraxberger, 1994). Behaviours that fall into this category include failure to use condoms, excessive sunbathing, excessive or yo-yo dieting, consumption of harmful substances (including alcohol and tobacco), use of steroids, failure to exercise, and cosmetic surgery (Leary et al., 1994). All these behaviours are self-enhancing, either through the image they project (for instance, excessive alcohol consumption is deemed "cool" by many adolescents) or by their effects (for instance, increased muscle mass from use of steroids, or weight-loss through dieting). However, as is apparent, the positive, self-enhancement effects are in most cases overshadowed by the potential threats these behaviours pose to the person's health.

For our purposes it might be more interesting to see how self-enhancement motives might influence people's actual interaction with health-services. This notion is addressed by (Martin, Leary, & Rejeski, 2000) who propose that failure to seek help for various health-problems can be explained, at least in part, by self-presentation concerns. Here, the embarrassment associated with examinations or procedures involving intimate body parts (i.e., genitals, breasts, et cetera) might lead people to avoid or delay these procedures. Also, threats to our self-image might influence help seeking for a number of other illnesses or conditions, when these are seen as stigmatizing or socially unacceptable. Many mental disorders fall under this category, as do sexually transmitted diseases, and to some extent illnesses attributed to lifestyle (obesity, diabetes, and so on).

Strategic Self-Presentation

It is interesting then that new communication technologies offer us increased flexibility with regards to how we present ourselves to others. Early writings about the social aspects of CMC noted the possibilities that mediated contexts offer for identity and self exploration (Rheingold, 1993; Turkle, 1995). Central to these notions were manipulation of self-presentation, for instance by presenting oneself as the opposite gender. Also, mere physical appearance (e.g., gender, ethnicity, (un)attractiveness) communicates a lot about ourselves to others, whether we like it or not. Appearances, also called "gating features" (McKenna et al., 2002) trigger expectations, sometimes in form of stereotypes. These features, which are inoperative online, can undermine bonds based on more substantive features of the encounter. Increased control over how we present of ourselves to others in CMC, has been addressed by several authors (e.g., McKenna & Bargh, 1999; O'Sullivan, 2000; Walther, 2007) and is central to an understanding of health related CMC.

O'Sullivan's studies (2000) suggest that mediated channels are unique in their ability to allow management of self-relevant information, and that people's awareness of this fact influences preferences and choices of communication channels in social situations. Mediated channels appear to be preferred in "confess" situations. These are described as situations where the information shared is self-oriented and the valence is negative. Returning to the notion of help seeking for health-problems, we see that these properties (self-orientation and negative perceived outcomes) might be typical for many types of health scenarios. Moral objections or social stigmatization are still attached to many illnesses. Examples include the teenager seeking information about sexually transmitted diseases. This person might feel threatened not only by the health-problem and possible outcomes, but also, and perhaps more so, by issues of morality. Similarly, the patient seeking information on how to cope with obsessive thoughts might feel stigmatized and prone to be misunderstood. For them, relating to the findings of O'Sullivan, choosing a text-based communication medium would address these threats effectively. The evidence suggests that the sharing of health-issues corresponding to the notion of the confess scenario is quite common in an online self-help context. Davison, Pennebaker, & Dickerson (2000), for instance, characterize online support as "(...) oriented around conditions poorly understood and somewhat overlooked by the medical community" (pp. 214).

Again, awareness of these findings may prove crucial in designing e-health services that augment healthcare in a patient-centred manner. It would appear that certain modalities of ICT makes it possible for people to manage presentations of themselves in a more controlled manner or more strategically than would be the case face-to-face. O'Sullivan's self-presentation scenarios make it possible to analyse the behaviour currently seen online (in relation to health) in greater detail and more theoretically, specifically in terms of understanding how self-enhancement motives have driven the spontaneous use of e-health. This knowledge might be a key to developing and offering truly patient-centred health services.

Equally important, when trying to describe the possible significance of strategic self-presentation in the healthcare setting, might be the proposition that "human goals and motivations are not likely to be much different regardless of whether interactions are mediated or not" (O'Sullivan, 2000, pp. 428). People's motivations and needs with regards to health services and health-related communication will not be radically different just because communication is taking place within the context of new media. The difference is simply that technologies offer people new options for how to achieve their goals. This should be of comfort to those who suspect that the online setting would be conducive to high degrees of manipulative behaviour, or simply constitute counterproductive thinking (e.g., how can people with social anxiety benefit from being further "isolated" by communicating online?). How then can communication strategies, similar to those explored earlier, be beneficial to health, and what health-goals can they be said to address?

LOWERING THRESHOLDS FOR HELP-SEEKING

It is well known that many neglect seeking appropriate healthcare (Oliver, Pearson, Coe, & Gunnell, 2005). For many, sickness and need of help can be embarrassing, regardless of how taboo-laden ones health complaints may be. The process of making an appointment, sitting in filled waiting-rooms, and then having to "spill ones guts out" to a stranger, can represent thresholds that outweigh the perceived need for help. Describing our subjective "cost-benefits assessments" for help seeking might be attempted along the lines of the expected utility analysis (von Neuman & Morgenstern, 1944). When we seek help for a health problem our goal is to have this problem resolved through the intervention of the healthcare system. At the same time, help seeking through face-to-face channels might be associated with considerable subjective costs. In the end, these (subjective) costs will be weighed against the patient's beliefs regarding the seriousness of the problem, and how probable it is that the healthcare system will be able to assist the individual. If this analysis leads to conclusions such as, "this is not a very serious problem" or "the healthcare system will not be able to help me," the threshold for approaching healthcare professionals would have to be very low. If the subjective costs of face-to-face communication are high, for instance in the case of stigmatizing illnesses or "confession" scenarios, avoidance may be expected even for serious problems.

Providing patients with a "less costly" venue for seeking help might make help minimize such behaviours. Thus, the process that gives people the ability to conduct more strategic self-presentation, might lead people to more readily seek help for a problem. Especially for young people, seeking help or support when confronted with a stressful event appears to be of fundamental importance to the mental health and well being (Rickwood, Deane, Wilson, & Ciarrochi, 2005), and, as we have seen, avoidance of embarrassment might serve as a motivator against seeking help (Martin, Ginis, & Leary, 2004). A premise of O'Sullivan's research is that people have rather clear preferences for the communication channels they would like to utilize in a given situation. Thus, people should be able to choose communication channels based on the self-presentational aspects of the situation, also for health-purposes.

The apparent popularity of online self-help arenas may be explained by viewing them as extreme low threshold situations. Concretely, these settings offer both the information processing advantages of text, and the anonymity and unaccountability afforded by communication with peers rather than healthcare professionals. The experience of having successfully disclosed ones problems to others might, over time, facilitate the inclination to seek help from official channels, despite the fact that these settings can never offer participants complete anonymity.

However, an interesting notion is the idea that control over information flow and content might make anonymity a less important concept, since anonymity is probably most relevant when we fear being misinterpreted or misunderstood. People that doubt their ability to present problems accurately face-to-face, and therefore shy away from seeking help in a traditional sense, might be swayed by the possibility of writing about their problems in a controlled environment. This writing-process could have many manifestations: spontaneously and acutely, as problems occur, or over a period of time (as would be the case for chronic diseases). In both cases, the possibilities of reprocessing and rehearsing content is equally relevant. This would constitute a type of information "quality-control" that is difficult to achieve, at least within the traditional doctor-patient consultation. Here, elicitation and responding to the patients concerns and information is highly contingent upon the effectiveness of doctors' and patients' verbal/listening skills within of the typical office visit timeframe of less than 20 minutes. While electronic information systems enabling information exchange between patients and health professionals are being introduced into medical practice (van den Brink, Moorman, de Boer, Pruyn, Verwoerd, & van Bemmel, 2005)—mainly aimed at increasing efficiency - we believe that lowered threshold and disclosure issues should be incorporated in system design for clinical objectives.Some may be concerned that lowering the threshold for help through online interaction may inadvertently reinforce certain health complaints (e.g., social anxiety). We would argue that the validity of "paternalistic attitudes" of this type needs to be verified empirically before they are given authority. From a patient-centred perspective, technologies that can aid patients in voicing their agendas should be pursued. Concerns that a lowered threshold for contact will flood professionals appear unfounded (Bergmo, Kummervold, Gammon, & Dahl, 2005). Rather, focus should be on designing systems that channel patient communication in ways that facilitate positive involvement and appropriate response.

GROUP PROCESSES: IMPLICATIONS FOR SELF-HELP

The Social Identity Model of Deindividuation Effects (SIDE) (Reicher, Spears, & Postmes, 1995) has provided researchers with a theoretical tool for studying online group processes. SIDE, as many other theories, sees anonymity as a strong force in shaping CMC. Specifically, SIDE sees anonymity as an enhancer of normative behaviour by means of reducing the cues available for signalling individual differences. Anonymity in this context is not a precursor of necessarily deviating or regressive behaviours. Formerly, Internet phenomena such as "flaming" were often taken as evidence of the detrimental effects of anonymity on online interaction (Lea, O'Shea, Fung, & Spears, 1992), where people, because they did not have to face the consequences of their online antics, would behave in quite antinormative ways. In contrast to this view, SIDE proposes that available (in most cases normative) group norms will be made extra salient when the individuals are no longer identifiable (as would be the case for face-to-face groups). As a result, the communication process (or behaviour) is more likely to stay within the confinements of these norms (e.g., Postmes, Spears, & Lea, 2000; Postmes, Spears, Sakhel, & de Groot, 2001). In cases such as the online self-help movement, it might be interesting to view the strong supportive foundations of the activities as strong normative forces (or as norms in their own right). It is well founded to talk about such groups, not as providing self-help (individual), but as providing mutual aid (interindividual). The foundations or norms common to these groups and organizations might be said to be member participation and the expectation of receiving emotional support, sharing personal experiences, and finding new ways to help themselves cope with their shared problems. Also, the guidelines or rules governing many real-life self-help groups are very much norms that are to be followed in an online setting (for instance, the twelve step program of Alcoholics Anonymous (AA)).

Indeed, research that taps the content of the interaction of similar online groups has consistently uncovered what appears to be very stringently supportive interaction patterns (Johnsen et al., 2002; Kummervold et al., 2002). The importance of establishing sensible norms in terms of health-promotion, for instance through professionals serving as role models, has also been noted (Johnsen, Steinsvik, & Gammon, 2004). Many similarities might be argued to exist between sharing stories online and, for instance, narrative therapeutic approaches. In essence, participating in an online setting is writing one's life-story, having others comment and reflect upon these experiences, and revising them as time goes by. Within this lies the potential for learning how to lead one's future life by reinterpreting the past.

IMPLICATIONS FOR HEALTH-SERVICES

The above sections have examined some of ways people use ICT outside the traditional healthcare channels, along with ways CMC research may help explain these uses. In what ways might this knowledge help in improving healthcare services? In the current section we discuss implications that this research can have for the design and evaluation of e-health services. Our focus is not on the more obvious practical contributions ICT can have for access and effectiveness. Rather, the implications of CMC for clinical communication (e.g., diagnosis and treatment) and relationships (e.g., patient-physician, client-therapist) are examined. In doing so, it is useful to first step back and look at some of the challenges of traditional face-to-face clinical communication.

Patient-Centeredness Face-to-Face

Naturally, the large body of research on clinical communication and relationships is based on traditional face-to-face communication. Any assessment of CMC in clinical communication will implicitly or explicitly be compared with what we know based on this research. It is well documented that effective clinical communication is decisive for developing good working relationships, patient satisfaction, adherence, and health outcomes (Beck, Daughtridge, & Sloane, 2002; Griffin, Kinmonth, Veltman, Gillard, Grant, & Stewart, 2004)

Much of this research shows that face-to-face clinical communication suffers from numerous challenges that are relevant in discussions of how CMC may improve clinical communication. In particular, studies show that physicians often fail to address what has been called the "patients' agenda" (Levenstein, McCracken, McWhinney, Stewart, & Brown, 1986). This concept encompasses all the reasons for the consultation including the ideas, concerns and expectations of the patient. For example, Levenstein and colleagues found that physicians failed to elicit 45% of patients worries and 54% of their reasons for consulting (Levenstein et al., 1986). Another study found that social and emotional issues are the issues most likely to be neglected in the consultation (Campion, Butler, & Cox, 1992).

Studies also indicate that physicians tend to talk more that listen. For example, Marvel and colleagues found that 72% of the doctors interrupted the patient's opening statement after an average of 23 seconds (Marvel, Epstein, Flowers, & Beckman, 1999). Patients, who were allowed to state their concerns without interruption, only used an average of six more seconds to complete expressing their concerns. Similarly, Waitzkin found that doctors tend underestimate the amount of information patients want and overestimate how much they in fact give (Waitzkin, 1984). In their study of 20-minute office visits, doctors spent about one minute per visit informing patients, but believed they were spending nine minutes per visit doing so. Not only do these studies give cause for concern about the quality of treatment. Doctors who lack communications skills are more likely to be sued. For example, an analysis of 45 malpractice cases found that many of the doctors being sued delivered information poorly and devalued the patient's views (Beckman, Markakis, Suchman, & Frankel, 1994). Studies such as these may help explain why a large portion—some experts claim up to 50%—of the health system's resources are tied up in face-to-face consultations which neither patients nor physicians believe are worthwhile (Berwick, 2003).

Efforts to improve clinical communication typically build on models of patient-centeredness (e.g., Little, Everitt, Williamson, Warner, Moore, Gould, Ferrier, & Payne, 2001). Although patient-centred models of clinical consultations are widely advocated, their uses in practice are probably limited. Explanations for failure to eliciting the patient's agenda include the characteristics of the biomedical model (Malterud, 2001), physician focus on medical notes rather than the patient (Njølstad & Aaraas, 1992), and time limitations (Little et al., 2001). Some suggest that possible causes might lie in the nature of face-to-face consultations (Gammon & Rosenvinge, 2000; Kummervold et al., 2002; Wright, 2002), although this has yet to be examined in controlled studies. In any case, we argue that face-to-face communication should not be viewed as an ideal. Rather, we should view it as a variable that can have positive and negative implications in given circumstances.

CMC in Facilitating Patient-Centeredness

Clinicians who express deep scepticism towards e-health claim that lack of physical proximity undermines the compassion and trust necessary in maintaining the moral integrity of clinical relationships (Bird, 2003; Curtis, 2000). Such (undocumented) claims need to be investigated thoroughly and seriously. Meanwhile, we have a lot to learn from people who prefer to use CMC for communicating about their health issues. Probably the most obvious lesson is that peoples' health needs, and their abilities to connect with others about those needs, are far more diverse than traditional healthcare is designed to accommodate.

More specifically, we have seen that people use media strategically in the ways they disclose their personal issues to others, and that CMC interplays with self-perceptions and self-regulation—processes at the heart of diagnosis and healing processes. Also, for those who are confused and/or embarrassed about their health complaints, CMC can reduce barriers for accessing others who can help them. The textual nature of CMC invites us to re-look at narrative approaches to diagnosis and treatment. Writing about the nuances of life and mood is viewed as equivalent to the "the culture of taking care of oneself" (Foucault, 1982), and is probably reflected in the popularity of text-based media for self-expression.

As a comfort to clinicians, who might balk at the idea of patients bombarding them with emotionally laden narratives, the sharing of these texts with someone else does not appear critical for obtaining the observed health effects (Pennebaker, 2004). Nevertheless, clinicians may find that legitimising the patient's voice through text may promote health processes that also provide insights useful for doing a better job. The challenge lies in designing systems that organise the writing process and the resulting insights effectively for the respective roles of patients and clinicians.

Future clinicians will be armed with an arsenal of tools for helping patients help themselves outside of the traditional clinical contexts. For instance, future "prescriptions" might include secure access to evidence-based psycho-educational and self-help programs, cognitive therapies, interactive narrative support and lifestyle monitoring/feedback. These types of tools *can be* used as an acknowledgement of—and in alliance with—the patients' own resources.

CHALLENGES AND FUTURE RESEARCH

Obviously in some circumstances, face-to-face will remain the only feasible and/or ethically acceptable mode of communication for people struggling with health issues (e.g., terminal or acute). Hopefully we will gain the knowledge necessary to discern under which circumstances it is superior, and under which circumstances other modes are more conducive in facilitating healing processes and building good clinical relationships. A good place to start may be patient-clinician dyads struggling with medically unexplained disorders, chronic conditions and risk-related lifestyles. For these types of health complaints, the communication issues addressed in this chapter are core aspects of any progression towards common understandings of problems and solutions.

Moore's Law" (Moore, 1965) suggests a future a future with processing power and bandwidth that enable a limitless range of multimedia applications to all aspects of healthcare—from prevention, to diagnosis, treatment and care. Faced with such dazzling potentials, it is prudent to remind ourselves that human beings—our capabilities and needs - are relatively stable, despite cultural nuances and differing manifestations through different time periods. Nevertheless, we are still scratching the surface of the role of communication in the complex interplay of psychological, social, and physical dimensions of "health and well-being." We need only remind ourselves of our failure to predict the popular role played by "poor" media in conveying extremely intimate thoughts and emotions, particularly among younger generations. As we have seen for some people and some health issues, "rich" multimedia applications such as real-time video, may hamper important relational processes that we have seen unfold through "poor" media. This is important to keep in mind as advancements in multimedia e-health technologies can distract us from a focus on basic human needs and capabilities.

It is, therefore, encouraging that health authorities increasingly acknowledge the need for better understanding the interface between health and CMC. As the U.S. Office of Disease Prevention and Health Promotion (ODPHP) point out in their report Healthy People 2010: "One of the main challenges in the design of effective health communication is to identify the optimal contexts, channels, content, and reasons that will motivate people to pay attention to and use health information" (ODPHP, 2000, pp. 11-5–11-6).

This chapter offers possible explanations for why some people are motivated to choose "poor" media for communicating about their health. These ideas may be equally relevant in helping healthcare service providers acknowledge the needs of those they are trying to help It represents another important reminder of the diversity of users' needs, motivations and capabilities, and how this must be reflected in a diversity of e-health tools to ensure access to health services for all.

The range of issues needing attention and acknowledgement is wide.From the psychological perspective outlined in this chapter, we believe that uniting forces between health psychology and CMC research can be particularly fruitful. Promising examples include the work being done on tailoring (for instance, Wangberg, 2007), approaches to studying online social support and disease self-management (Barrera, Glasgow, McKay, Boles, & Feil, 2002), and work to leverage the ubiquitous nature of mobile phones for supporting health-related behaviours (Kaplan, 2006; Fogg, 2003). All such efforts will need to be guided by consumer-centred approaches in order to ensure both use, ethical practices and positive health outcomes.

CONCLUDING REMARKS

In this chapter, we have examined psychological aspects of communicating about ones health through technology. We have argued that patient-centred e-health will depend upon a better understanding of why people use CMC for communicating about their health. It has been suggested that efforts to design "rich" e-health systems in order to impersonate in-person encounters is not necessarily such a good idea. Assumptions about the invariable superiority of face-to-face communication in building supportive relationships may inadvertently bypass valuable relational features of "faceless" and "old-fashioned" modes of communication (e.g., voice and text). The communicational paradox "less-is-more" should be explored in the context of facilitating self-reflection and self-presentations that more fully reflect the needs and resources of those with health concerns.

REFERENCES

Andreassen, H.K., Bujnowska-Fedak, M.M., Chronaki, C.E., Dumitru, R.C., Pudule, I., Santana, S., Voss, H., & Wynn, R. (2007). European citizens' use of e-health services: A study of seven countries [Electronic version]. *BMC Public Health*. Retrieved May 13, 2008, from http://www.biomedcentral.com/1471-2458/7/53

Barrera, M. Jr., Glasgow, R.E., McKay, H.G., Boles, S.M., & Feil, E.G. (2002). Do Internet-based support interventions change perceptions of social support? An experimental trial of approaches for supporting diabetes self-management. *American Journal of Community Psychology, 30*(5), 637-654.

Beck, R.S., Daughtridge, R., & Sloane, P. (2002). Physician-patient communication in the primary care office: A systematic review. *Journal American Board of Family Practice, 15*, 25-38.

Beckman, H.B., Markakis, K.M., Suchman, A.L., & Frankel, R.M. (1994). The doctor-patient relationship and malpractice. Lessons from plaintiff depositions. *Archives of Internal Medicine, 154*(12), 1365-1370.

Bem, D.J. (1972). Self-perception theory. In L. Berkowitz (Ed.), *Advances in experimental social psychology* (pp. 1-62). New York: Academic Press.

Bergmo, T.S., Kummervold, P.E., Gammon, D., & Dahl, L.B. (2005). Electronic patient-provider communication: Will it offset office visits and telephone consultations in primary care? *International Journal of Medical Informatics, 74*, 705-710.

Berwick, D. (2003). *Escape fire: Lessons for the future of healthcare*. New York: Commonwealth Fund.

Bird, J. (2003). "I wish to speak to the despisers of the body." The Internet, physicality, and psychoanalysis. *Journal for the Psychoanalysis of Culture & Society, 8*(1), 121-126.

Cameron, L.D., & Nicholls, G. (1998). Expression of stressful experiences through writing: Effects of a self-regulation manipulation for pessimists and optimists. *Health Psychology, 17*(1), 84-92.

Campbell, R.S., & Pennebaker, J.W. (2003). The secret life of pronouns: Flexibility in writing style and physical health. *Psychological Science, 14*(1), 60-65.

Campion, P.D., Butler, N.M., & Cox, A.D. (1992). Principle agendas of doctors and patients in general practice consultations. *Family Practice, 9*(2), 181-190.

Cech, C.G., & Condon, S.L. (1998). Message size constraints on discourse planning in synchronous computer-mediated communication. *Behavior Research Methods, Instruments, & Computers, 30*(2), 255-263.

Christensen, H., Griffiths, K.M., & Jorm, A.F. (2004). Delivering interventions for depression using the internet: Randomised controlled trial. *British Medical Journal, 328*, 265.

Curtis, A. (2000). *Through the WEB and what Alice found there: The impact of the Internet on the therapeutic alliance.* Paper presented at the 35th Annual Australian Psychological Society Conference, Canberra.

Daft, R.L., & Lengel, R.H. (1986). Organizational information requirements, media richness and structural design. *Management Science, 32*(5), 554-571.

Davison, K.P., Pennebaker, J.W., & Dickerson, S.S. (2000). Who talks? The social psychology of illness support groups. *American Psychologist, 55*(2), 205-217.

Deci, E.L., & Ryan, R.M. (1985). *Intrinsic motivation and self-determination in human behavior.* New York: Plenum.

Dennis, A.R., & Valacich, J.S. (1999). *Rethinking media richness: Towards a theory of media synchronicity.* Paper presented at the 32nd Hawaii International Conference on System Sciences, Hawaii.

Ferriter, M. (1993). Computer aided interviewing and the psychiatric social history. *Social Work and Social Sciences Review, 4*, 255-263.

Fiske, S.T., & Taylor, S.E. (1991). *Social cognition (second edition).* New York: McGraw-Hill, Inc.

Fogg, B.J. (2003). *Persuasive technology: Using computers to change what we think and do.* San Francisco: Morgan Kaufmann Publishers.

Foucault, M. (1982). *Technologies of the self.* Retrieved May 13, 2008, from http://scholar.google.com/scholar?hl=en&lr=&q=cache:ZaTVbZuQ6xEJ:www.sp.uconn.edu/~en109vc/Old/S2002/Technologies.pdf+Foucault+Birth+of+the+clinic

Gammon, D., & Rosenvinge, J. (2000). Can Internet aid persons with serious mental disorders? *Journal of the Norwegian Medical Association, 120*, 1890-1892.

Greenberg, M.A., Wortman, C.B., & Stone, A.A. (1996). Emotional expression and physical health: Revising traumatic memories or fostering self-regulation? *Journal of Personality and Social Psychology, 71*(3), 588-602.

Greist, J.H., Klein, M.H., & VanCura, L. (1973). A computer interview by psychiatric patient target symptoms. *Archives of General Psychiatry, 29*, 247-253.

Griffin, S.J., Kinmonth, A.-L., Veltman, M.W.M., Gillard, S., Grant, J., & Stewart, M. (2004). Effect on health-related outcomes of interventions to alter the interaction between patients and practitioners: A systematic review of trials. *Annals of Family Medicine, 2*(6), 595-608.

Griffiths, K.M., Christensen, H., Jorm, A.F., Evans, K., & Groves, C. (2004). Effect of Web-based depression literacy and cognitive-behavioral therapy interventions on stigmatising attitudes to depression. *British Journal of Psychiatry, 185*, 342-349.

Guastella, A.J., & Dadds, M.R. (2006). Cognitive-behavioral models of emotional writing: A validation study. *Cognitive Therapy and Research, 30*, 397-414.

Harkness, J. (2005). *What is patient-centred healthcare? A review of definitions and principles.* London: International Alliance of Patients' Organisations.

Isaacs, E., Whittaker, S., Frohlich, D., & O'Conaill, B. (1994). Informal communication re-examined: New functions for video in supporting opportunistic encounters. In K.E. Finn, A.J. Sellen, & S.B. Wilbur (Eds.). *Video-Mediated Communication* (pp. 459-485). Mahwah, NJ: Lawrence Erlbaum.

Johnsen, J.-A.K. (2007). Constraints on message size in quasi-synchronous computer mediated communication: Effect on self-concept accessibility. *Computers in Human Behavior, 23*, 2269-2284.

Johnsen, J.-A.K., Rosenvinge, J.H., & Gammon, D. (2002). Online group interaction and mental health: An analysis of three online discussion forums. *Scandinavian Journal of Psychology, 43*, 445-449.

Johnsen, J.-A.K., Steinsvik, O.O., & Gammon, D. (2004). Health-care professionals' participation in an online discussion forum: The impact on structure, content, and interaction. *Journal of Technology in Human Services, 22*, 31-44.

Joinson, A.N. (1999). Anonymity, disinhibition and social desirability on the Internet. *Behavior Research Methods, Instruments, & Computers, 31*, 433-438.

Joinson, A.N. (2001a). Knowing me, knowing you: Reciprocal self-disclosure on the Internet. *CyberPsychology & Behavior, 4*, 587-591.

Joinson, A.N. (2001b). Self-disclosure in computer-mediated communication: The role of self-awareness and visual anonymity. *European Journal of Social Psychology, 31*, 177-192.

Joinson, A.N. (2004). Self-esteem, interpersonal risk, and preference for e-mail to face-to-face communication. *CyberPsychology & Behavior, 7*(4), 472-478.

Joinson, A.N., McKenna, K.Y.A., Postmes, T., & Reips, U.-D. (Eds.). (2007). *The Oxford handbook of Internet psychology.* Oxford: Oxford University Press.

Kam, L.E., & Chismar, W.G. (2003). *A self-disclosure model for personal health information.* Paper presented at the 36th Hawaii International Conference on System Sciences, Hawaii.

Kaplan, W.A. (2006). Can the ubiquitous power of mobile phones be used to improve health outcomes in developing countries? [Electronic version]. *Globalization and Health*. Retrieved May 13, 2008, from http://www.globalizationandhealth.com/content/2/1/9

King, S.A., & Moreggi, D. (1998). Internet therapy and self-help groups—The pros and cons. In J. Gackenbach (Ed.). *The psychology of the Internet: Intrapersonal, interpersonal and transpersonal implications* (pp. 77-109). San Diego, CA: Academic Press.

Kummervold, P.E., Gammon, D., Bergvik, S., Johnsen, J.-A.K., Hasvold, T., & Rosenvinge, J.H. (2002). Social support in a wired world: Use of online discussion forums in Norway. *Nordic Journal of Psychiatry, 56*(1), 59-65.

Laurenceau, J.-P., Barrett, L.F., & Pietromonaco, P.R. (1998). Intimacy as an interpersonal process: The importance of self-disclosure, partner disclosure, and perceived partner responsiveness in interpersonal exchanges. *Journal of Personality and Social Psychology, 74*(5), 1238-1251.

Lea, M., O'Shea, T., Fung, P., & Spears, R. (1992). "Flaming" in computer-mediated communication: Observations, explanations and implications. In M. Lea (Ed.). *Contexts of computer-mediated communication* (pp. 89-112). London: Harvester-Wheatsheaf.

Lea, M., & Spears, R. (1995). Love at first byte? Building personal relationships over computer networks. In J.T. Wood & S. Duck (Eds.). *Understudied relationships: Off the beaten track* (pp. 197-233). Newbury Park, CA: Sage.

Leary, M.R., Tchividjian, L.R., & Kraxberger, B.E. (1994). Self-presentation can be hazardous to your health: Impression management and health risk. *Health Psychology, 13*, 461-470.

Levenstein, J.H., McCracken, E.C., McWhinney, I.R., Stewart, M.A., & Brown, J.B. (1986). The patient-centred clinical method, 1: A model for the doctor-patient interaction in family medicine. *Family Practice, 3*(1), 24-30.

Little, P., Everitt, H., Williamson, I., Warner, G., Moore, M., Gould, C., Ferrier, K., & Payne, S. (2001). Observational study of effect of patient centredness and positive approach on outcomes of general practice consultations. *British Medical Journal, 323*(7318), 908-911.

Littrell, J. (1998). Is the re-experience of painful emotion therapeutic? *Clinical Psychology Review, 18*(1), 71-102.

Malterud, K. (2001). The art and science of clinical knowledge: Evidence beyond measures and numbers. *Lancet, 358*, 397-400.

Martin Ginis, K.A., & Leary, M.R. (2004). Self-presentational processes in health-damaging behavior. *Journal of Applied Sport Psychology, 16*, 59-74.

Martin, K.A., Leary, M.R., & Rejeski, W.J. (2000). Self-presentational concerns in older adults: Implications for health and well-being. *Basic and Applied Social Psychology, 22*(3), 169-179.

Marvel, M.K., Epstein, R.M., Flowers, K., & Beckman, H.B. (1999). Soliciting the patient's agenda: Have we improved? *Journal of the American Medical Association, 281*(3), 283-287.

McKenna, K.Y.A., & Bargh, J.A. (1998). Coming out in the age of the internet: Identity demarginalization through virtual group participation. *Journal of Personality and Social Psychology, 75*(3), 681-694.

McKenna, K.Y.A., & Bargh, J.A. (1999). Causes and consequences of social interaction on the Internet: A conceptual framework. *Media Psychology, 1*, 249-269.

McKenna, K.Y.A., Green, A.S., & Gleason, M.E.J. (2002). Relationship formation on the Internet: What's the big attraction? *Journal of Social Issues, 58*(1), 9-31.

Moore, G.E. (1965). Cramming more components onto integrated circuits. *Electronics, 38*(8), 114-117.

Nardi, B., Whittaker, S., & Bradner, E. (2000). *Interaction and outeraction: Instant messaging in action.* Paper presented at the CSCW 2000, Philadelphia, PA, USA.

Njølstad, I., & Aaraas, I. (1992). Look at the patient, not the notes. *Lancet, 340*(8816), 413.

O'Sullivan, P.B. (2000). What you don't know won't hurt me: Impression management functions of communication channels in relationships. *Human Communication Research, 26*(3), 403-431.

Office of Disease Prevention and Health Promotion (ODPHP). (2000). *Healthy people 2010: Volume 1 (Second edition).* Washington, DC: Health and Human Services Dept.

Oliver, M.I., Pearson, N., Coe, N., & Gunnell, D. (2005). Help-seeking behaviour in men and women with common mental health problems: Cross-sectional study. *British Journal of Psychiatry, 186*(4), 297-301.

Parks, M.R., & Floyd, K. (1996). Making friends in cyberspace. *Journal of Communication, 46*(1), 80-97.

Parks, M.R., & Roberts, L.E. (1998). "Making mOOsic": The development of personal relationships on-line and a comparison to their off-line counterparts. *Journal of Social and Personal Relationships, 15*(4), 517-537.

Parsons, T. (1951). *The social system.* London: Routledge.

Pennebaker, J.W. (1997). *Opening up: The healing power of expressing emotions (second edition).* New York: The Guilford Press.

Pennebaker, J.W. (2004). Theories, therapies, and taxpayers: On the complexities of the expressive writing paradigm. *Clinical Psychology: Science and Practice, 11*, 138-142.

Pennebaker, J.W., & Beall, S.K. (1986). Confronting a traumatic event: Toward an understanding of inhibition and disease. *Journal of Abnormal Psychology, 95*, 274-281.

Pennebaker, J.W., & Francis, M.E. (1996). Cognitive, emotional and language processes in disclosure. *Cognition and Emotion, 10*, 621-626.

Pennebaker, J.W., Mayne, T.J., & Francis, M.E. (1997). Linguistic predictors of adaptive bereavement. *Journal of Personality and Social Psychology, 72*, 863-871.

Peterson, M.C., Holbrook, J.H., Von Hales, D., Smith, N.L., & Staker, L.V. (1992). Contributions of the history, physical examination, and laboratory investigation in making medical diagnoses. *Western Journal of Medicine, 156*(2), 163-165.

Postmes, T., & Spears, R. (1998). Deindividuation and anti-normative behavior: A meta-analysis. *Psychological Bulletin, 123*, 238-259.

Postmes, T., Spears, R., & Lea, M. (2000). The formation of group norms in computer-mediated communication. *Human Communication Research, 26*(3), 341-371.

Postmes, T., Spears, R., Sakhel, K., & de Groot, D. (2001). Social influence in computer-mediated communication: The effects of anonymity on group behavior. *Personality and Social Psychology Bulletin, 27*(10), 1243-1254.

Reicher, S.D., Spears, R., & Postmes, T. (1995). A social identity model of deindividuation phenomena. In W. Stroebe & M. Hewstone (Eds.). *European Review of Social Psychology* (Vol. 6, pp. 161-198). Chichester, U.K.: Wiley.

Rheingold, H. (1993). *The virtual community: Homesteading on the electronic frontier.* New York: Perseus Books.

Rickwood, D., Deane, F.P., Wilson, C.J., & Ciarrochi, J. (2005). Young people's help-seeking for mental health problems [Electronic version].

Australian e-Journal for the Advancement of Mental Health. Retrieved May 13, 2008, from http://www.auseinet.com/journal/vol4iss3suppl/rickwood.pdf

Robinson, R., & West, R. (1992). A comparison of computer and questionnaire methods of history-taking in a genito-urinary clinic. *Psychology and Health, 6*, 77-84.

Schlenker, B.R. (2003). Self-presentation. In M.R. Leary & J.P. Tangney (Eds.). *Handbook of self and identity* (pp. 492-518). New York: The Guilford Press.

Schliemann, T., Asting, T., Følstad, A., & Heim, J. (2002). *Medium preference and medium effects in person-person communication.* Paper presented at the CHI 2002, Minneapolis, MN, USA.

Smyth, J.M. (1998). Written emotional expression: Effect sizes, outcome types, and moderating variables. *Journal of Consulting and Clinical Psychology, 66*(1), 174-184.

Spears, R., Lea, M., & Postmes, T. (2001). Social psychological theories of computer-mediated communication: Social pain or social gain. In W.P. Robinson & H. Giles (Eds.). *The New Handbook of Language and Social Psychology.* Chichester, U.K.: John Wiley & Sons Ltd.

Stensland, P., & Malterud, K. (1997). New gateways to dialogue in general practice: Development of an illness diary to expand communication. *Scandinavian Journal of Primary Healthcare, 15*, 175-179.

Suler, J.R. (2000). Psychotherapy in cyberspace: A 5-dimensional model of online and computer-mediated psychotherapy. *CyberPsychology & Behavior, 3*(2), 151-159.

Tidwell, L.C., & Walther, J.B. (2002). Computer-mediated communication effects on disclosure, impressions, and interpersonal evaluations: Getting to know one another a bit at a time. *Human Communication Research, 28*(3), 317-348.

Turkle, S. (1995). *Life on the screen: Identity in the age of the Internet.* New York: Simon & Schuster, Inc.

van den Brink, J.L., Moorman, P.W., de Boer, M.F., Pruyn, J.F.A., Verwoerd, C.D. A., & van Bemmel, J.H. (2005). Involving the patient: A prospective study on use, appreciation and effectiveness of an information system in head and neck cancer care. *International Journal of Medical Informatics, 74*, 839-849.

von Neuman, J., & Morgenstern, O. (1944). *The theory of games and economic behavior.* Princeton, NJ: Princeton University Press.

Waitzkin, H. (1984). Doctor-patient communication. Clinical implications of social scientific research. *Journal of the American Medical Association, 252*(17), 2441-2446.

Walther, J.B., & Burgoon, J.K. (1992). Relational communication in computer-mediated interaction. *Human Communication Research, 19*, 50-88.

Walther, J. B. (2007). Selective self-presentation in computer-mediated communication: Hyperpersonal dimensions of technology, language, and cognition. *Computers in Human Behavior, 23*, 2538-2557.

Wangberg, S.C. (2007). An Internet-based diabetes self-care intervention tailored to self-efficacy [Electronic Version]. *Health Education Research.* Retrieved May 13, 2008, from http://her.oxfordjournals.org/cgi/content/full/cym014v1

Wangberg, S., Gammon, D., & Spitznogle, K. (2007). In the eyes of the beholder: Exploring psychologists' attitudes towards and use of eTherapy in Norway. *CyberPsychology & Behaviour, 10*(3), 418-423.

Wichowski, H.C., & Kubsch, S.M. (1997). The relationship of self-perception of illness and compliance with healthcare regimens. *Journal of Advanced Nursing, 25*, 548-553.

Wright, J. (2002). Online counselling: Learning from writing therapy. *British Journal of Guidance & Counselling, 30*(3), 287-298.

ENDNOTES

1. Deindividuation is defined as a state of reduced self-awareness through immersion and anonymity within the group, with accompanying deregulated behaviour (Postmes & Spears, 1998).
2. Anonymity is used here broadly, even though many different distinctions could conceivably be made. For instance, visual anonymity, perceived anonymity, et cetera.
3. Often *impression management* is used interchangeably with self-presentation, although this normally refers to activities where the impressions that are controlled are those of other people or entities (Schlenker, 2003).

Chapter IV
Personal Health Records: Patients in Control

Ebrahim Randeree
Florida State University, USA

Melinda Whetstone
Florida State University, USA

ABSTRACT

An increasing focus on e-health and a governmental push to improve healthcare quality while giving patients more control of their health data have combined to promote the emergence of the personal health record (PHR). The PHR addresses timeliness, patient safety, and equity, goals that the Institute of Medicine has identified as integral to improving healthcare. The PHR is vital to the National Health Information Network (NHIN) that is being developed to give all Americans access to electronic health records by 2014. Despite increasing public access to PHRs via employers, insurance companies, healthcare providers, and independent entities, it is unclear whether the PHR will be successfully implemented and adopted by the public. This chapter looks at how PHRs address the needs, desires, and expectations of patients, explores the data quality concerns regarding patient-generated information (data capture, sharing and integration with other systems), discusses social implications of adoption, and concludes with a discussion of the evolving role that PHRs play in the growth of patient-centered e-health.

INTRODUCTION

The ongoing transition toward the electronic medical record (EMR), initially referred to as computerized patient record or electronic patient chart (Tang & McDonald, 2001), was spurred by concerns over medical errors and rising costs in healthcare. As EMR systems became more robust, they proved themselves to be beneficial to healthcare providers in many ways. The EMR reduced information duplication (Ewing & Cusick, 2004), improved utilization of lab and radiology results (Ewing & Cusick, 2004; Wang, Middleton, Prosser, Bardon, Spurr, Carchidi, et al., 2003), increased the efficiency of coding and billing (Menachemi & Brooks, 2006; Schmitt & Wofford, 2002), and provided healthcare personnel with quicker access to patient records (Sandrick, 1998; Wang et al., 2003).

Yet, patients and their caregivers share EMR benefits only indirectly. Patients continue to be viewed by EMR developers as passive participants who should not have direct access to or control of health data that are contained within the EMR. At the same time, patients want to be more engaged in their own healthcare and are seeking information online (Ball, Smith, & Bakalar, 2007). Use of the Internet to gather information about healthcare has increased substantially in recent years (Clark, Williams, Clark, & Clark, 2002; Gerber & Eiser, 2001; Lenhart, Horrigan, & Fallows, 2004), and the Pew Internet & American Life Project estimates the number of Americans searching for online health information at 113 million (Fox, 2006). As a result, patients have been undergoing a role change that is facilitated by Internet technology. The traditional paradigm of the patient as a passive recipient of physician diagnosis and instruction is evolving toward the patient becoming the driver of healthcare relationships. Patients have more options for receiving care, such as newly-created "store front" clinics being offered by major retailers to provide basic care (Wal-Mart, 2007). In addition, the Internet has greatly improved access to health information (Greenberg, D'Andrea, & Lorence, 2004), allowing patients to explore new treatments, to access current research journals, and to utilize increasingly sophisticated interactive and individually tailored programs through the Internet and Internet-enabled devices for health behavior change and chronic disease management (Ahern, 2007).

The personal health record (PHR) has emerged as a mechanism for patients to participate directly in the benefits of electronic records and integrated e-health delivery. Proposed benefits of the PHR include secure online access, comprehensive personal health history, means to become one's own health advocate, benchmarks and prompts for health maintenance, fluid communication between patient and provider, and automatic data entry (Morrissey, 2005). As patients manage their own personal health records using a PHR, it is hoped that this will help them make more informed choices about available options and give them the ability to exercise greater control over their own healthcare (Tsiknakis, Katehakis, & Orphanoudakis, 2002), in effect converting patients from passive information recipients to proactive consumers and generators of health information.

Leading health informatics groups in the U.S.—the American Health Information Management Association (AHIMA) and the American Medical Informatics Association (AMIA)—note that PHRs empower patients by providing a means for collecting, tracking, and sharing important, up-to-date health information for them or those in their care (AHIMA, 2006). Additionally, PHRs can promote patients' health management by providing cues for health issues (e.g., weight control or diabetes management), delivering reminders for medical test scheduling, and supporting entry of information—such as blood pressure or blood glucose levels—that may increase compliance to treatment protocols.

Patients have increasing opportunities to use a PHR, but many current initiatives offer only a partial PHR solution, are difficult to use, or raise privacy concerns. Typical offerings by employers and national insurers implement partially complete PHR designs that are limited in the scope of information that is readily included. For example, the PHR offered by Aetna, Inc. primarily provides information that is found in insurance records, such as billing and coding (Havenstein, 2007), and Kaiser's PHR contains only limited types of medical information (Hines, 2007). Although third-party PHRs have the potential to contain more complete healthcare documentation, the amount of manual data entry that users are required to perform and concerns over unauthorized secondary usage and privacy have dampened interest.

Despite positive news coverage of PHRs and their proposed benefits, nearly half of all Americans are still unaware of PHRs (Sprague, 2006). Adoption has been encouraged via legislation, with the premise that empowered consumers will help to decrease healthcare costs. However, the implications of further adoption—financial, social, and health-wise—are unknown. This chapter looks at how PHRs address the needs, desires, and expectations of patients, explores the data quality concerns regarding patient-generated information (data capture, sharing and integration with other systems), discusses social implications of adoption, and concludes with a discussion of the evolving role that PHRs play in the growth of patient-centered e-health.

BACKGROUND

PHRs have emerged as a new option for patients to become active participants in the federal push towards widespread digitized healthcare in the U.S. National Committee on Vital and Health Statistics (NCVHS, 2001) has identified the individual (personal health) as a key stakeholder in a technological National Health Information infrastructure, along with communities (population health) and healthcare providers. PHRs are seen as a critical component of an effective healthcare system, as they promote the patient-centeredness aspect of the six aims for improving healthcare called for by the Institute of Medicine, including safety, effectiveness, patient-centeredness, timeliness, efficiency, and equity (IOM, 1999, 2001).

The drive toward PHRs gained momentum in 2004 when the U.S. President signed Executive Order 13335, calling for "the development and nationwide implementation of an interoperable health information technology infrastructure to improve efficiency, reduce medical errors, raise the quality of care, and provide better information for patients, physicians, and other healthcare providers" (Brailer, 2005). This momentum is continuing in the U.S. with a steady flow of bills promoting a National Health Information Network (NHIN), overall health information technology adoption (S.1408, 2007; S.1455, 2007; S.1693, 2007), physician grants for EMR purchases (HR 2377, 2007), and physician reimbursement for each PHR that is provided to a patient.

Privacy and Security

As the push for PHRs increases and more companies provide access to them, the federal government will need to consider implications for health information privacy and security. Currently, personal health information is protected under the Health Insurance Portability and Accountability Act (HIPAA) of 1996, Public Law 104-191 (HIPAA, 1996). In addition to protecting personal health information, HIPAA ensures portability of medical records while governing the ability to disclose information contained within the records. HIPAA provides for sharing personal health information when "covered entities" have "reasonable safeguards and minimum necessary policies and procedures" in place (HHS OCR, 2003). A covered entity as defined by HIPAA is a health plan, healthcare clearinghouse, or healthcare provider who transmits protected health information in electronic form in connection with a transaction covered by the HIPAA transactions regulation (HIPAA PL 104-191, Sec 1172(a)). Under HIPAA, covered entities are expected to "maintain reasonable and appropriate administrative, technical, and physical safeguards" in order to "ensure the integrity and confidentiality of the information; to protect against" data or disclosure breaches and "ensure compliance with this part by the officers and employees of such person." Many security issues relating to the transmission and storage of PHR data have yet to be worked out, especially in the context of online PHRs, and this could slow the progress of PHR initiatives.

The concept of the PHR continues to evolve; its purpose and definition is still changing in step with technology advances and consumer demands (NCVHS, 2006). However, it is envisioned as an integral health resource that will promote informed health decisions as a consequence of increased health literacy, improved knowledge of healthcare practices, and expanded healthcare choices (AHIC, 2007). Optimally, the PHR will interrelate with other types of medical records, primarily the electronic medical record (EMR) and the electronic health record (EHR).

Electronic Medical Records and Electronic Health Records

The EMR is considered to be the legal record created in hospitals and ambulatory environments (Garets & Davis, 2006), and is the encompassing concept for health information (Stead, Kelly, & Kolodner, 2005). The EHR is a subset of the EMR that spans episodes of care across multiple healthcare providers and is designed specifically to be a resource for patients (Garets & Davis, 2006). Both records are generated as by-products of the healthcare provider's EMR system (Stead et al., 2005), the computerized system used by a healthcare provider to collect and manage detailed medical information (Connecting for Health, 2003; Garets & Davis, 2006). In effect, the EMR encompasses the various pieces of information collected and managed by the EMR system, and the EHR represents portions of the EMR that are most relevant to patients, potentially integrating documentation of care that is received from multiple providers. Although much of this information is only useful for administrative, financial, and billing parts of a healthcare practice, the EMR and EHR also contain patient encounter information which is highly relevant to the PHR.

Personal Health Information Management

Patients are not new to searching, retrieving, and storing health information. They have historically gathered personal medical information, including stacks of receipts, journal clippings, and lab results which are then organized to support ongoing management of health conditions or according to personal conceptions of future need. Moen and Brennan (2005) report that individuals use a wide range of media to manage health information for themselves and their families, including calendars, phonebooks, medical histories, and independent paper documents containing information about procedures, medication side effects, and medical instructions. These nondigital "personal health records" often are stored under refrigerator magnets, in shoeboxes, or simply piled in a drawer (Moen & Brennan, 2005). Only infrequently is a personal computer or personal digital assistant (PDA) used to manage personal health information at the present time.

Approaches to the PHR

Vendors of new PHR products strive to provide an efficient cataloging and health information management system that can replace *ad hoc* methods which patients have come to use. These new PHRs are intended to provide affordable, easy to use, life-long health and medical histories that are complete and accurate and can be generated and maintained effectively by patients or their caregivers (AHIC, 2007; AHIMA, 2005). Specific contents of PHRs vary, but these typically include the information that is normally filled out on a standard new patient questionnaire, such as personal identification, emergency contacts, prior healthcare providers, and insurance documentation. PHRs also frequently include documentation relating to immunizations, allergies and adverse drug reactions, prescribed medications (including dose and how often taken), over-the-counter medications and herbal remedies, incidents of illness and hospitalization, surgeries and other medical procedures, laboratory test results, and family histories. Additional information that may be encompassed by the PHR includes living wills and advance directives, organ donor authorization, physical examination results, physician opinions, eye and dental records, permission forms, and lifestyle information (AHIMA, 2005; Connecting for Health, 2004). As a complete and life-long record, the PHR should be designed to contain health information from all organizations and providers that serve patients (Connecting for Health, 2003). Additionally, the PHR should be maintained within a private, secure, and confidential environment (Connecting for Health, 2003).

Standards for data transfer and interoperability are supported by America's Health Insurance Plans (AHIP), a national association representing 1300 health insurers, and the Blue Cross and Blue Shield Association (BCBSA), a national federation of health coverage providers (MNT, 2006). Current standards primarily support data-driven PHRs, as described below. However, new standards have been proposed that will apply to all PHRs (Health Level Seven, 2007).

The three primary approaches to creating a PHR are as independent and personal applications, as transaction data-driven applications, and as EHR-integrated applications. Creation methods and security characteristics vary substantially among these approaches:

- **Independent and personal:** These PHRs are created manually by the individual user using commercially available applications and are unbound from any specific healthcare provider. They are categorized as stand-alone (independent) or Web-based types. When these PHRs are used as standalone systems, they offer high levels of security and privacy. However, they also require the most time to create and maintain, and standalone PHRs may not offer the level of "anyplace-anytime" access that is available with Web-based PHRs.
- **Transaction data-driven:** These PHRs are automatically created and typically maintained using transaction data from sources such as a healthcare provider, a health plan, or a pharmacy. As a result, they will typically be limited to automatically providing only information that is specific to the source, for example, an insurance company may only provide information pertaining to office visit dates, diagnoses, and costs related to covered providers. This type of PHR is sometimes referred to as "tethered" due to linkage with and control by a specific source entity. At least 70 million Americans have some form of access to a transaction data-driven PHR (Sprague, 2006), yet actual usage is estimated to be low, based on overall PHR use patterns (Denton, 2001).
- **EHR-integrated:** These are considered to be the "holy grail" among PHRs, as they are automatically populated with data from a healthcare provider's EHR, potentially providing the most complete collection of relevant patient information that can be made available (Tang & Lansky, 2005, pp. 1292). EHR-integrated PHRs often include additional functionality, such as secure email messaging, prescription renewal, appointment scheduling, and the ability for the user to add supplemental information (Sprague, 2006; Tang, Ash, Bates, Overhage, & Sands, 2006). Limited versions of the EHR-integrated PHR simply provide a view of the provider's EHR data. Several large organizations, such as the Pal Alto Medical Foundation (PAMF) (Tang, Black, Buchanan, Young, Hooper, & Lane, et al., 2003), Kaiser Permanente and the Veterans Health Administration (Sprague, 2006) currently provide this type of limited access. Until a greater proportion of healthcare providers adopt EHRs, however, availability of EHR-integrated PHRs will be constrained.

Each approach described above presents trade-offs. For example, the standalone PHR ensures high levels of privacy, but requires a high personal labor cost for creation and maintenance. While PHRs that are automatically populated with data from healthcare provider systems may appear to be optimal in that they require the patient to invest less startup effort, there are higher costs associated with this PHR approach as it requires the healthcare provider to use an EHR and to pay for the PHR to be integrated with it.

DATA QUALITY CONCERNS

We have discussed the importance of ease of use and interoperability in gaining patients' acceptance of PHRs. Ensuring data quality and relieving patients' concerns in this area are also important. High quality health information can reduce medical errors, avoid duplicating services, and give patients and their providers reliable information on which to base decisions. Quality issues are inherently multifaceted, and attention must be given to a number of dimensions in order to comprehensively address data quality issues and mitigate patients' concerns for data quality in PHRs:

- **Relevant content:** The most important criteria of a PHR is content (i.e., its informational and transactional capabilities) (Agarwal & Venkatesh, 2002). Relevant content promotes usage, especially where the content fosters self-education (Walter & Tung, 2002). This makes it important for PHR designers to learn which types of content are essential to patients and develop interfaces that allow quick access to this content while minimizing distractions. This is not a trivial exercise, as the relevance of content can be affected by numerous variables, including motivation, reading level, culture, primary language, technical knowledge, and background experiences of software users (Calongne, 2001).
- **Accuracy:** Accuracy (including completeness) of health information is very important for PHR users and their healthcare providers, as inaccurate information can lead to medical errors and practitioner liability. As the volume of electronic data increases, there is always the potential to overlook or aggregate relevant information. Of the various types of data entry methods employed by PHRs, approaches that rely on guided or automated entry of data elements abstracted from primary source documents may promote more accurate entry (Kim & Johnson, 2004). An additional concern for information that is provided to patients is the need to avoid descriptions that patients are likely to misinterpret. It is not in the best interests of patients or their physicians to provide health information with insufficient structure, patient education, or guidance to make it understandable to them (Walter & Tung, 2002).
- **Privacy/Security:** Security and privacy issues are of concern to both PHR users and developers. Patients using Web-based PHRs must be aware of the potential for misuse, unauthorized secondary usage, and other dangers that come with online transmission and remote data storage. Striking a balance between privacy concerns and the need for access can be difficult (Kelly & Unsal, 2002). Web-based data must be secured by the PHR provider, and patients should be confident that their data is secured and encrypted during online transmission. PHR providers should attempt to meet all HIPAA standards for protection of patient health information, even where these are not directed explicitly toward online operations. Currently, many providers of Web-based PHRs operate outside of HIPAA rules, as they are not covered entities as defined by

HIPAA and are not regulated by HIPAA privacy rules (Conn, 2006). Nevertheless, health records contain information that is highly sensitive, and patients have a strong expectation that such information will be used only in the context of providing effective care (Rindfleisch, 1997). Privacy and confidentiality issues are primary concerns underscoring the reluctance of administrators, physicians, and patients to completely embrace Internet technologies (Kerwin & Madison, 2002).

- **Authority:** Qualification of the author is crucial in determining the credibility of health information in PHRs. Physicians receive and process large amounts of data. If they allow patients to bring in PHR data, there must be checks and balances to support its interpretation. Similarly, patients who import EHR data into a PHR database must be able to verify who has provided the information. Authority has been recognized as the underlying theme in source credibility (Rieh & Belkin, 1998), and trust is established when the information is presented by a recognized author (Lin & Umoh, 2002). Authority criteria should include author identification (physician identification if the information is collected from an EHR). Identification of the author promotes perceptions of legitimacy and accountability of the information.
- **Timeliness:** Availability of timely health information is essential to improving the quality of healthcare. In addition, it is important that medical decisions be based upon correctly sequenced health information. For this reason, PHR entries should be accompanied by the dates and times the information was created, modified, and added to the PHR in order to inform judgments as to the value and relevance of the information. In addition, the PHR should be updated following medical encounters or to reflect changes in the patient's health status.
- **Usability:** Ease of use has been extensively researched across the IT domain (Agarwal & Venkatesh, 2002), and the general IT findings suggest usability is a key driver of PHR usage. Presence of design elements that support usability is an important determinant of whether visitors are likely to return to Web sites (Klein, 1998). A recent study of health records reports that attention to navigation, context, and information design is critical to the usability of a system (Rose, Schnipper, Park, Poon, Li, & Middleton, 2005). PHR developers should conduct usability testing to support patients in obtaining quality access to health data.
- **Information audits:** Given the critical nature of health information contained in the PHR, patients must have the ability to audit the information in order to identify and correct any discrepancies or to update information. Where the PHR is integrated with a provider's EHR, giving patients a moderated ability to review and update data could make both health records more robust. Auditing capabilities give patients control over the information dissemination and, by providing access histories, may help allay patients' concerns for privacy and security.

SOCIAL CONCERNS

Historically, one unfortunate side effect of the diffusion of new technology has been increased disparity for the socioeconomically disadvantaged (Rogers, 2003). The PHR is multifaceted in that it can operate as a data repository, a health information management tool, or an educational dissemination portal. The PHR is also a developing technology, and vendors generally have objectives toward using PHRs to support equitable and patient-centered healthcare. However, if efforts are not made ensure equitable access and to develop the appropriate levels of health literacy and technology competence for all potential users, the PHR may further alienate populations that have the most to gain from using it, such as chronically ill patients who have difficulty affording healthcare. Despite developers' intentions, PHRs may act to highlight and even exacerbate social inequities in healthcare. These social concerns can be broadly represented by the digital divide phenomenon with a secondary focus on literacy:

- **Digital divide:** Focusing on those with access to technology and those without will be a challenge for any PHR developer to overcome. The traditional racial and socioeconomic disparities of access to financial means, to computers, and to the healthcare system in general become more apparent in a PHR designed for Web access. While some may see public Internet access, at the library, for example, as a means to overcome barriers, a challenge still remains in how to provide PHR access to those who do not have medical insurance. Although "free" PHR access is available, these products typically offer limited functionality and still require extensive access to a computer.
- **Literacy:** Concerns of literacy relating to PHRs can be subdivided into three distinct areas: technology literacy (ability to understand and use the technology such as Web portals, Web forms, and so on), information literacy (ability to understand the information presented and the instructions provided), and health literacy (ability to understand the medical content provided sufficient o make basic health decisions). Use of PHRs is hindered by a range of barriers including lacking access to computers or devices, cognitive disabilities, physical disabilities, low computer skills or reading literacy, and low health literacy (Lober, Zierler, Herbaugh, Shinstrom, Stolyar, Kim, & Kim, 2006).

CONCLUSION

The national focus on applying health information technologies to improve healthcare delivery quality and lower costs has created momentum for patient-centered solutions. Increasing patient demand and a changing healthcare market now make it likely that Internet-based communication between providers and patients could soon be an everyday part of healthcare throughout the Internet-connected world (Wilson, 2003). The true benefits of PHRs become apparent when they are fully integrated with the healthcare provider's EHR or EMR. Using integrated PHRs, patients will not only gain access to their medical records but also will have the ability to update, correct, or add to the records. This will allow patients to become more engaged with their medical histories, plans of care, and options for treatment. While issues of data quality exist, inclusion of the patients will allow for these primary stakeholders in the healthcare process to be active participants in their own care. Potential benefits include better compliance with care protocols (translating to lower costs for insurers and patients), increased patient literacy, increased convenience for patients and their providers (translating to service improvements and better coordination of care), and better quality outcomes.

The monitoring of chronic conditions is an ideal fit for PHRs. The movement to involve patients stems to a large degree from the desire to engage patients in managing chronic diseases, along with selecting care based on quality characteristics, improving the quality of the care delivery system, and making healthcare more market-driven by increasing patients' share of costs (Fowles, Kind, Craft, Kind, Mandel, & Adlis, 2004). Chronic conditions require long term treatment plans and provide an opportunity for cost reduction if the care is coordinated effectively between the physician and the patient. Incorporating home monitoring and self-reporting features offers some of the most interesting opportunities for PHRs (Heubusch, 2007).

PHRs have potential to transform the healthcare setting: they can replace or augment existing care processes, provide interactive communication, support information exchange, initiate consumer activity, and increase convenience and efficiency of healthcare services (Hartman, 2006). In order for PHR benefits to be realized, however, several criteria must be addressed in the areas of PHR standards, interoperability, and system functionality:

- **Standards:** Current PHR systems are either linked to an EMR/EHR or are stand-alone systems that lack national standards. These heterogeneous systems will need to coalesce towards a shared standard that allows for simplified data transfer among systems. Records must be of sufficient size and scope to include both clinical and nonclinical data. Data standards should also determine the sources of information that is allowed to flow into and out of the PHR.
- **Interoperability with Privacy/Security:** The current focus in health information exchange initiatives is to connect electronic medical records among healthcare providers to allow sharing of data among physicians and healthcare facilities. The proprietary nature of health information systems presents a barrier to health information exchange in its current form. As patients interact with multiple providers and multiple systems, the creation of a national standard for electronic records will facilitate the exchange. The Certification Commission for Healthcare Information Technology (CCHIT) is a recognized certification body for electronic health records and their networks, and an independent, voluntary, private-sector initiative (www.cchit.org). CCHIT is working to accelerate the adoption of health information technology by creating an efficient, credible and sustainable certification program. The certification allows for development of interoperability standards among vendors that market electronic medical records.
- **Functionality:** Use of PHRs will be directly related to the benefits that patients perceive from usage. In this case, the functionality of the PHR and its ability to reduce costs increase the likelihood of quality outcomes. The ability to easily view and enter health information will help to increase use, as will automated integration of information between the PHR and the healthcare provider's EHR or EMR. Additional benefits of reduced insurance premiums for chronic condition management as well as participation in the management of care decisions could incentivize PHR usage.

As PHR vendors compete for market share, new models will need to be developed. PHR vendors must move toward providing more complete integration and access to medical records for patients to become fully empowered. PHR vendors must also integrate their services with traditional EMR and EHR vendors. For physicians to support these efforts, the PHR must not interfere with the workflow of the office and must be interoperable with existing systems so data can move seamlessly among systems, assuming adequate privacy and security protections are in place.

The growth of patient empowerment initiatives will continue to drive the direction of healthcare. Studies on how the Internet affects patients' experience of empowerment within the clinical encounter have shown mixed outcomes. While patients' desire to use the Internet for health information is increasing generally, many patients are reluctant to discuss information from the Internet in the clinical encounter for fear of challenging the physician's authority, and some physicians express frustration in dealing with patients who arrive with health information they obtain online (Jacobson, 2007). In contrast, PHRs tend to empower patients in their personal healthcare and in interactions with healthcare providers. In a comparison of effects of computer-generated medical record summaries and written PHRs on patients' attitudes, knowledge and behavior concerning health promotion, researchers found that patients receiving summaries as part of mail recruitment were significantly more likely to attend for a health check; those receiving both PHR and summaries were more likely to keep and use the record; and those receiving PHR improved their knowledge of health promotion, became more aware of lifestyle issues, and were more likely to change their lifestyle (Liaw, Lawrence, & Rendell, 1996).

The growth of patient self-management tools for remote monitoring will fuel PHR adoption, if tools and standards are developed that make clinical information understandable to and usable by patients (Ball et al., 2007). As a caveat, it must be recognized that not all patients will be excited to adopt PHRs. The use of a PHR to empower patients with their medical records will be beneficial to early adopters and those with chronic conditions. However, some patients, such as those who experience a rare acute incident, may not be attracted to PHRs. Patients also exist at varying levels of literacy, and not all will be eager to delve into their medical records without support.

For PHRs to have a future, the healthcare industry must determine the public's needs and interests and provide flexible tools that offer a range of data and resources that can be used to satisfy these needs and interests (Heubusch, 2007). In addition, physicians must be willing to share information with their patients through PHRs. In many cases, physicians concerns for negative impacts of information sharing are overblown and based on anecdotal sources, as empirical research in this area is limited and dated (Fowles et al., 2004). Much of the value of PHRs lies in shared information and shared decision-making in support of the continuity of care (Ball et al., 2007).

REFERENCES

Agarwal, R., & Venkatesh, V. (2002). Assessing a firm's Web presence: A heuristic evaluation procedure for the measurement of usability. *Information Systems Research, 13*(2), 168-186.

Ahern, D.K. (2007). Challenges and opportunities of eHealth research. *American Journal of Preventive Medicine, 32*(5), 75-82.

AHIC. (2007). *Community meeting: Consumer empowerment workgroup.* Mountain View, CA: American Health Information Community.

AHIMA. (2005). The role of the personal health record in the EHR. *Journal of American Health Information Management Association, 76*(7), 64A-D.

AHIMA. (2006). The value of personal health records. A joint position statement for consumers of healthcare. *Journal of American Health Information Management Association, 77*(9), 22-24.

Ball, M., Smith, C., & Bakalar, R.S. (2007). Personal health records: Empowering consumers. *Journal of Health Information Management, 21*(1), 76-86.

Brailer, D.J. (2005) *Is there a doctor in the mouse?: Using information technology to improve healthcare.* Testimony before the U.S. House of Representatives, Committee on Government Reform, Subcommittee on Federal Workforce and Agency Organization. Retrieved May 14, 2008, from http://www.hhs.gov/healthit/t050727.html

Calongne, C.M. (2001). Designing for Web site usability. *Journal of Computing in Small Colleges, 16*(3), 39-45.

Clark, R., Williams, J., Clark, J., & Clark, C. (2002). Assessing Web site usability: Construction zone. *Journal of Healthcare Information Management, 17*(2), 51-55.

Conn, J. (2006). Personal and (maybe) confidential. *Modern Healthcare, 36*, 28-31.

Connecting for Health. (2003). *The personal health working group final report*. Markle Foundation. Retrieved May 14, 2008, from http://www.markle.org/downloadable_assets/final_phwg_report1.pdf

Connecting for Health. (2004). *Connecting Americans to their healthcare: Final report*. Markle Foundation. Retrieved May 14, 2008, from http://www.connectingforhealth.org/resources/wg_eis_final_report_0704.pdf

Denton, I.C. (2001). Will patients use electronic personal health records? Responses from a real-life experience. *Journal of Healthcare Information Management, 15*(3), 251-259.

Ewing, T., & Cusick, D. (2004). Knowing what to measure. *Healthcare Financial Management, 58*(6), 60-63.

Fowles, J.B., Kind, A.C., Craft, C., Kind, E.A., Mandel, J.L., & Adlis, S. (2004). Patients' interest in reading their medical record: Relation with clinical and sociodemographic characteristics and patients' approach to healthcare. *Archives of Internal Medicine, 164*(7), 793-800.

Fox, S. (2006). *Online health search 2006*. Pew Internet & American Life Project. Retrieved May 14, 2008, from http://www.pewinternet.org/PPF/r/190/report_display.asp

Garets, D., & Davis, M. (2006). Electronic medical records vs. electronic health records: Yes, there is a difference. *HIMSS Analytics*. Retrieved May 14, 2008, from http://www.himssanalytics.org/docs/WP_EMR_EHR.pdf

Gerber, B.S., & Eiser, A.R. (2001). The patient physician relationship in the Internet age: Future prospects and the research agenda. *Journal of Medical Internet Research, 3*(2), E15.

Greenberg, L., D'Andrea, G., & Lorence, D.P. (2004). Setting the public agenda for online health search: A white paper and action agenda. *Journal of Medical Internet Research, 6*(2), 1-10.

Hartman, M.J. (2006). Personal health records and electronic health records: Navigating the intersections. *Health Policy Newsletter, 19*, 1.

Havenstein, H. (2007). Aetna clients to get access to online health data. *Computerworld*. Retrieved May 14, 2008, from http://www.computerworld.com/action/article.do?command=viewArticleBasicandarticleId=278859

Health Level Seven. (2007). *HL7's EHR technical committee opens public comment on personal health record system (PHR-S) functional model*. Retrieved May 14, 2008, from http://www.hl7.org/documentcenter/public/pressreleases/HL7_PRESS_20070827.pdf

Heubusch, K. (2007). Piecing together the PHR. *Journal of American Health Information Management Association, 78*(4), 28-32.

Hines, L. (2007). Healthcare targets paper trail. *Press Enterprise*. Retrieved May 14, 2008, from http://www.pe.com/localnews/inland/stories/PE_News_Local_D_medicalrecords31.27afdf2.html

HIPAA. (1996). *Health insurance portability and accountability act of 1996 (public law 104-191)*. Retrieved May 14, 2008, from http://aspe.hhs.gov/admnsimp/pl104191.htm

IOM. (1999). *To err is human: Building a safer health system*. Washington, DC: Institute of Medicine, National Academies Press.

IOM. (2001). *Crossing the quality chasm: A new health system for the 21st century*. Washington, DC: Institute of Medicine, National Academies Press.

Jacobson, P. (2007). Empowering the physician-patient relationship: The effect of the Internet. *Partnership: The Canadian Journal of Library and Information Practice and Research, 2*(1). Retrieved May 14, 2008, from http://journal.lib.uoguelph.ca/index.php/perj/issue/view/31

Kelly, E.P., & Unsal, F. (2002). Health Information privacy and e-healthcare. *International Journal of Healthcare Technology and Management, 4*(1/2), 41-52.

Kerwin, K.E., & Madison, J. (2002). The role of the Internet in improving healthcare quality. *Journal of Healthcare Management, 47*(4), 225-236.

Kim, M.I., & Johnson, K.B. (2004). Patient entry of information: Evaluation of user interfaces. *Journal of Medical Internet Research, 6*(2), e13.

Klein, L.R. (1998). Evaluating the potential of interactive media through a new lens: Search versus experience goods. *Journal of Business Research, 41*(3), 195-203.

Lenhart, A., Horrigan, J., & Fallows, D. (2004). Content creation online. *Pew Internet & American life project*. Retrieved May 14, 2008, from http://www.pewinternet.org/pdfs/PIP_Content_Creation_Report.pdf

Liaw, T., Lawrence, M., & Rendell, J. (1996). The effect of a computer-generated patient-held medical record summary and/or a written personal health record on patients' attitudes, knowledge and behaviour concerning health promotion. *Family Practice 13*(3), 289-293.

Lin, B., & Umoh, D. (2002). E-healthcare: A vehicle of change. *American Business Review, 20*(2), 27-32.

Lober, W., Zierler, B., Herbaugh, A., Shinstrom, S., Stolyar, A., Kim, E. & Kim, Y. (2006). Barriers to the use of a personal health record by an elderly population. In Proceedings of *2006 AMIA Annual Symposium Proceedings* (pp. 514-518).

Menachemi, N., & Brooks, R.G. (2006). Reviewing the benefits of electronic health records and associated patient safety technologies. *Journal of Medical Systems, 30*(3), 159-168.

Moen, A., & Brennan, P.F. (2005). Health@Home: The work of health information management in the household (HIMH): Implications for consumer health informatics (CHI) innovations. *Journal of the American Medical Informatics Association, 12*(6), 648-656.

Morrissey, J. (2005). But what does the public think? For consumers to adopt PHRs, they need reasons that hit home. *Journal of American Health Information Management Association, 76*(10), 42-44.

MNT. (2006). AHIP, BCBSA issue standards for personal health records. *Medical News Today.* Retrieved May 14, 2008, from http://www.medicalnewstoday.com/articles/59052.php

NCVHS. (2001). A strategy for building the national health information infrastructure. *National Committee on Vital and Health Statistics.* Washington DC: U.S. Department of Health and Human Services.

Rieh, S.Y., & Belkin, N.J. (1998). Understanding judgment of information quality and cognitive authority in the www. *Journal of the American Society for Information Science, 35*, 279-289.

Rindfleisch, T.C. (1997). Privacy, information technology, and healthcare. *Communication of the ACM, 40*(8), 92-100.

Rogers, E.M. (2003). *Diffusion of innovations (fifth edition).* New York: The Free Press.

Rose, A.F., Schnipper, J.L., Park, E.R., Poon, E.G., Li, Q., & Middleton, B. (2005). Using qualitative studies to improve the usability of an EMR. *Journal of Biomedical Informatics, 38*, 51-60.

Sandrick, K. (1998). Calculating ROI for CPRs. *Health Management Technology, 19*(6), 16-20.

Schmitt, K.F., & Wofford, D.A. (2002). Financial analysis projects clear returns from electronic medical records. *Healthcare Financial Management, 56*(1), 52-57.

Sprague, L. (2006). *Personal health records: The peoples' choice?* (Publication No. 820). Washington D.C.; National Health Policy Forum. Retrieved May 14, 2008, from http://www.nhpf.org/pdfs_ib/IB820_PHRs_11-30-06.pdf

Stead, W.W., Kelly, B.J., & Kolodner, R.M. (2005). Achievable steps toward building a National Health Information infrastructure in the United States. *Journal of the American Medical Informatics Association, 12*(2), 113-120.

Tang, P.C., Ash, J.S., Bates, D.W., Overhage, J.M., & Sands, D.Z. (2006). Personal health records: Definitions, benefits, and strategies for overcoming barriers to adoption. *Journal of the American Medical Informatics Association, 13*(2), 121-126.

Tang, P.C., Black, W., Buchanan, J., Young, C.Y., Hooper, D., Lane, S.R., et al. (2003). *PAMFOnline: Integrating EHealth with an electronic medical record system.* Paper presented at the 2003 AMIA Annual Symposium Proceedings.

Tang, P.C., & Lansky, D. (2005). The missing link: Bridging the patient-provider health information gap. *Health Affairs, 24*(5), 1290-1295.

Tang, P.C., & McDonald, C.J. (2001). Computer-based patient-record systems. In E.H. Shortliffe & L.E. Perreault (Eds.). *Medical informatics: Computer applications in healthcare and biomedicine* (Second edition, pp. 327-358). New York: Springer-Verlag.

Tsiknakis, M., Katehakis, D.G., & Orphanoudakis, S.C. (2002). An open, component-based information infrastructure for integrated health information networks. *International Journal of Medical Informatics 68*, 3-26.

Wal-Mart. (2007). *400 health clinics to open in Wal-mart stores during next three years.* Retrieved May 14, 2008, from http://www.walmartfacts.com/articles/default.aspx?id=4973

Wang, S.J., Middleton, B., Prosser, L.A., Bardon, C.G., Spurr, C.D., Carchidi, P.J., et al., (2003). A cost-benefit analysis of electronic medical records in primary care. *The American Journal of Medicine, 114*(5), 397-403.

Walter, Z., & Tung, Y.A. (2002). E-healthcare system design: A consumer preference approach. *International Journal of Healthcare Technology and Management, 4*(1/2), 53-70.

Wilson, E.V. (2003). Asynchronous healthcare communication. *Communications of the ACM, 46*(6), 79-84.

Chapter V
Disability Determinations and Personal Health Records

Elaine A. Blechman
University of Colorado at Boulder, USA

ABSTRACT

Newly disabled workers are often unemployed, uninsured, and indigent. They are in desperate need of Social Security OASDI monthly benefits, and the Medicare health insurance that follows 24 months after benefits begin. Applicants must prove that their medical conditions (excluding drug and alcohol abuse) have resulted in severe functional limitations that prevent them from any gainful employment. Delays and denials of benefits result when applicants cannot find or retrieve medical records from providers familiar with their medical history, health status, and functional limitations. The disability application workflow is complex, particularly for applicants with cognitive and mental health impairments. Health information technology (HIT) has been used to automate care delivery workflow through provider-controlled, electronic health record systems (EHRs). Disability applicants' workflow could, just as well, be automated through consumer-controlled, unbound, and intelligent personal electronic health record systems (PHRs), which are not tethered to a health plan or employer network, and which automatically exchange information updates with authorized providers' EHRs. Applicants' PHRs may later prove helpful with self-management of chronic conditions prior to Medicare coverage and with periodic reevaluations of their medical status.

INTRODUCTION

"A 20-year-old worker has a 3 in 10 chance of becoming disabled before reaching retirement age" (http://www.socialsecurity.gov) by a condition that prevents work or that limits the kind or amount of possible work (Burkhauser & Houtenville, 2006). In 2004, an estimated 7.9% (or about one in 13) civilian noninstitutionalized, men and women, aged 18-64 in the United States reported a disability that limits work; about one in four people with disabilities lived in families with incomes below the poverty line (Houtenville, Erickson, & Lee, 2005).

About 46.6 million people or 15.9 percent of the U.S. population have no health insurance (Hadley, 2007). Approximately 18,000 Americans die prematurely each year because they lack health insurance (DeNavas-Walt, Proctor, & Lee, 2006). A telephone survey of people with disabilities found that those who were uninsured were more likely than others to do without or delay necessary care, including prescription drugs and preventive healthcare services that would reduce their future need for healthcare (Hanson, Neuman, Dutwin, & Kasper, 2003). Newly disabled and unemployed workers who no longer have private health insurance coverage are exceptionally vulnerable to deteriorating health and untimely death. If they qualify for Social Security disability benefits, they get a modest income for themselves and their dependents and, after 24 months, Medicare Part A (http://www.socialsecurity.gov/disability/3368).

Disability benefits have expanded and contracted since their institution during the Great Depression (http://www.ssa.gov/history/briefhistory3.html). In 1935, President Roosevelt signed the Social Security Act (SSA), creating a contributory system in which workers prepared for their retirement through taxes that they paid while employed. In 1956, an amendment to the Act provided benefits to disabled workers aged 50-64 and disabled adult children. In 1960, President Eisenhower signed an amendment permitting SSA disability benefits for disabled workers of any age and their dependents. In 1996, President Clinton signed a bill (P.L. 104-121) that changed eligibility for SSA disability benefits from a medical condition that prevents work, to a medical condition other than drug addiction or alcoholism that prevents work.

About 48.4 million people received Old Age, Survivors, and Disability Insurance (OASDI) monthly benefits in December 2005. Disabled workers and their dependents were 17% of OASDI beneficiaries, their average monthly benefits were $938. In 2005, OASDI payments exceeded $44 billion a month, approached $521 billion for the year, and represented 4.2% of the U.S. gross domestic product. At the same time, employees, self-employed workers, and employers contributed $593 billion to the OASDI trust funds (SSA, 2007).

Two recent studies indirectly suggest the importance of SSA disability benefits. In Sweden, 197 individuals granted disability pensions reported less illness, larger social networks, and less work and family role limitations than 96 individuals who did not receive disability pensions (Ydreborg, Ekberg, & Nordlund, 2006). In the U.S., a survey of 4,918 veterans found that their odds of impoverishment were reduced considerably if they applied for and received VA benefits for posttraumatic stress disorder (Murdoch, van Ryn, Hodges, & Cowper, 2005).

The findings of a third study (McWilliams, Meara, Zaslasvky, & Ayanian, 2007) are directly relevant to the impact of Medicare coverage following (by 24 months) qualification for SSA disability benefits. McWilliams et al. (2007) used longitudinal data from the nationally representative Health and Retirement Study to assess self-reported healthcare use and expenditures from 1992 through 2004 among 5,158 adults who were privately insured or uninsured before age 65 and of Medicare eligibility. Previously uninsured Medicare beneficiaries with hypertension, diabetes, heart disease, or stroke required more intensive and costly healthcare, and died earlier than previously insured Medicare beneficiaries with these same chronic conditions. There were no differences in morbidity or mortality between previously uninsured and insured Medicare beneficiaries without chronic conditions.

Chapter Overview

Newly disabled workers are often unemployed, uninsured, and indigent. They are in desperate need of Social Security OASDI monthly benefits and the Medicare health insurance that follows 24 months after benefits begin. Applicants must prove that their medical conditions (excluding drug and alcohol abuse) have resulted in severe functional limitations that prevent them from any gainful employment. Delays and denials of benefits result when applicants cannot find or retrieve medical records from providers familiar with their medical history, health status, and functional limitations. The disability application workflow is complex and obscure (Pransky & Dempsey, 2004), particularly for applicants with cognitive and mental health impairments (Banks & Lawrence, 2005).

Health information technology (HIT) has been used to automate care delivery workflow through provider-controlled, electronic health record systems (EHRs). For example, providers can use capabilities of their EHR systems to automate scheduling of patient encounters, e-prescribing, ordering of laboratory tests and import of laboratory results, and production and export of health insurance claims for reimbursement of their services.

Disability applicants' workflow could, just as well, be automated through consumer-controlled, unbound, and intelligent personal electronic health record systems (PHRs), which are not tethered to a health plan or employer network and which automatically exchange information with authorized providers' EHRs. For example, consumers could use their PHRs to automate transmission of requests for medical records, autofilling of SSA forms, importing of requested data and documents from providers' EHRs, and exporting of the completed application portfolio to SSA interviewers and evaluators in formats they require. Applicants' PHRs may later prove helpful with self-management of chronic conditions prior to Medicare coverage, and with periodic reevaluations of their medical status.

In the remainder of this chapter, I suggest how newly disabled workers could use PHRs to ease the disability benefits application process. First, I describe some of the workflow requirements confronting newly disabled workers applying for SSA benefits. Next, I present the conventional assumption that a National Health Information Network (NHIN), scheduled for rollout in 2014, should be composed of provider-controlled EHRs networked in regional health information exchanges (HIEs) with limited consumer access via tethered PHRs.

A provider-controlled NHIN simply cannot satisfy the workflow requirements of low-income, unemployed consumers with chronic conditions, such as applicants for SSA benefits. And so, I recommend that the NHIN architecture make room for consumer-controlled, unbound, intelligent personal electronic health record systems (PHRs), which are capable of automating data exchange across the NHIN with provider-controlled EHRs, are not tethered to employer or health plan networks, and automate the workflow required to compile, update, and selectively share an electronic disability benefits application portfolio.

PROBLEM: APPLYING FOR SSA DISABILITY BENEFITS

The applicant for SSA disability benefits must satisfy SSA's five-step disability application process. Applicants must meet an earnings requirement including a duration-of-work test to show sufficient length of work under Social Security. And, they must prove that they are unable to work due to limitations associated with medical conditions other than drug addiction or alcoholism. Decisions about eligibility, according to various SSA documents, can take from three months (for applicants with confirmed disabilities on the SSA list) to five years (for applicants who contest denial of their initial application and await the ruling of an administrative law judge). The application process, with its various permutations, is depicted on the SSA Web site in a 15-page-long flow chart.

SSA deems applicants eligible for benefits if they:

1. Are not working or have monthly earning in an acceptably low range;
2. Have a severe medical condition that "significantly limits your ability to do basic work activities—such as walking and remembering—for at least one year";
3. Have medical conditions on the SSA list of impairments (http://www.ssa.gov/disability/professionals/bluebook/AdultListings.htm) that are automatically considered disabilities as defined by law; or
4. Have medical conditions that the state agency decides prevents applicants from being able to do the work they did before; and
5. Are judged by a state agency unable to do other work than before.

SSA 3368: The process usually begins at the applicant's local Social Security office where the applicant, assisted by an SSA interviewer, completes SSA Disability Application 3368, Adult Disability and Work History Report (http://www.socialsecurity.gov/disability/3368). SSA 3368 includes 275 data fields covering illnesses, injuries, conditions; work; medical records; medications; tests; education and training; vocational rehabilitation; and employment. SSA 3368 is available online so that applicants can print it out and use it to prepare for the interview at the local SSA office. (Although the SSA Web site indicates that online submission is an option, my several attempts to initiate an online submission failed).

Other applicant forms: In addition to the basic SSA 3368 application form, applicants must complete other forms which describe their medical conditions and explain how it affects their ability to work, and which give permission to doctors, hospitals, and other healthcare professionals to release applicant information and records to the SSA. (These forms are mentioned on the SSA Web site, but my repeated attempts to find these forms failed).

Supporting documents and medical records: SSA requires applicants to supply documents and medical records that support claims made in SSA 3368 forms including:

- The Social Security number and birth certificate or other proof of age for each person applying for benefits (including your spouse and children, if they are applying for benefits);
- Names, addresses, and telephone numbers of doctors, hospitals, clinics, and institutions that treated you and dates of treatment;
- Names and prescribed dosage of all medications you are taking;
- Medical records from your doctors, therapists, hospitals, clinics, and caseworkers;
- Laboratory and test results;
- A summary of where you worked in the past 16 years (company names, addresses, supervisors' telephone numbers) and the kind of work you did;
- A copy of your W-2 Form (Wage and Tax Statement), or if you are self-employed, your federal tax return for the past year; and
- Dates of your current and any prior marriages, if applicable

The SSA Blue Book (SSA, 2006a) recommends that applicants request medical records documenting their medical condition (including prescribed medications and lab test results) from healthcare providers who are familiar with them and able to provide *a detailed longitudinal picture of the claimant's impairments.* Many applicants cannot retrieve medical records from the healthcare providers who diagnosed and treated them in the past. Their past providers may be unresponsive to requests for medical records. Or, they may not be able to recall the identity or location of the many past providers with whom they have had diagnostic and treatment encounters. Applicants who are unable to retrieve sufficient documentation from their own healthcare providers must submit to a one-time examination by an SSA-appointed examiner. SSA examiners are unfamiliar with applicants' medical history and health status; and, they are probably less inclined than applicants' own physicians to find in the applicant's favor.

If an applicant's claim is denied by the state agency, the applicant may request a hearing before an administrative law judge involving reconsideration of application evidence by a vocational or medical expert. The waiting time for hearings ranges from 90 days to 18 months. When a judge issues a partially favorable or unfavorable decision, the claimant may appeal to Social Security's Appeals Council, whose response time ranges from 12 weeks to three years.

The SSA disability application process requires applicants to procure, store, and share a comprehensive and up to date portfolio of medical records, lab tests, and evaluation reports. Applicants must make copies of items in this portfolio available to any number of SSA employees and subcontractors involved in the applicant's case for as many as five years from start to finish of the application process. Most applicants who are awarded benefits must be prepared for periodic re-evaluations of their status by continuously updating their medical records portfolios.

The SSA publishes annual statistical reports (e.g., SSA, 2007) enumerating the proportion of applicants who are denied benefits and the reasons for denial such as "Impairment is not severe." An unknown number of applicants pay doctors and lawyers to prepare, submit, and appeal their applications. It is not clear how many applicants are improperly denied benefits, because they lack the human or financial resources required for continuous, long-term exchange of records and information with providers, vocational and medical experts, lawyers, administrative law judges, and appeals councils. Nor, is it clear how many applicants make substantial investments in this process, but die before they become eligible for benefits.

It seems likely that a substantial number of genuinely eligible applicants cannot find and supply the required data and supporting documents, due to the presence of medical conditions (such as traumatic brain injury) and associated cognitive and mental health disabilities (such as dementia and PTSD), and due to the absence of capable, informed family caregivers. Many beneficiaries, similarly unprepared for SSA reevaluation of their status, may lose their benefits.

Controversy: A Provider-Centered National Health Information Network

For about two decades, health information technology (HIT) has been employed to automate healthcare providers' workflow, including records management, scheduling of patient encounters, and submission of claims to health insurance payers. No noticeable attention has been directed to automation of workflow of consumers with chronic conditions and their family caregivers who spend hours each week managing health-care records, scheduling appointments with providers, and contending with healthcare financing problems. Lessons learned from automation of providers' workflow could readily be applied to consumers such as SSA disability benefits applicants or SSA beneficiaries undergoing reevaluation of status. HIT might just as well be used to automate the SSA disability application workflow, making it easier for deserving applicants to speedily and successfully submit applications and qualify for benefits.

Health Information Technology Policy Recommendations

The Institute of Medicine (IOM) of the National Academies of Science is a nongovernmental body established to advise the U.S. Congress about healthcare policy. The IOM has repeatedly recommended the use of HIT to automate the workflow of healthcare providers with the expectation that the results would benefit consumers, particularly those with chronic illnesses and disabilities.

In 1991, the IOM proposed, "The Computer-Based Patient Record," as an essential technology solution for inadequacies in U.S. healthcare (IOM, 1991). In 2000, the IOM reported that, "More people die in a given year as a result of medical errors than from motor vehicle accidents (43,458), breast cancer (42,297), or AIDS (16,516)" (IOM, 2000, pp. 1), and in 2001, recommended the use of HIT to make healthcare more safe, effective, patient-centered, timely, efficient, and equitable (IOM, 2001). In 2003, the IOM described the key care delivery functions with which an electronic health record system or EHR could promote patient safety in hospitals, ambulatory care settings, nursing homes, and the community (IOM, 2003). In 2006, the IOM recommended the use of HIT to improve the coordination of care for cancer survivors (IOM, 2006). In 2007, the IOM recommended e-prescribing in order to prevent an estimated 1.5 million adverse drug events each year (IOM, 2007).

Building a National Health Information Network

The U.S. is a decade or so behind other economically developed countries in the design and deployment of a nationwide health information network and in network inclusion of disabled, uninsured, and indigent individuals (Anderson, Frogner, Johns, & Reinhardt, 2006).

With bipartisan support, President Bush, in 2004, ordered nationwide implementation of an interoperable health information technology infrastructure to improve the quality and efficiency of healthcare by 2014. David Brailer (2005), the first national health information technology coordinator, predicted that a National Health Information Network (NHIN) composed of interoperable electronic health records (EHRs) would "not only transform but become healthcare," with regional health information organizations (now called health information exchanges or HIEs) as likely local NHIN hubs (Halamka, Aranow, Ascenzo, Bates, Debor, Glaser, Goroll, Stowe, Tripathi, & Vineyard, 2005).

Kaushal, Blumenthal, Poon, Jha, Franz, Middleton, Glaser, Kuperman, Christino, Fernandopulle, Newhouse, Bates, and the Cost of National Health Information Working Group (2005) estimated NHIN roll out over five years would cost $156 billion, assuming that physicians, hospitals, skilled nursing facilities, home health agencies, laboratories, payers, and pharmacies acquire interoperable EHRs. Walker, Pan, Johnston, Adler-Milstein, Bates, and Middleton (2005) estimated the costs of interoperability between physicians, hospitals, laboratories, radiology centers, pharmacies, payers, and public health departments at $320 billion if nonstandardized (i.e., dependent on customized adapters to translate data between EHRs), and at $276 billion if standardized (i.e., based on common standards for data exchange).

Efforts are underway to build sustainable business models (e.g., Yasnoff, Humphreys, Overhage, Detmer, Brennan, Morris, Middleton, Bates, & Fanning, 2004) that would leverage private healthcare enterprise funding for the NHIN with federal contributions for research and development but not for ongoing operations. Private funding for the NHIN would come from providers who adopt interoperable EHRs and from regional HIEs, which provide the infrastructure for data exchange among EHRs across the NHIN. How a private enterprise NHIN business model would impact uninsured, unemployed, and indigent consumers has been given little consideration to date.

So far, only 9-15% of physician offices have adopted EHRs (Kaushal et al., 2005). To motivate provider adoptions, vendors are enhancing EHRs in ways presumed to build patient loyalty and simplify practice workflow. One such EHR enhancement gives consumers limited views of their records through patient portals or tethered personal electronic health record (PHRs). Tethered PHRs ease the workflow of providers and office staff by encouraging consumers to report information (e.g., allergies, family medical history, complaints), schedule appointments, and otherwise self-manage their healthcare—online. For healthy, employed, and insured consumers, who encounter their primary care providers perhaps once a year, tethered PHR are a pleasant convenience.

For disabled, unemployed, and uninsured consumers, who frequently visit many providers, tethered PHRs are not particularly convenient because they display partial views of fragments of consumer information and do not permit aggregation of data across tethered PHRs or exchange of aggregate data with other EHR systems. Applicants for disability benefits need both options. Regardless of the capabilities of tethered PHRs, disabled workers are unlikely to encounter many publicly funded providers who are equipped with EHRs and associated tethered PHRs.

Efforts are underway to select and harmonize technical standards (Hammond, 2005) for information exchange across the NHIN. The search for interoperability standards is largely focused on the exchange of patient information among provider-controlled EHRs within and across regional HIEs. The expected result is that the NHIN will be implemented as a network of networks that joins national technical interoperability standards to state or local control and funding.

In order to implement the NHIN, the Office of the National Coordinator of Health information technology (ONC), in the U.S. Department of Health and Human Services, established the American Health Information Community (AHIC) and the Health information technology Standards Panels (HITSP). AHIC's role is to develop high-level use cases related to information exchange across the NHIN. The role of HITSP's four technical committees—public health, care delivery (EHRs), consumer empowerment (PHRs), and security and privacy—is to develop interoperability standard specifications for the AHIC use cases.

How the architecture of the NHIN will impact uninsured, unemployed, and indigent consumers, who are not profitable customers of privately financed healthcare, has been given little consideration to date.

Recommendation: Room at the NHIN for Consumers with Disabilities

There needs to be room at the NHIN for consumers without primary-care provider advocates. Newly disabled workers exemplify the consumers who most need NHIN data-exchange capabilities but who are least able to get what they need for their disability benefits applications from provider-controlled EHRs.

Delays and denials of benefits result when applicants cannot find or retrieve medical records from providers familiar with their medical history, health status, and functional limitations. The disability benefit application workflow is complex, particularly for applicants with cognitive and mental health impairments. Health information technology (HIT), which is routinely used to automate care delivery workflow through provider-controlled EHRs might just as well be used to automate the workflow of benefit applicants through consumer-controlled PHRs. For this purpose, applicants would need unbound, intelligent PHRs.

Unbound PHR systems are not tethered to a health plan or employer network; they supply the utility infrastructure services required for current point-to-point exchange with diverse providers' EHRs and for future participation in the NHIN. Intelligent PHRs automate the workflow of applicants including the automated exchange of new and updated information with authorized providers' EHRs, eliminating the necessity for manual data entry, without reimbursement, by providers' office staff.

Tethered PHRs, which give consumers selected glimpses into providers' EHRs, represent the first generation of PHRs. Consumer-controlled and unbound PHRs, which enable consumers to control the exchange of data with providers' EHRs represent the second generation of PHRs. Consumer-controlled, unbound, and intelligent PHRs (or smart PHRs), which automate consumers' healthcare workflow such as applying for SSA disability benefits, represent the third-generation of PHRs (see for example, http://www.thesmartphr.com).

For disability applicants, smart PHRs would seem to offer several advantages including facilitation of the initial benefits application and of periodic reevaluations of their medical status, self-management of chronic conditions prior to Medicare coverage, and ongoing preparedness for medical emergencies and Hurricane Katrina-like disasters.

Instead of prolonged speculation about potential advantages, we need randomized field trials with large samples of disability applicants. The first research step would be to examine usage rates, and self- and provider-perceived utility for various PHR types with and without assistance from patient navigators. (What type of PHR with what kind and amount of assistance is used most and perceived as most useful by all or some applicants?) The next step would be to examine impact on the disability application process of a frequently used, and apparently useful PHR. (Are PHR-equipped applicants more successful at getting benefits than PHR-unequipped applicants?) A third, and particularly important, research step would be to examine the impact of PHR usage on perceived and objective measures of applicant health. (Do beneficiaries with high rates of PHR usage evidence better health in the two years before Medicare coverage than beneficiaries with lower rates of PHR usage, controlling for pre-existing differences between high-usage and low-usage beneficiaries?)

FUTURE TRENDS

Due to Google, consumers expect to have information about every imaginable topic immediately available. Yet, consumers' own medical records are inaccessible, locked away in providers' paper and electronic files. Educated and affluent consumers, aware of the fallibility of the healthcare establishment, are primed for advances in information technology that give them increased control over the healthcare workflow. The purchasing decisions of these opinion leaders may make consumer-controlled PHRs as ubiquitous as cell phones and affordable even to newly disabled workers applying for SSA benefits.

CONCLUSION

A National Health Information Network can be accessible to providers via interoperable EHRs supported by regional HIE networks and to consumers via interoperable, unbound, and intelligent PHRs with HIE infrastructure inside. Disabled workers applying for SSA benefits or undergoing periodic reevaluations of their status could use this consumer-centered information technology to avoid delays and denials of essential income and Medicare coverage. Evaluations of adoptions, usage, and consequences of this technology among SSA applicants and beneficiaries are in order. At the end of the day, health information technology has value only if it benefits the disabled consumers who "pay the price for America's healthcare crisis" (Cohn, 2007).

REFERENCES

Anderson, G.F., Frogner, B.F., Johns, R.A., & Reinhardt, U.E. (2006). Healthcare spending and use of information technology in OECD countries. *Health Affairs, 25,* 819-831.

Banks, P., & Lawrence, M. (2005). Transparent or opaque? Disabled people in Scotland describe their experience of applying for disability living allowance. *Journal of Social Work, 5,* 299-317.

Brailer, D.J. (2005). Interoperability: The key to the future healthcare system. *Health Affairs, Web Exclusive, W5-19-W5-21.*

Burkhauser, R.V., & Houtenville, A.J. (2006). A guide to disability statistics from the current population survey. *Annual Social and Economic Supplement (March CPS).* Rehabilitation Research and Training Center on Disability Demographics and Statistics, Cornell University, Ithaca, NY. Retrieved May 21, 2008, from http://digitalcommons.ilr.cornell.edu/edicollect/1233/

Bush, G.W. (2004). *Executive order: Incentives for the use of health information technology and establishing the position of the national health information technology coordinator.* Washington D.C.: The White House.

Cohn, J. (2007). *Sick: The untold story of America's healthcare crisis---and the people who pay the price.* NY: Harper Collins.

DeNavas-Walt, C., Proctor, B.D., & Lee, C.H. (2006). U.S. census bureau, current population reports, P60-231, *Income, poverty, and health insurance coverage in the United States: 2005.* Washington D.C.: U.S. Government Printing Office.

Hadley, J. (2007). Insurance coverage, medical care use, and short-term health changes following an unintentional injury or the onset of a chronic condition. *Journal of the American Medical Association (JAMA), 297,* 1073-1084.

Halamka, J., Aranow, M., Ascenzo, C., Bates, D., Debor, G., Glaser, J., Goroll, A., Stowe, J., Tripathi, M., & Vineyard, G. (2005). Healthcare IT collaboration in Massachusetts: The experience of regional connectivity. *Journal of American Medical International Association (JAMIA), 12,* 596-601.

Hammond, W.E. (2005). The making and adoption of health data standards. *Health Affairs, 24*(5), 1205-1213.

Hanson, K.W., Neuman, P., Dutwin, D., & Kasper, J.D. (2003). Uncovering the health challenges facing people with disabilities: The role of health insurance. *Health Affairs, Web Exclusive, W3-552-565.*

Houtenville, A.J., Erickson, W.A., & Lee, C.G. (2005). *Disability statistics from the current population survey (CPS).* Cornell University Rehabilitation Research and Training Center on Disability Demographics and Statistics, Ithaca, NY (StatsRRTC). Retrieved May 21, 2008, from www.disabilitystatistics.org

Institute of Medicine (IOM). (1991). In R.S. Dick & E.B. Steen (Eds.), *The computer-based patient record: An essential technology for healthcare.* Washington D.C.: National Academy Press.

Institute of Medicine. (2000). *To err is human: Building a safer health system.* In L.T. Kohn, J.M. Corrigan, & M.S. Donaldson (Eds.). Washington D.C.: National Academy Press.

Institute of Medicine. (2001). Crossing the quality chasm: A new health system for the 21st century. *Committee on Quality of Healthcare in America.* Washington D.C.: National Academy.

Institute of Medicine. (2003). *Key capabilities of an electronic health record system.* Committee on Data Standards for Patient Safety. Washington D.C.: National Academy Press.

Institute of Medicine. (2006). *From cancer patient to cancer survivor. Lost in transition.* In M. Hewitt, S. Greenfield, & E. Stovall (Eds.). Washington D.C.: National Academy Press.

Institute of Medicine. (2007). *Preventing medication errors.* In P. Aspden, J. Wolcott, J.L. Bootman, & L.R. Cronenwett (Eds.). Washington D.C.: National Academy Press.

Kaushal, R., Blumenthal, D., Poon, E.G., Jha, A.K., Franz, C., Middleton, B., Glaser, J., Kuperman, G., Christino, M., Fernandopulle, R., Newhouse, J.P., Bates, D.W., & the Cost of National Health Information Working Group. (2005).The costs of a National Health Information Network. *Annals of Internal Medicine, 143*, 165-173.

McWilliams, J.M., Meara, E., Zaslavsky, A.M., & Ayanian, J.Z. (2007). Use of health services by previously uninsured Medicare beneficiaries. *New England Journal of Medicine, 357,* 143-153.

Murdoch, M., van Ryn, M., Hodges, J., & Cowper, D. (2005). Mitigating effect of department of veterans affairs disability benefits for posttraumatic stress disorder on low income. *Military Medicine, 170*, 137-140.

National Health Interview Survey. (2006). *Public use data release. NHIS survey description.* Division of Health Interview Statistics. National Center for Health Statistics Hyattsville, Maryland Centers for Disease Control and Prevention U.S. Department of Health and Human Services. Retrieved May 21, 2008, from http://www.cdc.gov/nchs/about/major/nhis/quest_data_related_1997_forward.htm

Pransky, G.S., & Dempsey, P.G. (2004). Practical aspects of functional capacity evaluations. *Journal of Occupational Rehabilitation, 14*, 217-229.

Social Security Administration (SSA). (2006a). *Social Security disability benefits.* SSA Publication No. 05-10029. ICN 456000. Retrieved May 21, 2008, from http://www.ssa.gov/pubs/10029.html#part2

Social Security Administration. (2006b). *Disability evaluation under social security. Blue book.* SSA Publication No. 64-039 ICN 468600. Retrieved May 21, 2008, from http://www.ssa.gov/disability/professionals/bluebook/

Social Security Administration. (2007). *Annual statistical supplement to the Social Security bulletin.* SSA Publication No. 13-11700. Social Security Administration, Office of Policy, Office of Research, Evaluation, and Statistics: Washington D.C. Retrieved May 21, 2008, from http://www.socialsecurity.gov/policy/docs/statcomps/supplement/2006/supplement06.pdf

Walker, J., Pan, E., Johnston, D., Adler-Milstein, J., Bates, D.W., & Middleton, B. (2005). The value of healthcare information exchange and interoperability. *Health Affairs Web Exclusive, W5-10-W5-18.*

Yasnoff, W.A., Humphreys, B.L., Overhage, J.M., Detmer, D.E., Brennan, P.F., Morris, R.W., Middleton, B., Bates, D.W., & Fanning, J.P. (2004). A consensus action agenda for achieving the national health information infrastructure. *Journal of American Medical International Association, 11*(4), 332-228.

Ydreborg, B., Ekberg, K., & Nordlund, A. (2006). Health, quality of life, social network and use of healthcare: A comparison between those granted and those not granted disability pensions. *Disability and Rehabilitation, 28*, 25-32.

Chapter VI
E-Health Marketing

Muhammad F. Walji
University of Texas Dental Branch at Houston, USA

John A. Valenza
University of Texas Dental Branch at Houston, USA

Jiajie Zhang
University of Texas School of Health Information Sciences at Houston, USA

ABSTRACT

In this chapter, we review key concepts, using the marketing mix framework, to identify the needs of healthcare consumers, and the tools and services that can fulfill these needs. Unlike traditional healthcare delivery, patient-centered e-health (PCEH) involves the consumer as a partner and has a number of marketing implications. A more informed understanding of PCEH will help practitioners and researchers to formulate marketing strategies that improve healthcare outcomes and are acceptable to patients.

INTRODUCTION

Over 100 million Americans use the Internet for healthcare purposes (Fox, 2006b). Consumers not only find and read information related to their health, but also purchase medications, choose their providers, and in some cases engage in virtual discussions with doctors and fellow patients.

Healthcare providers now have direct access to consumers; bringing great opportunities and responsibilities. Practitioners marketing their services or promoting healthy lifestyles to consumers need to stay abreast of the changing needs of patients, the most current evidence base for diagnostic and treatment decision-making, and the rapidly developing technologies. They must also understand the dangers of the unregulated nature of the Internet and provide safeguards to prevent harm to patients.

In this chapter, we critically review patient-centered e-health (PCEH) marketing efforts by examining the current state of the science and exploring real world applications. We also review social and ethical implications of the technology and provide suggestions for future opportunities.

WHAT IS E-HEALTH MARKETING?

Marketing is the study of how to optimally communicate information to consumers about a product, service, or idea (Berkowitz, 2006). Marketing theory highlights the roles of product, place, promotion and pricing, also called the *marketing mix* (Kotler & Keller, 2005). Marketing is an essential strategy to inform consumers about the availability of a product or service to satisfy their needs.

In healthcare, marketing is widely used to increase awareness and adoption of healthcare services for patients. Many physicians, dentists and other providers use marketing strategies to attract patients to their practices, and pharmaceutical companies spend billions of dollars annually in direct-to-consumer advertising, carefully crafting their marketing campaigns to increase sales of their medicines. Hospitals use marketing to inform patients about the availability of services and to direct patients to practitioners credentialed at their institution. Marketing can assist in meeting business goals of healthcare organizations, but it also can have repercussions. Recently, pharmaceutical companies have come under question for the practice of *disease mongering* (i.e., manufacturing the need for problems that consumers may not previously have been aware that they suffered) (Healy, 2006; Lexchin, 2006). In response, Web sites such as nofreelunch.org and pharmedout.org have been created to educate clinicians about the dangers of accepting pharmaceutical company gifts.

Marketing on the Internet is different from traditional offline marketing. First, the Internet has attracted a demographic group that is relatively affluent, educated, and homogeneous, although people with more diverse characteristics are joining the online community in increasing numbers. Second, the Internet is a unique marketing medium in that computer programs can customize interactions to meet individual preferences.

Healthcare providers necessarily target PCEH to serve and retain current patients, but PCEH can also be applied to other purposes that include recruiting new patients, enhancing public relations, and providing community service. This range of functions implies many opportunities to apply marketing principles. In this chapter, our focus is to address how PCEH marketing can help patients and other consumers leverage the Internet to gain health benefits.

WHO WILL USE PCEH?

Defining a target market is a critical component of marketing. It is estimated that almost 100 million Americans have used the Internet to search for health information (Fox, 2006b). All these individuals are potential users of PCEH delivered by their healthcare provider. However, they are not currently representative of the broader population. Internet users are more educated, younger, and have higher incomes on average. More females than males use the Internet for health-related searches, and individuals with a disability or chronic disease are much less likely to use the Internet than healthier individuals (Fox, 2006a; Fox, 2007). As computer technology becomes more affordable and access to the Internet more prevalent, Internet user demographics are likely to become increasingly inclusive.

In the meantime, for PCEH to have the largest effect it must be accessible to those with the greatest need: individuals with limited means who are afflicted with chronic diseases. Marketing strategies that account for limited health and e-health literacy are likely to be key in assisting these groups to participate in PCEH, especially where these initiatives can tailor information and functionality to serve individual preferences.

THE PCEH MARKETING MIX

We use the marketing mix of *product, place, promotion,* and *price* factors as a framework to describe the important issues related to PCEH. In addition, we explore four supplementary factors that have been proposed as relevant for marketing on the Internet. These are *personalization, participation, peer-to-peer,* and *predictive modeling* (Mootee, 2004). For each factor in this extended marketing mix, we describe the general concept, specifics relating to PCEH, and examples of applications.

Product

In healthcare, products may be tangible goods (such as pharmaceuticals or medical devices), services, or even behaviors. Services are normally provided by licensed healthcare practitioners such as a physician, dentist, nurse, or pharmacist. In addition to products and services, behaviors may also be marketed. Interventions to reduce smoking or promote healthy eating are examples of marketable behaviors. In the context of PCEH, we define a product as a tangible good, service, or behavior that is delivered by the healthcare provider via the Internet with the goals of supporting patients' healthcare knowledge and decisions, and/or fulfilling other purposes that are supportive to the healthcare provider, such as patient recruitment.

Place

PCEH will be delivered either exclusively or in part over the Internet and World Wide Web (Web). The Internet is a highly distributed global network of computer networks that serves as a platform for delivery of the information contained in the Web (Berners-Lee, 2000). Individuals may use PCEH on a desktop, laptop, cell phone, or other device connected to the Internet. PCEH applications may be used from dedicated Internet connections at home or work, or in public places that offer Internet access.

Price

In the marketing mix, price refers to the payment that is exchanged by the consumer for the product. While healthcare products are traditionally exchanged through payment in hard currency, such a model may be antithetic in an online environment, where individuals are accustomed to paying little or nothing for Web-based services and tools. On the Internet, individuals often agree to purchase goods and/or services in exchange for viewing advertising or providing personal information that can be monetized in some fashion.

The Stages of Internet Engagement Model (McGoldrick & O'Dell, 2000) provides a useful perspective to determine the development of PCEH and pricing models. The five normative stages are (1) publishing, (2) interacting, (3) transacting, (4) integrating, and (5) transforming. To date, voluminous health-related content has been published on the Internet, serving as a valuable resource for patients. In addition, patients and providers are also beginning to interact on the Internet, mainly as a supplement to traditional healthcare services. It has been suggested that the initial stages of publishing and interaction "do not radically reduce costs or contribute to the development of new revenue streams" (McGoldrick & O'Dell, 2000); however, they may improve customer relationships. PCEH applications have been touted as one piece in the drive towards greater efficiency and accountability in the healthcare system. Yet, there should not be expectations that these services will increase revenue for providers, or substantially reduce inefficiencies until they are fully integrated into the delivery system.

Promotion

Promotion refers to advertising and gaining publicity for a product. An organizational Web site is the most common online example of a promotional strategy. For the primary strategy of promoting PCEH to current patients, healthcare providers have numerous options, including target mailings and handing out brochures during office visits. For secondary marketing purposes, such as recruiting new patients, many healthcare providers have a Web site that lists information about their practice in an attempt to increase "office traffic in an increasingly competitive environment" (Sanchez, 2002). This aspect of PCEH promotion is similar to other forms of Internet marketing.

One of the most effective ways to promote a Web site's offerings is through listings on search engines. When individuals seek out health information they normally go to a search engine and input keywords rather than going to a particular Web site. Being listed on the first few pages of search results is crucial for those who want to provide information and services to a patient (Eysenbach & Kohler, 2002). However, attaining a high rank on a search engine is becoming increasingly competitive, and each search engine uses a proprietary algorithm to rank Web sites. Google.com, for example, uses the PageRank algorithm, which give priority to Web pages that have numerous incoming links (Page, Brin, Motwani, & Winograd, 1998). Similar to academic papers, this algorithm assumes that those that are of high quality will be highly cited. Web sites that have numerous links to their sites from other highly linked sites would rank even higher. In response, a new industry known as search engine optimization has been created to help Web site owners become highly ranked based upon the algorithmic characteristics of search engines (Vence, 2007).

Another way to ensure top listing on a search results page is to pay to be listed on the search engine's sponsored results section. These are highly visible sections that appear at the beginning of the search listings. Sponsored listings are bought on a pro-rated where advertisers are charged only when a user clicks on their advertisement. The sponsored search industry has grown rapidly and accounts for billions of dollars in revenue (Haire, 2007). However, the effectiveness of sponsored search results may be due, in part, because users cannot differentiate between the organic search results and paid search listings. In order for individuals to be fully informed about the services they choose, full disclosure is critical.

Personalization

Internet applications, unlike other types of media such as television, can be programmed to be highly personal. There are many levels in which a site can be customized for individual users. Personalizing information in PCEH is beneficial for both patient and provider. For the patient, it increases the likelihood that information will be relevant, meaningful, and potentially adopted or accepted. For the provider, personal information can be used to guide developing future services that enhance value to patients.

Levels of Personalization

There are three levels of information customization: personalized, targeted, and tailored. Personalized information has the patient's name on the message (Revere & Dunbar, 2001). For example, a provider may send an e-mail newsletter that contains standard content but addresses the patient by name. A targeted message seeks to differentiate or segment groups of patients. For example, a provider would target an e-mail newsletter regarding diabetes management only to patients with diabetes. Tailored messages are those that are designed specifically for an individual rather than the group based upon relevant individual characteristics. Tailoring is thought to be the most effective form of information customization as it reduces redundancy and cognitive load required to process information (Brug, Campbell, & van Assema, 1999).

Information Prescriptions

In order to guide patients toward credible sources of health information on the Internet, providers are beginning to write information prescriptions that contain a URL or Web link for a particular health information need. Such interventions have been reported to improve patient-physician dialog during a clinical encounter, assist patients in effective Internet use, and enhance the patient education process (Siegel, Logan, Harnsberger, Cravedi, Krause, Lyon, Hajarian, Uhl, Ruffin, & Lindberg, 2006).

Information prescriptions are one type of information therapy, the delivery of highly personalized and relevant health information to patients through the use of technology. Mettler and Kemper (2005) suggest that for information to be considered therapeutic, it must be decision-focused, evidence-based, reviewed by experts, referenced, up-to-date and free from commercial bias. In order for information therapy to be patient-centered it must be a starting point for a meaningful and engaging discussion between the patient and provider rather than a unidirectional directive.

Participation

Participation by patients is a key concept in PCEH. Active patient involvement shifts the burden of healthcare delivery solely from the provider to a shared responsibility with the patient. In this section, we focus technologies that promote participation by patients in PCEH.

E-Mail

Electronic mail is one of the most widely used tools on the Internet, yet it is used infrequently for practitioner-patient communication (Beckjord, Finney Rutten, Squiers, Arora, Volckmann, Moser, & Hesse, 2007). There is evidence that patients would like to communicate with their doctors through e-mail (Houston, Sands, Jenckes, & Ford, 2004). Some patients claim that they would even switch physicians in order to realize this benefit. There are several barriers to communication via e-mail, such as reimbursement issues and privacy concerns (Patt, Houston, Jenckes, Sands, & Ford, 2003). Clinicians see e-mail communications as an added service they provide in which they should be reimbursed (Brooks, 2006), but most patients are not willing to pay much for the added benefit of electronically communicating with their doctors (Adler, 2006). Privacy concerns remain a barrier to adoption, due to the ease in which unencrypted e-mail can be intercepted, read, and altered. In response to these concerns, many practices require communication to occur within a secure or encrypted portal. However, usability is reduced by forcing patients to log in to yet another system in order to send and receive e-mail. Another barrier is fear by clinicians that they will be deluged with e-mail requests from their patients. Studies suggest that this may actually not be the case, and that patients who use e-mail tend to use it infrequently and reduce the number of telephone calls they make to the practice.

E-mail is unlikely to replace patients' face-to-face clinic visits with a provider. However, there are many benefits to an asynchronous technology such as e-mail. Following a clinic visit, patients can be automatically e-mailed a summary of the clinic visit with links to supporting material. This allows patients to review and contemplate information in the comfort of their home and at their leisure. As a follow-up to prescriptions, patients can be asked to report by e-mail how well they are tolerating a particular medication and thereby be approved for refills.

Blogs

Blogs (shortened from Web logs) are personal Web sites in which entries are updated frequently, akin to a diary or journal. Unlike a private diary, they invite readership from others around the Internet and allow readers to become involved in a conversation through the posting of comments. Blogs have increasingly become popular, and some have very large readerships similar to some broadcast media. The ease of use in creation and maintenance of a blog and its relatively low cost has catalyzed the popularity of this Internet medium (Boulos, Maramba, & Wheeler, 2006; Mathieu, 2007).

Patients have begun to use blogs to dialogue with other patients and update their family members about their health conditions. Examples of Web sites that allow patients to share their experiences include carepages.com and caringbridge.org. It is currently unclear as to the extent to which physicians, dentists or other healthcare providers will use blogs as a communication vehicle with their patients.

Wikis

Wikis allow a diverse group to contribute, edit and manage a body of knowledge. The most widely used wiki is Wikipedia.com. Wikipedia contains a multitude of health-related information. Although it is not clear who exactly contributes to the health content, interested patients clearly play an important role. Some have questioned how accurate health information can be on a relatively unregulated content platform such as Wikipedia (Taylor-Mendes, 2007). In response, such groups as Scholarpedia.org and Citizendium.org have begun to develop wikis, in which content is moderated by verified experts.

Virtual Environments and Simulation

Online virtual environments, such as SecondLife.com, are becoming popular for users to interact digitally in simulation of real world interactions. In a virtual environment, users can develop their own persona and appearance through a graphical image or avatar. The virtual environment is appealing for PCEH research and applications as it allows patients to request information and explore decisions in relatively nonthreatening environment. In a study that provided education about hallucinations, a survey of Second Life users who experienced the virtual interaction reported that most users had improved understanding about the condition (Yellowlees & Cook, 2006). Other studies have explored use of simulations to mitigate conditions such as phobia of flying (Wallach & Bar-Zvi, 2007).

Virtual environments also allow users to model behaviors and determine the consequences, which can be effective in influencing and changing behavior (Fogg, 2002). As computer processing power increases and costs decline, virtual environments are likely to become more sophisticated. When patients are exploring various treatment options, rather than reading information or watching a video they could be immersed in a near-real environment to learn how a procedure may feel and experience the consequences after completion. Such a scenario could also be used for prevention. For example, patients who are borderline diabetic can be asked to model life as a "real" diabetic to motivate behavior change.

Peer-to-Peer

Individuals are greatly empowered by communication with their peers. Peer-to-peer communication services including discussion forums, social networking, and consumer rating services have spurred the ability of patients to communicate with each other. Providers can promote and participate in peer-to-peer interactions in a number of ways. Physicians and dentists may suggest to their patients that they join virtual support groups in order to increase a sense of camaraderie and sharing. In addition, peer-to-peer interactions can be used for health education and to increase health literacy by providing support for moderated environments and encouraging participation as mentors by patients who have had experience with the particular health condition or treatment protocol.

Discussion Forums

Discussion forums are online locations where conversations on specific topics can be discussed by a wide group of users. A patient who has a health question can pose a query to a discussion forum, and members or browsers of the community who have an interest in that topic can then comment with advice and/or sharing of personal experiences.

There are various levels of discussion forums. Some are created and run by individuals, while health professionals moderate others. Netwellness.org is a popular site where patients can pose questions to healthcare professionals. The questions and answers are posted to aid all participants who may have similar problems.

There are concerns that individuals who participate in discussion groups without experts or healthcare facilitators may fall victim to misinformation, ultimately leading to real harm. However, research suggests that individuals have the capacity to self correct and self police online information (Esquivel, Meric-Bernstam, & Bernstam, 2006). Further, analysis of a weight loss forum found that most advice given in such as setting was not harmful or erroneous (Hwang, Farheen, Johnson, Thomas, Barnes, & Bernstam, 2007). Despite some preliminary studies, however, the overall impact of discussion forums on actual health outcomes is not yet known (Etter, 2006).

Social Networking Sites

Social networking is an emerging Web phenomenon that allows individuals to maintain a virtual presence among a social network. Examples of popular social networking sites include facebook.com and myspace.com. Users keep their social network appraised of occurrences in their live using a variety of methods, such as posting messages to a friend's "wall" (i.e., a Web page where invited members can post comments). Other examples include sharing photos on flickr.com and videos on youtube.com. Both of the latter Web sites have posted voluminous health and medical content ranging from images about health conditions to videos of actual patient surgeries. In the context of PCEH, social networking can exploit the power of the network to help providers and patients create new content, share resources and experiences, and organize the content through collaborative "tagging."

Viral Marketing

Viral marketing is a term used to describe the circumstance in which a small group of individuals who are 'infected' with a marketing message can then serve as hosts and pass on this message to others in their social network. A common example of viral marketing occurs when individuals forward an e-mail to their network. Healthcare information is reportedly the third most popular category of information that is frequently forwarded by individuals (Pamben, 2007).

The Centers for Disease Control (CDC) initiated an innovative viral marketing campaign called Verbnow to encourage increased physical activity in children. They devised a campaign where a group of kids are provided with a yellow ball. They are instructed to play with it and then logon to the verbnow.com Web site and blog about their experiences. Each group is encouraged to keep the ball 'alive' by giving it to other children who would in turn play and blog with the yellow ball (Pamben, 2007). Initial media reports suggest that this viral marking campaign was effective in boosting physical activity in spite of its simplicity and low cost.

Patients' Ratings of Their Healthcare Providers

Choosing a healthcare practitioner is an important task for patients (Davis, Collins, Schoen, & Morris, 1995; Hsu, Schmittdiel, Krupat, Stein, Thom, Fireman, & Selby, 2003; Schmittdiel, Selby, Grumbach, & Quesenberry, 1997). Although patients have many sources to help them make decisions about providers, the Internet is becoming increasingly important. The Internet already provides a wealth of information about provider personnel, including qualifications, professional certifications, experience, and disciplinary records (Krumholz, Rathore, Chen, Wang, & Radford, 2002; Narins, Dozier, Ling, & Zareba, 2005). This type of information may be provided by health plans, report cards, state boards, professional associations or even the provider's own Web site. However, a new trend is emerging in which patients are contributing and sharing their own subjective ratings and feelings regarding healthcare providers that they have encountered, supported by Web sites such as ratemds.com or doctoroogle.com. Patient-generated ratings and reviews of providers may be a particularly appealing source of information to individuals who are searching for a new provider.

Predictive Modeling

Predictive modeling is the field of inquiry that uses information about consumers to predict how they will react to some particular aspect of marketing, such as a product or advertising approach. Predictive modeling is relevant in PCEH as it potentially allows for customization of e-health services targeted to the specific group of patients who are most likely to accept and benefit from the services. Patient relationship management (PRM), electronic health records (EHR) and personal health records (PHR) are examples of health information systems that are beginning to amass large amounts of patient health information.

PRM is a data driven approach focused on determining and targeting services toward current and prospective patients' needs and preferences (Benz & Paddison, 2004). Providers can apply patient information to predict, for example, a choice for treatment that each patient is most likely to accept based on their individual profile. It is important to note that the ethics of such an approach may be questionable. For example, is it appropriate to present to a patient who needs dental treatment a primary option that other patients with similar needs have opted for, or should the provider give the patient and unbiased presentation of all relevant treatment options?

These types of ethical dilemmas raise an interesting issue for providers considering when and how to market services both online and offline. Should only information be provided to patients, or should doctors provide information that is persuasively framed towards a particular decision? The appropriateness of persuasive marketing campaigns in healthcare will likely depend on the situation. In some cases a persuasive campaign may convince a patient to stop a risky health behavior, such as smoking. However, in other cases, persuasion may be inappropriate. Worden and Flynn (2001) suggest that persuasive messages should be used when one course of action is clearly preferred over another. Influencing a patient's treatment decision and advocating surgery while a noninvasive procedure may be equally beneficial is undoubtedly questionable.

If predictive modeling techniques are used for PCEH, patients should be informed about why certain information is being promoted to them. They need to be able to opt out of these techniques. Deceptive practices, even when the intent is good, can diminish confidence in the provider and be detrimental in the long run. Providers should approach patient relations with goals to empower, support, and guide patients towards appropriate healthcare decisions. Fully informing patients is an effective way to achieve those goals.

SUMMARY

PCEH marketing is the study of how to identify the needs of a provider's patients, prospective patients, and community and to provide tools and services to help fulfill these needs. Unlike traditional healthcare delivery, PCEH involves the patient as a partner. Similarly, there are great opportunities to involve patients in the process of marketing and developing PCEH applications. In this chapter, we describe technologies that currently exist to help market PCEH within an extended marketing mix framework.

The most likely users of PCEH in the near-term are those that have the means, knowledge, and desire to access the Internet. However, it is likely that the Internet will become increasingly ubiquitous with time, providing great opportunities for PCEH applications to reach those populations with the greatest need, such as the elderly and poor.

Revenue models for PCEH remain unclear. Individuals are accustomed to receiving information and services on the Web for free. In order for PCEH to be fully integrated, third party payers, policy makers, and others with financial interests in patients' needs and choices will need to be convinced that this is an appropriate means of delivering and supporting healthcare. Researchers and developers will play an important role in informing these decisions by continuing to evaluate and report on the outcomes of PCEH implementations.

As more and more aspects of our everyday lives become computerized, there will be greater value placed on those things that cannot be automated, such as personal touch and emotion. Therefore the relationship between patients and providers is likely to remain a key point where value is created; however, we argue that caring relationships can be encouraged and nurtured through effective marketing practices within PCEH. Healthcare providers who can adapt from the paternalistic model of care to one of shared decision-making and responsibility are likely to flourish. Providing caring advice, encouragement and counsel via Internet technologies will be a key element for providers of the future.

REFERENCES

Adler, K.G. (2006). Web portals in primary care: An evaluation of patient readiness and willingness to pay for online services. *Journal of Medical Internet Research, 8*(4), e26.

Beckjord, E.B., Finney Rutten, L.J., Squiers, L., Arora, N.K., Volckmann, L., Moser, R. P., & Hesse B.W. (2007). Use of the internet to communicate with healthcare providers in the United States: Estimates from the 2003 and 2005 health information national trends surveys (HINTS). *Journal of Medical Internet Research, 9*(3), e20.

Benz, G., & Paddison, N.V. (2004). Developing patient-based marketing strategies. *Healthcare Executive, 19*(5), 40-42.

Berkowitz, E.N. (2006). *Essentials of healthcare marketing.* Sudbury, MA: Jones & Bartlett.

Berners-lee, T. (2000). *Weaving the Web: The original design and ultimate destiny of the world wide Web (first edition).* New York: HarperCollins Publishers.

Boulos, M.N., Maramba, I., & Wheeler, S. (2006). Wikis, blogs and podcasts: A new generation of Web-based tools for virtual collaborative clinical practice and education. *BMC Medical Education, 6*, 41.

Brooks, R.G., M.D. (2006). Physicians' use of e-mail with patients: Factors influencing electronic communication and adherence to best practices. *Journal of Medical Internet Research, 8*(1), e2.

Brug, J., Campbell, M., & van Assema, P. (1999). The application and impact of computer-generated personalized nutrition education: A review of the literature. *Patient Education and Counseling, 36*(2), 145-156.

Davis, K., Collins, K.S., Schoen, C., & Morris, C. (1995). Choice matters: Enrollees' views of their health plans. *Health Affairs, 14*(2), 99-112.

Esquivel, A., Meric-Bernstam, F., & Bernstam, E.V. (2006). Accuracy and self correction of information received from an internet breast cancer list: Content analysis. *British Medical Journal, 332*(7547), 939-942.

Etter, J.F. (2006). Internet-based smoking cessation programs. *International Journal of Medical Informatics, 75*(1), 110-116.

Eysenbach, G., & Kohler, C. (2002). How do consumers search for and appraise health information on the world wide Web? Qualitative study using focus groups, usability tests, and in-depth interviews. *British Medical Journal, 324*(7337), 573-577.

Fogg, B.J. (2002). *Persuasive technology: Using computers to change what we think and do.* San Francisco, CA: Morgan Kaufmann.

Fox, S. (2006a). *Can the health informatician help seniors cross the digital divide?* Paper presented at the meeting of the American Medical Informatics Association, Washington, D.C.

Fox, S. (2006b). Online health search 2006. *Pew Internet & American Life Project.* Retrieved May 22, 2008, from http://www.pewinternet.org/PPF/r/190/report_display.asp

Fox, S. (2007). MyHealth, circa 2007. *Pew Internet & American Life Project Presentation.* Retrieved May 22, 2008, from http://www.pewinternet.org/PPF/r/87/presentation_display.asp

Haire, T. (2007). Search marketing comes into its own. *Response Magazine, 15*(7), 48-52.

Healy, D. (2006). The latest mania: Selling bipolar disorder. *PLoS Medicine, 3*(4), e185.

Houston, T.K., Sands, D.Z., Jenckes, M.W., & Ford, D.E. (2004). Experiences of patients who were early adopters of electronic communication with their physician: Satisfaction, benefits, and concerns. *The American Journal of Managed Care, 10*(9), 601-608.

Hsu, J., Schmittdiel, J., Krupat, E., Stein, T., Thom, D., Fireman, B., & Selby, J. (2003). Patient choice. A randomized controlled trial of provider selection. *Journal of General Internal Medicine, 18*(5), 319-325.

Hwang, K.O., Farheen, K., Johnson, C.W., Thomas, E.J., Barnes, A.S., & Bernstam, E.V. (2007). Quality of weight loss advice on internet forums. *The American Journal of Medicine, 120*(7), 604-609.

Kotler, P., & Keller, L. (2005). *Marketing management.* Upper Saddle River, NJ: Pearson.

Krumholz, H.M., Rathore, S.S., Chen, J., Wang, Y., & Radford, M.J. (2002). Evaluation of a consumer-oriented internet healthcare report card: The risk of quality ratings based on mortality data. *Journal of the American Medical Association, 287*(10), 1277-1287.

Lexchin, J. (2006). Bigger and better: How Pfizer redefined erectile dysfunction. *PLoS Medicine, 3*(4), e132.

Mathieu, J. (2007). Blogs, podcasts, and wikis: The new names in information dissemination. *Journal of the American Dietetic Association, 107*(4), 553-555.

McGoldrick, C., & O'Dell, S. (2000). The road to e-health: Marketing implications. *Marketing Health Services, 20*(4), 32-34.

Mettler, M., & Kemper, D.W. (2005). Information therapy: The strategic role of prescribed information in disease self-management. *Studies in Health Technology and Informatics, 8*(2), 69-76.

Mootee, I. (2004). *High intensity marketing.* Toronto, ON: SA Press.

Narins, C.R., Dozier, A.M., Ling, F.S., & Zareba, W. (2005). The influence of public reporting of outcome data on medical decision making by physicians. *Archives of Internal Medicine, 165*(1), 83-87.

Page, L., Brin, S., Motwani, R., & Winograd, T. (1998). The PageRank citation ranking: Bringing order to the Web. *Stanford Digital Library Technologies Project.* Retrieved May 22, 2008, from http://dbpubs.stanford.edu:8090/pub/1999-66

Pamben, D. (2007). Spreading the message. *Cabinet Maker, 5536*, 10.

Patt, M.R., Houston, T.K., Jenckes, M.W., Sands, D.Z., & Ford, D.E. (2003). Doctors who are using e-mail with their patients: A qualitative exploration. *Journal of Medical Internet Research. 5*(2), e9.

Revere, D., & Dunbar, P.J. (2001). Review of computer-generated outpatient health behavior interventions: Clinical encounters "in absentia." *Journal of the American Medical Informatics Association, 8*(1), 62-79.

Sanchez, P.M. (2002). Refocusing Web site marketing: Physician-patient relationships. *Health Marketing Quarterly, 20*(1), 37.

Schmittdiel, J., Selby, J.V., Grumbach, K., & Quesenberry, C.P., Jr. (1997). Choice of a personal physician and patient satisfaction in a health maintenance organization. *Journal of the American Medical Association, 278*(19), 1596-1599.

Siegel, E.R., Logan, R.A., Harnsberger, R.L., Cravedi, K., Krause, J.A., Lyon, B., Hajarian, K., Uhl, J., Ruffin, A., & Lindberg, D.A. (2006). Information Rx: Evaluation of a new informatics tool for physicians, patients, and libraries. *Information Services and Use, 26*(1), 1-10.

Taylor-Mendes, C. (2007). Proceed with caution: Using Wikipedia as a reference. *Neonatal Network, 26*(3), 140-141.

Vence, D.L. (2007). SRO SEO. *Marketing News, 41*(13), 4.

Wallach, H.S., & Bar-Zvi, M. (2007). Virtual-reality-assisted treatment of flight phobia. *The Israel Journal of Psychiatry and Related Sciences, 44*(1), 29-32.

Worden, J.K., & Flynn, B.S. (2001). The case for persuasive health messages. *Effective Clinical Practice, 4*(2), 73-75.

Yellowlees, P.M., & Cook, J.N. (2006). Education about hallucinations using an Internet virtual reality system: A qualitative survey. *Academic Psychiatry, 30*(6), 534-539.

Chapter VII
Privacy Management of Patient-Centered E-Health

Olli P. Järvinen
Finnish Game and Fisheries Research Institute, Finland

ABSTRACT

This chapter introduces the privacy management framework as a means of studying patient-centered e-health. The chapter raises some important issues in regards to the privacy domain of e-health and offers a privacy framework to look at the issue that addresses some of the concerns people and industries have regarding privacy. The framework does not neglect the important distinction between the different interests affected by e-health. It acknowledges the voluntary nature of the way in which individuals have surrendered control over personal information in exchange for the benefits that information technology brings. Because the applications of information technology are logically malleable, there are sufficient strategic reasons to suggest that privacy management as a concept and practice will survive, and that to ignore privacy issues might be fatal for the success of PCEH.

INTRODUCTION

Transactional and interactive patient-centered e-health (PCEH) has many direct impacts on health service. Most e-health Web sites are pitched publicly as tools that give individuals greater control over their lives and their healthcare. Electronic health information on the Internet can be easily accessible to many different people. A health provider's ability to quickly access a customer's entire medical record, assembled from various sources, can facilitate diagnosis and eliminate medical errors, such as prescribing incompatible medications. Health records are kept and shared for diagnosis and treatment of the customer, payment of healthcare services rendered, public health reporting, research, and even for marketing and use by the media. Individuals can interact with doctors and other participants in chat rooms and by e-mail, and they can obtain healthcare services, such as second opinions and medical consultations, and products such as prescription drugs, online (Choy, Hudson, Pritts, & Goldman, 2001).

Unfortunately, such information practices may conflict with individuals' desires to be shielded from unauthorized use of their personal information. All of these activities involve the exchange of information with or without the consent of the individual, and with or without their knowledge. Mouse clicks and keystrokes are frequently recorded by online health organizations. That means information about which Web sites he or she visits, how long he or she stays there, and where he or she goes afterward are recorded. The majority of data exchange is visible to the individual, but there are many methods through which a Web site can gather information without the individual being aware, including cookies and data-mining. Whenever he or she visits a Web site, a large amount of information may easily become available to the Web site. When transactions are stored and exchanged using electronic services, personally identifiable information become more widely accessible and potentially vulnerable. Even when a customer orders a medicine from an online pharmacy, transactional information about the purchase is recorded, and information about that particular transaction can be (and frequently is) used for future business decisions and actions (Järvinen, 2005).

The ability to provide differentiated, consistently superior service on the Internet will be crucial to the survival of healthcare providers and affiliated organizations, and the customer vulnerability is exceptionally high, due to the sensitive nature of information. The protection of individuals' personal health information is not an option but a necessity, but the study of 39 U.S. health providers' privacy policies submits that health providers' Web sites are still at relatively early stages in their privacy issue evolution (Järvinen, 2005). Many practices suggest privacy is not a fundamental priority for those organizations. Most Web sites do not meet fair information practices—such as providing adequate privacy notice, giving customers some control over their information, and holding business partners to the same privacy standards. Every analyzed Web site had a privacy policy, but the responsibility is left to the customer to read and understand the entire privacy policy at every visit. Many of the analyzed privacy policies contained technical and confusing language (i.e., unnatural language) that makes it difficult for the customers to fully understand what they are agreeing to.

When the ethical problems involving e-health are considered, none is more paradigmatic than the issue of privacy. Given the ability of information technology to widely gather, endlessly store, cheaply transfer, efficiently sort, and effortlessly locate information, we are justifiably concerned that e-health may provide the means to invade our privacy and reveal information that is harmful to us. Information and knowledge easily cross cultural, institutional, organizational, and many other boundaries, and e-health application and its context may be so novel that there are no convenient customs or laws established anywhere to cope with privacy issues. A vacuum in terms of privacy practice may occur in every culture. The key detail of the Internet is that there is no such thing as "absolute privacy." There is no central authority or management, and no one to install the technology or establish network-wide security and privacy policies. We are, however, reluctant to give up the advantages and the services of the Web technology. We appreciate the easy access to the Web site services when checking health information, buying the drugstore items, and many other things. The number and kinds of PCEH applications increase dramatically each year, and the impact of the Web technology is felt around the planet.

The widespread use of personally identifiable information (PII) and the complexity of Web infrastructure is a combination that makes solitude and privacy more essential to the individual. Privacy has emerged as a central policy concern as more people go online every day. Not surprisingly, a great many people are fretful about the things that could happen online and the way in which data about them might be gathered and used. A strong sense of distrust shadows individuals' view of the online world, and the uneasiness has grown. An overwhelming majority of customers are concerned about businesses or people they don't know getting personal information about themselves or their families. (Fox, Rainie, Horrigan, Lenhart, Spooner, & Carter, 2000b). Customers are afraid of Web sites selling or giving away information about them, about insurance companies learning what they have done online and making coverage decisions based on that, and about their employers learning what they have done (Fox & Rainie, 2000a).

Privacy concerns can pose a serious impediment to expanded growth of PCEH in the future. Even the most convenient PCEH services may function ineffectively, because sharing personal medical and health information requires a certain leap of faith—or at least a strong sense of privacy and trust (Fox & Fallows, 2003). Trust is a critical factor in any relationship in which the individual does not have direct control over the actions of company, the decision is important, and the environment is uncertain (Mayer, Davis, & Schoorman, 1995).

This chapter concentrates on privacy issues and problems in two main interests; namely, the online customer and the online health provider. Customers of PCEH are active and involved participants, and therefore, our target is to consider individual needs and capabilities as the primary criteria for designing PCEH services and privacy practices. In this chapter, a framework for PCEH privacy management is presented. The framework balances the rights of individuals to privacy against the possibility of companies to use this technology opportunistically. This understanding is critical, because individuals are becoming increasingly privacy aware and more interested in knowing how to protect their own privacy. At the same time, individuals desire a wide range of new PCEH services.

BACKGROUND

Perspectives on Privacy

Privacy, which is often associated with, and sometimes described in terms of liberty, autonomy, solitude, and secrecy is a concept that is not easily defined (Tavani, 1999a, pp. 137). "Unlike privacy, secrecy appears to have a tight connection to information" (Thompson, 2001, pp. 15). If something is secret, there is at least one person to whom the information is not known. "While confidentiality continues to be an important ethical problem for computer professions, and while security is an increasingly important technical issue, privacy is a red herring" (Thompson, 2001, p. 14).

The term "privacy" is sometimes used to designate a situation in which people are protected from intrusion or observation by natural or physical circumstances. Natural privacy rights are intended to protect a sphere of activity, often a physical place but sometimes an interpersonal relationship, from intrusion by government and other third parties, *the right to be let alone* (Warren & Brandeis, 1890).

Many analysts use the expression "informational privacy" or "information privacy" to refer to a distinct category of privacy concern. Informational privacy is a category of privacy with a set of issues that are distinguishable from privacy concerns related to intrusion and interference (Tavani, 1999a; Tavani, 1999b). When we consider informational privacy "one often finds oneself in a conceptual muddle", because "the issues are not trivial matters of semantics" (Moor, 1998, pp. 16). There are cases when general knowledge of private matters does not breach persons' privacy in any morally significant way. A person's health information may be widely known, but that in no way makes them less private. Having information about a person's sensitive matters may make it possible for someone to violate that person's privacy by discriminating for or against them in an inappropriate way. Such information is widely available in most societies, and "the significance of such information lies not in simple knowledge of it, but in its further use [...] Medical information can be used to deny employment and other opportunities to which a person is entitled, and embarrassment is a form of emotional harm that can have extreme consequences in certain situations" (Thompson, 2001, pp.15). "Many Americans know that violation of copyright is a crime, and many believe that violation of their privacy should be a crime too. Why is distributing a corporation's software without its permission called 'piracy,' while distributing a person's information without permission is called 'sharing'?" (Fox et al., 2000b, pp. 11).

A normatively private situation is a situation protected by ethical, legal, or conventional norms. When we frame the debate simply in terms of how to balance privacy interests as an individual good against interests involving the larger social good, support for those interests believed to benefit the latter good will likely override concerns regarding individual privacy (Regan, 1995, pp. 213). There is almost a paradox about our feelings in the personal and social costs of sabotage and the concomitant personal and social benefits of tight security. For the sake of my safety, I would like all others' e-mails monitored to eliminate any possibility that they will be able to damage society. At the same time, I would prefer that my e-mails not be monitored. My wish to maintain privacy for my personal e-mails is, however, unreasonable against the generalization of everyone's wish for their safety. "In isolation my desire for privacy is reasonable; it only becomes unreasonable in the contemporary social context" (McArthur, 2001, pp. 125). If the monitoring of e-mails would add security in a community or would raise that community's standard of living, then a decision to add monitoring would likely be perceived as yielding a greater overall good than would a decision to protect the privacy of individuals. Theorists working in sociological traditions have tended to interpret the emergence of computerized information technology as something that enables an evolution in social power relations that favors governmental and commercial organizations against the interests of individual citizens (Johnson, 1994; Gotlieb, 1995). And it includes elements of the threat of overly broad normative law that contains the possibility for misinterpretations. Human nature has also shown that security fears can be used to hurt a community with big brother style invasions of privacy used to support one social group over another.

There are two main solutions to deal with the legitimate rights of informational privacy. The more common is to use the regulatory powers of the state. This practice is predominant in the EU, which uses very strict directives concerning the privacy matter[1]. The other solution is the voluntary basis. That practice is very predominant in the U.S., where the greatest likelihood is that industry will be left to develop voluntary guidelines[2], rather than Congress imposing regulations.

There was little legal protection for health information—online or off-line—until the release of HIPAA regulation in the U.S.[3] But while HIPAA regulation is an important step, its application is limited. The regulation does not cover a significant portion of the health-related activities that take place online. The HIPAA analysis of Choy et al. (2001) shows that many who engage in online health activities will fall outside the scope of the regulation. "People often believe they are invisible and anonymous online, but they are often exposing their most sensitive health information to online healthcare sites that are not required by law to protect the information or keep it confidential. The potential for abuse is enormous" (Choy et al., 2001, pp. 25).

If we put conceptions of privacy together with distinction between normative and natural privacy, we get a situation-dependent issue of privacy: "An individual or group has normative privacy in a situation with regard to others if and only if in that situation the individual or group is normatively protected from intrusion, interference, and information access by others" (Culver, Moor, Duerfeldt, Kapp, & Sullivan, 1994, pp. 6). The general term "situation" is useful because it is broad enough to cover many kinds of informational privacy: private locations such as a medicine delivery record in a database; private relationships such as an electronic prescription to one's pharmacy, and private activities such as the utilization of computerized health information. Privacy situation covers also role, time, and place-dependant issues.

If an unauthorized entry is made into a normatively private situation, "privacy has not only been lost, it has been breached or invaded" (Moor, 1997, pp. 30). If a worker uses an online system for the delivery of a medicine and processes a customer's healthcare treatment using the older information of the medicine deliveries, then the worker is not invading the individual's privacy. She is allowed in this situation and working role to investigate the customer's medicine history. However, if that same worker were to "open" that same customer's case record after hours just to browse around, then the worker would be breaching the individual's privacy although the worker may gain no new information. The worker has legitimate access in the first situation but not the in the second.

Value of Privacy

The Internet technology has created a "universal" technology platform, and to justify the importance of privacy more exactly in the global setting we can continue by asking whether informational privacy has instrumental and intrinsic value. Instrumental values are those values that are good because they lead to something else which is good. Intrinsic values are values that are good in themselves (Moor, 1997).

Privacy has instrumental value, because privacy offers us protection against harm, but "to justify the high instrumental value of privacy we need to show that not only does privacy have instrumental value but that it leads to something very, very important" (Moor, 1997, pp. 28) One of the most well-known attempts to do this has been given by James Rachels. In a 1975 article, Rachels lists several cases where "information about a person might provide someone with a reason for mistreating him in some way" (Rachels, 1975, pp. 351). Rachels suggests that such cases are misleading when they are taken to indicate why privacy is important. Privacy is valuable because it enables us to form varied relationships with other people. Privacy also enables us to form intimate bonds with other people that might otherwise be difficult to form and maintain in public. In a society where individuals have no privacy, friendships, intimacy, and trust cannot develop (Fried, 1970). If we want such relationships, we must have privacy. However, the need to relate to others differently may not ground privacy securely "because not everyone may want to form varied relationships and those who do may not need privacy to do it" (Moor, 1997, pp. 28). This view is based on the principle that some people simply do not care how others perceive them.

Some arguments tie privacy more tightly to autonomy, because privacy is understood to be not just a means of autonomy but a part of the very meaning of this term. We don't seek privacy in order to get autonomy, but "autonomy is inconceivable without privacy." (Johnson, 1994, p. 89). Autonomy is not just one among many values (i.e., autonomy is fundamental to what it means to be human and to our value as human beings). Privacy is necessary for diversity of relationships, and privacy is an essential aspect of autonomy. Assuming that autonomy is intrinsically valuable and privacy is a necessary condition for autonomy we have the strong and attractive claim that privacy is a necessary condition for an intrinsic good. But, is it true that autonomy is inconceivable without informational privacy? Suppose an online pharmacy collects information about customer purchases into database. Normally, customers recognize the collection process when they fill medicine prescriptions online. Consider the situation in which the online pharmacy does not share the information with anyone else or take advantage of customer in any way whatsoever. Customers have complete autonomy, just no privacy (Moor, 1997, pp. 28). Thus, it follows that privacy is not an essential condition for autonomy on PCEH services. It is conceivable to have autonomy without privacy.

We can continue by asking whether privacy is a core value. Core values are set of values that are shared by most, if not all, humans and are familiar to all of us. They are shared and fundamental to human evaluation, for example, life and happiness are two of the most obvious. It is possible to test for a core value by asking whether it a value that is found in all human cultures. The core values provide standards with which to evaluate the rationality of our actions and policies. They give us reasons to prefer some courses of action over others. They provide a framework of values for judging the activities of others as well (Moor, 1997; Moor, 1998).

It seems that privacy is not a core value per se, because "the concept of privacy has a distinctly cultural aspect which goes beyond the core values. Some cultures may value privacy and some may not" (Moor, 1997, pp.29). Maybe privacy is not a core value per se, but it is deeply linked to the value of security. Gotlieb (1995, pp. 168) points out that "what must be secured in every civilized and free society is, of course, security of person." Protection from strangers who may have goals antithetical to our own is sought, and all cultures need security of some kind because without protection species and cultures don't survive and flourish. "As societies become larger, highly interactive, but less intimate, privacy becomes a natural expression of the need for security." (Moor, 1997, pp. 29). In particular, a highly computerized culture where lots of personally identifiable information is manipulated, stored, and transferred, it is almost inevitable that privacy will emerge as an expression of the core value, security.

In summary, the justification of privacy is firm because privacy can be grounded instrumentally and intrinsically—instrumentally, in support of the core values, and intrinsically, as an expression of security and more. Because privacy is instrumental in support of the core values, it is instrumental for important matters. Moreover, because privacy is an expression of the core value of security, it is a critical, interlocking member of our systems of values in our increasingly electronic culture. If an online company collects a lot of personally identifiable information without consent (which does not harm its customer when it collects, stores, and manipulates), it nevertheless seems to be doing something wrong intrinsically. The subjects' security is being violated by the company even if no other harm befalls the person. The seminal article of Warren and Brandeis (1890) initiated the view that privacy is a positive good, and that individuals have an interest in maintaining a political right to privacy. Privacy is also a necessary means of support in a networked electronic healthcare, and thus, privacy is well grounded for our consideration. People have a basic right to protection, which, from the viewpoint of the patient-centered e-health, includes privacy protection.

PRIVACY FRAMEWORK

Privacy seems to be something of very great importance and something vital to defend, but also a matter of individual preference and culturally relative. The attempt to find one general measure for global privacy policy fails—there are too many situation-dependant aspects to consider. Privacy matters are deeply situation-dependent issues and cannot be found by applying a predefined list without considering the situation widely. A privacy problem may arise in a specific situation, and it may occur as the result of an unpredictable incident. Privacy constantly includes a large number of evolving situations that are difficult to conceptualize clearly, and it is hard to find justified practices. Therefore, privacy involves more than rote application of existing norms.

This section presents existing privacy theories and consider how they apply to PCEH. Finally the privacy framework is presented. It acknowledges the voluntary nature of the way in which individuals have surrendered control over personal information in exchange for the benefits that information technology brings.

Privacy Theories

Two privacy theories, which relate to personal information, are the "control" and the "limitation" theories.

According to the control theory, one has privacy if and only if one has control over information about oneself. "Privacy is not simply an absence of information about us in the minds of others, rather it is the control we have over information about ourselves" (Fried, 1984, pp. 209). The control theory correctly recognizes the aspect of choice that an individual who has privacy enjoys in being able to grant, as well as to deny, individual access to information about oneself. Control theory has some weaknesses. No one is able to have complete control over every piece of information about oneself, although Michelfelder (2001, pp. 134) states that "because the richness of the lived world is not mirrored in the online world, there are fewer relevant privacy values to be concerned about." But still the control theory has that practical problem. It is highly desirable that we are able to control information about ourselves. However, in a highly networked society it is simply impossible. We are not able to control vast amounts of electronic information about ourselves. Personally identifiable information is well greased and slides rapidly through networks around the world, around the clock.

The needed amendment to the control theory is a situation dependence, which limits the matters to consider. A theory offering assistance in this area is called the limitation theory by Tavani (1999b). The limitation theory recognizes the importance of setting up zones of privacy. Privacy consists of the condition of having access to information about oneself limited or restricted in a certain situation. One important weakness of the limitation theory is that "it tends to underestimate the role of control or choice that is also required in one's having privacy" (Tavani, 1999b, pp. 267). Some variations of the limitation theory suggest that a person's privacy correlates with the extent to which information about a person is limited. Therefore privacy according to the limitation theory would seem to be very closely related to secrecy. It seems, however, that in some cases, the word "private" is virtually synonymous with the word "secret"; or "confidential." Thompson (2001, pp. 15) points out that when we say "They want to keep some aspect of their life private in order to avoid embarrassment," or "Medical records should be kept private," we can substitute the word "confidential" for "private" without altering the meaning of the statement.

Limitation theory has many good features, but the theory ignores the fact that someone who has privacy can choose to grant, as well as to limit or deny, others access to information about oneself, thus it needs some amendments to be adequate for online practices for PCEH. Control theory has that missing feature, but because it does not include the condition of having access to information about oneself limited or restricted in certain situations, its perspective is too wide and open-ended to be practical.

Moor (1997) presents a theory, the control and restricted access theory, that covers both the preceding weaknesses. The main thesis of the theory is in order to protect ourselves we need to make sure the right people and only the right people have access to relevant information at the right time. Basically it has the advantages of the control theory for giving individuals as much control (informed consent) over personal data as realistically possible. But it also incorporates the strength of the limitation theory in maintaining that privacy needs to be understood in terms of situations where access to individuals is limited or restricted. So it recognizes the importance of setting up zones of privacy. Finally it incorporates the strength of both theories in holding that individuals affected by a certain situation need to have some control or choice in determining whether that information will be kept private or not.

In our considerations, it is important that the customers can make the most convenient choices in terms of their own needs and values from a number of alternatives, because what one customer considers a privacy invasion may be a valued feature or service to another customer. Rather than regarding privacy as an all or nothing proposition, the control and restricted access theory acknowledges the situation in which information is authorized to flow to some people some of the time. Ideally, those who need to know have access and others do not.

The control and restricted access theory also helps explain some anomalies about private situations. So far we have discussed situations in which individuals possess damaging personally identifiable information they want to keep others from knowing. Moor (1997, pp. 31) points out that "situations can be private in other circumstances." Moor presents an example that occurs in a physician's waiting room where scores of customers are waiting for their appointments. A couple begins to argue loudly and eventually shouting to each other about a problem they are having. They go into excruciating detail about various events and catastrophes. Everyone can hear them and many customers feel uncomfortable as they sit there with nothing special going on. Finally, one customer, who thinks he can help, cannot stand it anymore. He asks whether they would like his advice. The couple in unison tells him, "No, it's a private matter."

As funny as couple's comment may be in that situation, it does make sense on several levels. It is not reasonable to claim that an invasion of privacy has occurred, since the couple was the original cause of the information's becoming public. But "in private situations the access to information can be blocked in both directions" (Moor, 1997, pp. 31). The couple did not want to allow information from the customer although they themselves had been rude in revealing details to everyone.

In our considerations, it is important that the access to information is possible to be blocked in both directions by the individual. Because the Internet is an effective tool for receiving and sharing information, e-health providers can use very large pools of data from multiple sources and suggest similar advice using e-mails and much more.

Privacy Principles

McArthur (2001, pp. 124) presents two useful principles that emerge from the preceding examples:

The Mischance Principle: We cannot reasonably expect to maintain privacy over that which another person could discover, overhear, or come to know without concerted effort on his/her part to obtain this information.

Arguing loudly in the waiting room would certainly fall into this category. The mischance principle works, as McArthur (2001, pp. 124) points out, "in a range of possible instances because it is relatively easy to figure out what precautions to take to maintain privacy against casual observation." And thus, "anything put by a person in the public domain could be viewed as public information" (Fulda, 1997, pp.28).

The Voluntary Principle: If I choose to decrease the relative amount of privacy for myself and information under my control by exposing it to view, I thereby decrease the reasonableness of any expectation that this privacy will be observed.

Decreasing the relative amount of privacy is accomplished by increasing the likelihood under the circumstances that the information will come to another's attention through mischance, and therefore our examples would certainly also fall into this category. McArthur (2001, pp. 125) points out that "one of the ways in which the voluntary principle is sometimes interpreted is that the failure to attempt to maintain privacy constitutes willingness for that information to become public." By arguing loudly in the place where people are gathered, the person is positively increasing the likelihood of that information becoming known. By arguing loudly in the room where no people are gathered, the person is negatively increasing the likelihood that the matter will become known. This principle is referred to as the negative voluntary principle. The extent to which expectations of privacy are reasonable takes into account the social norms governing the particular form of information may have as well as the context. Therefore, the interpretation of whether the person is positively or negatively increasing the likelihood of that information becoming known is not always easy to make.

As DeCew (1997, pp. 7) states, we should presume in favour of privacy and then develop ways that would "allow the individual to determine for themselves how and when that presumption should be overridden." Combined with the mischance and voluntary principles, application to PCEH of Moor's (1997, pp. 32) three principles, the Publicity Principle, the Justification of Exceptions Principle, and the Adjustment Principle enables us to do as DeCew states:

- *The Publicity Principle*: Rules and conditions governing private situations should be clear and known to the persons affected by them.
- *The Justification of Exceptions Principle:* A breach of a private situation is justified if and only if there is a great likelihood that the harm caused by the disclosure will be so much less than the harm prevented that an impartial person would permit breach in this and in morally similar situations.
- *The Adjustment Principle:* If special circumstances justify a change in the parameters of a private situation, then the alteration should become an explicit and public part of the rules and conditions governing the private situations.

The strength of Moor's principles is a very practical one because customers do not need to have absolute or unlimited control in order to have privacy on PCEH. The publicity principle suggests that we can plan to protect our privacy better if we know where the zones of privacy are and under what conditions and to whom information will be given. The publicity principle encourages informed consent and rational decision making, which are important factors for expanded growth of PCEH.

Once policies are established and known, circumstances sometimes arise which invite us to breach the privacy policy. Privacy policy breaches should be avoided as much as possible because they undermine confidence in the policy. However, exceptional circumstances sometimes occur in the cases related to special health issues, which are discussed later.

The adjustment principle normalizes the changed privacy situation. It is an important principle of PCEH where situation-dependant issues, possibilities of technological change and development of new services are pervasive.

Model of Privacy Management

The presented framework, including five principles and the control and restricted access theory, results in privacy responsibilities and advantages for both e-health customers and providers. The framework has the advantage that privacy and service functions can be fine tuned with consideration to the privacy situation.

Figure 1. Privacy management model

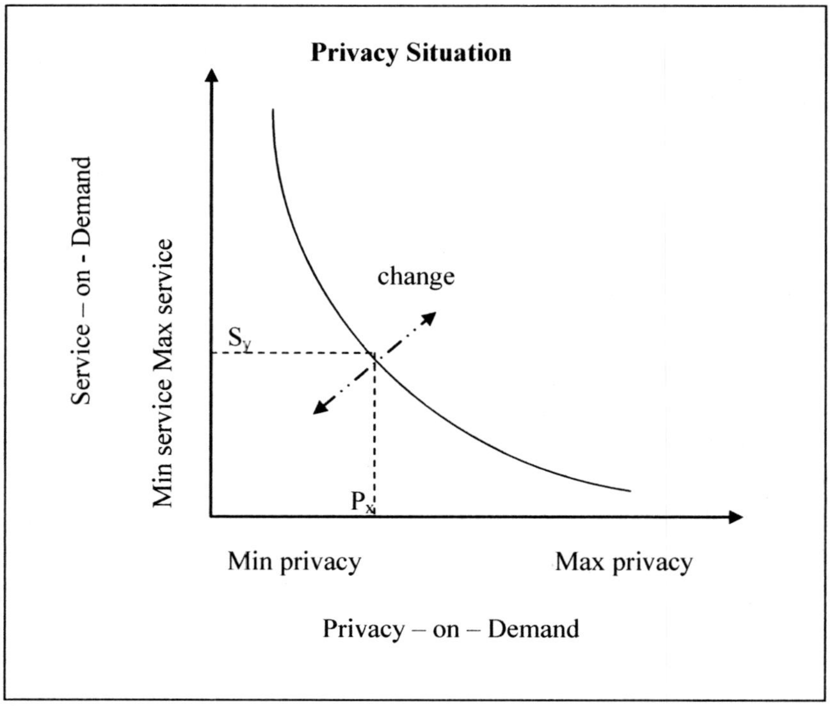

The idea of the privacy management model of PCEH is presented in the Figure 1, where customer privacy (Privacy-on-Demand function P_x) is related to the service (Service-on-Demand function S_y). Employing an interactive dialog by demanding or consenting, customers are able to choose from "max service" to "min service" to be polarized into the concept of privacy (i.e., "min privacy" or "max privacy" and vice versa).

The model does not downplay the voluntary nature of the way in which customers of PCEH have surrendered control over personal information in exchange for the benefits that information technology brings. This model is consistent with exchange theory (Thibaut & Kelley, 1959). According to exchange theory, individuals form associations on the basis of trust, and try to avoid exchange relationships that are likely to bring more pain than pleasure. "Developmentally, a relationship among parties who have not had prior association is expected to emerge incrementally and to begin with small actions that initially require little reliance on trust" (Jarvenpaa, Tractinsky, & Vitale, 2000, pp. 46). If the actions are reciprocated, trust tends to spiral upward. If they are not reciprocated, trust spirals downward (Sitkin & Roth, 1993). One of the consequences of trust is that it reduces the individual's perception of risk associated with opportunistic behavior by the organization (Ganesan, 1994).

Web site interactive content can add considerable value for both the company and its customer. In the model, the customer has the opportunity to choose and "manipulate" online health service and privacy practices. Typically, more services means less privacy and more privacy means less service possibilities. The interactivity possibilities of Web applications have the means to customize privacy and service functions more exactly to the needs of PCEH customers, thus enabling them to choose privacy practices and make more informed decisions concerning to whom they entrust their personally identifiable information and what kind of service they prefer or don't prefer. Employing an interactive dialog by demanding or consenting, customers are able to change Privacy-on-Demand and Service-on-Demand functions. If the company changes privacy situations without consent or demand by the customer, it is leaning toward opportunism.

One important aspect of the model is that it proposes possibilities and advantages for both customers and companies. The model proposes flexibility for PCEH privacy policy, but also demanding rules and principles. The model normally illustrates the situation where a customer is able to give informed consent and to make rational decisions—a customer is able to opt-in to (or opt-out of) privacy and service levels (Järvinen, 2005).

Almost 90 percent of Internet users are in favor of "opt-in" privacy policies that require Internet companies to ask people for permission to use their personal information. Online applications should ask individuals for permission to use their personal information, which is the kind of system has been adopted by the EU. However, this view challenges the policy negotiated by the Federal Trade Commission and a consortium of Web advertisers, which gives users of U.S.-based Web sites the right to "opt out." An "opt-out" scheme would compel individuals to take steps to protect their privacy (Fox et al. 2000b, pp. 3).

Example of Privacy Management Model

Next the data mining of genetic information is discussed to illustrate the use of the privacy management model in practice.

Advances in data mining techniques for large databases are a technological trend that heightens ethical concerns, because they enable companies to find out a lot of detailed personal information about individuals. Data mining causes privacy concerns because individuals are often not aware of data mining practices in advance. Data for which they may have given their consent for collection and use in one context is being mined in ways they had not explicitly authorized.

Suppose a customer decides to get tested for a breast cancer gene. Breast cancer runs in her family, and she wants to know whether she is genetically disposed to have breast cancer. She goes to the laboratory for tests for the gene and the results are positive. The laboratory results are stored in her electronic medical record so that the test results are available to medical researchers and physicians to encourage aggressive testing for the disease in the future. Because the information will be computerized, it means that many health providers and researchers may have access to the information. For example, if the customer's health insurance company gets access to it, then it could mean problems to the "owner of the information." Information of this kind could be detrimental to the individual when obtaining life insurance or future health insurance. Eventually, if the medical information slides through enough networks and information systems, it could be detrimental to the individual's relatives when obtaining insurance and applying for employment, even though they have shown no signs of the disease and have never been tested (Moor, 1997).

The model suggests that Web application should set up a zone of privacy for customers (P_X) who only want predictive testing done (S_Y) because there is, as Moor points out (1997, pp. 32):

a difference between predictive genetic testing in which the patient is tested for genetic information that may be indicative of future disease and diagnostic testing in which the patient is tested for genetic information that may confirm a diagnosis of an existing disease.

The health provider should establish a private situation for predictive testing so that the customer's analyst results were not incorporated into the regular medical file. If we think about privacy issues from the perspective of the privacy model, these medical records would be computerized but not accessible to all of those who have access to the general medical record. This practice (S_Y) allows adjustment of the access conditions to increase the level of privacy (P_X) for the customer.

According to the framework, it is clear that customers should be told what will happen to the analysis information. The customers can choose their privacy situation better if they know where the zones of privacy are and under what conditions and to whom information will be given. Rules and conditions governing private situations should be clear and known to the persons affected by them, so customers are able to determine service and privacy levels accordingly. The customers might prefer ("opt-in") to have the analysis information included in their regular medical record.

The genetic test gives us also an example that describes the nature of the justification of exceptions principle. Suppose that after some predictive genetic tests are run, new information about the consequences of the analysis results is uncovered by means of the data mining process. The customer's old health information in combination with the analysis results show that the customer surely must have transmitted a devastating disease to her offspring, but that the disease can be treated effectively if caught in time. The physician's duty to keep the customer's secrets confidential is an important protection of privacy and the values related to it, but it is by no means absolute in medical law or ethics generally (Somerville, 1999; Mason, McCall, & Smith, 1985).

In the context of genetic information, the most prominent reason for breaches of confidentiality is the harm inflicted on others by their ignorance [...] But the strength of arguments like this varies from case to case, depending on the specific nature of family relationships between the individuals involved (Häyry & Takala, 2001, pp. 408).

In such circumstances, it would seem that the health provider should notify not only the customer but also her adult offspring even though that was not part of the original privacy policy. The breach is justified because the harm caused by the disclosure will be so much less than the harm prevented. Using the justification of exception principle, a health provider may determine the change of privacy policy without the threat of opportunism. The ethical significance of beneficial outcomes should be included in discussions of privacy. We should not, however, presume that beneficial outcomes can always be used to counterbalance harmful outcomes in any straightforward manner. It should be avoided to override customers' wishes as much as possible because they undermine confidence. Using anonymity or fake names (Fox et al., 2000b; Uslaner, 2000) in the health service process is not a convenient practice because it might be even a threat to sufficient health operations.

To shield themselves from what they consider harmful and intrusive uses of their health information, customers have engaged in privacy-protective behaviors, such as providing incomplete information, thereby putting themselves at risk from undiagnosed, untreated conditions. The lack of complete and accurate health information on patients impacts the community as well. Healthcare information used for important research and public health initiatives downstream becomes unreliable and incomplete (Choy et al., 2001, pp. 1).

The adjustment principle in this example states that those who continued to have predictive genetic testing would know what information would be released in stated exceptional circumstances. They would know the possible consequences of their decision to have predictive genetic testing and could plan accordingly. According to the adjustment principle, the privacy policy should indicate the new service and privacy practice.

According to the model, it is important that the customerl is given the opportunity to decide what information is to be used and whether it may be used for new purposes after changes of practices. Normally privacy policies should provide assurance that previously gathered data won't be used in any new way before consent of the customer. If the customer does not accept the change, then the customer should be able to remove all data, update it, or freeze information usage at the level of the old service and privacy practice. Concerning the change of privacy and service functions customers should have possibility to choose as follows: (a) customers do not agree with the new practices at all and demand that their personal information be deleted; (b) customers want their personal information frozen at the previous state of practice; and (c) customers agree to the new practices.

When informed about the details of new practices, some customers would perhaps be inclined to choose Option A and elect not to participate in the company's processes at all in the future. Some customers elect to have their personal information used in older ways, because they are used to getting services based on that level, provided that they can be assured that information about them would not be used in new ways. Other customers might elect Option C and consent to their information being used in new ways, probably because of certain perceived new benefits they might receive.

The important point of the model is that through explicit and open notification and the opportunity to choose different alternatives, individuals could have a greater say or choice regarding how information about them is being used. The interactivity properties of Internet technology give us an efficient manner to deal with the proposed practice of the model (see Järvinen, 2005, pp. 139–147; 201–226).

FUTURE TRENDS

Today's Web-technology enables new means to provide services for knowledge-intensive industries such as insurance, banking and healthcare. A key characteristic of the Internet is that individuals are totally in control of which sites they visit and how long they stay and perceived risk negatively influences willingness to use Web-services. Therefore, trustworthy privacy and service management are obviously imperative sources of value creation and competitiveness. In the future, companies will compete to give individuals the services and the privacy they want. In that scenario, very strict normative privacy regulations according to the privacy framework mean that individuals may not receive satisfactory services. The industry in the U.S. has vowed to self-regulate, but privacy and service management of Web-based e-health services are underdeveloped in general. In that situation, from the perspective of privacy, confidentiality and trust, individuals need more comprehensible tools to gain control over Web-organizations' privacy and service practices. From the perspective of information and communication technology, service providers need more comprehensible methods for the design of Web-based privacy and service management.

It is relatively easy to set up a Web site, but far more difficult to create a Web-based business model. The medical establishment is beginning to recognize both the potential benefits and pitfalls of using electronic communications in healthcare (Fox & Fallows, 2003). As customer demands continue to increase and the availability of informational and interactive Web site content continues to proliferate, the bar for acceptable performance by health providers will continue to rise.

CONCLUSION

It seems that privacy is a broad and, in many ways, elusive concept. Privacy is a social, cultural, and legal concept, all three aspects of which vary from country to country. However, the justification of informational privacy is firm because privacy can be grounded instrumentally and intrinsically—instrumentally, in support of the core values, and intrinsically, as an expression of security and more. Thus, there is a presumption that privacy is a positive value that is worth protecting.

Concerns about informational privacy generally relate not to the collection of information itself, which many individuals would gladly give for appropriate use in a specific situation, but to the manner in which personal information is used and then disclosed. When a business collects information without the knowledge or consent of the individual to whom the information relates, or uses that information in ways that are not known to the individual, or discloses the information without the consent of the individual, information privacy is seriously threatened.

The situations that are normatively private can vary significantly from culture to culture, situation to situation, and time to time. This does not mean that the privacy standards are arbitrary or unjustified; they are just different. A safe retreat to a realm of pure facts, without any consideration of values is never possible, and that also includes privacy and service management of patient-centered e-health.

According to the privacy framework, the attempt to find one general measure for global privacy management fails—there are too many situation-dependant aspects to consider. In general, the amount of privacy individuals have, and can reasonably expect to have, is a function of the practices and laws of society and publicity and voluntary principles. Privacy matters of healthcare are deeply situation-dependent issues and cannot be found by applying a predefined list without considering the situation thoroughly. Information practices of e-health may conflict with individuals' desires to be shielded from unauthorized use of their personal information. The framework focuses on what we should be considering when developing privacy management for protecting our privacy in that situation. It does not neglect the important distinction between the different interests affected by PCEH. The strength of the framework is its ability to distinguish between the condition of privacy and the right to privacy and between a loss of privacy and a violation of privacy.

The privacy management model acknowledges the voluntary nature of the way in which individuals have surrendered control over personal information in exchange for the benefits that information technology brings. The interactivity features of the Internet provide health providers with many opportunities for online management so that the individuals can make the most convenient choices in terms of their own needs and values from a number of alternatives. What one customer considers a privacy invasion may be a valued feature or service to another customer. Interactive Web site content can provide considerable added value for both the health provider and its customer.

Because the applications of information technology are logically malleable, there are sufficient strategic reasons to suggest that privacy management as a concept and practice will survive, and that to ignore privacy issues might be fatal for the success of PCEH. If we naively regard the issues of privacy management as routine or, even worse, as unsolvable, then individuals are in the greatest danger of being harmed by information technology, or those services will not be used at all. If privacy is understood, not merely as a value involving the good of individuals, but as one that also contributes to the broader business and organizational good, then the concern for privacy might have a greater chance of receiving the kind of consideration it deserves.

ACKNOWLEDGMENT

The Foundation for Economic Education is acknowledged for their support. This support has been very important and it has enabled fluent progress of the privacy management project. Some anonymous reviewers of the manuscript have also contributed through constructive comments.

REFERENCES

Choy, A., Hudson, Z., Pritts, J., & Goldman, J. (2001). Exposed online: Why the new federal health privacy regulation doesn't offer much protection to Internet users. *Pew Internet & American Life Project*. Retrieved May 24, 2008, from http://www.pewInternet.org/pdfs/PIP_HPP_HealthPriv_report.pdf

Culver, C., Moor, J., Duerfeldt, W., Kapp, M., & Sullivan, M. (1994). Privacy. *Professional Ethics 3*(3-4), 3-25.

DeCew, J.W. (1997). *In pursuit privacy: Law, ethics, and the rise of technology*. Ithica, NY: Cornell University Press.

Federal Trade Commission (FTC). (1973). *The code of fair information practices*. U.S. Department of Health, Education and Welfare, Secretary's Advisory Committee on Automated Personal Data Systems, Records, Computers, and the Rights of Citizens, viii. Retrieved May 24, 2008, from http://www.epic.org/privacy/consumer

Federal Trade Commission. (1998). *Privacy online: A report to congress*. Federal Trade Commission. Retrieved May 24, 2008, from http//www.ftc.gov/reports/privacy3/

Federal Trade Commission. (2000). *Privacy online: Fair information practices in the electronic marketplace*. A report to congress. Federal Trade Commission. Retrieved May 24, 2008, from http://www.ftc.gov/reports/privacy2000/privacy2000.pdf

Fox, S., & Fallows, D. (2003). Internet health resources. *Pew Internet & American Life Project*. Retrieved May 24, 2008, from

http://www.pewInternet.org/pdfs/PIP_Health_Report_July_2003.pdf

Fox, S., & Rainie, L. (2000a). The online healthcare revolution: How the Web helps Americans take better care of themselves. *Pew Internet & American Life Project*. Retrieved May 24, 2008, from http://www.pewInternet.org/reports/toc.asp?Report=26

Fox, S., Rainie, L., Horrigan, J., Lenhart, A., Spooner, T., & Carter, C. (2000b). Trust and privacy online: Why Americans want to rewrite the rules. *Pew Internet & American Life Project*. Retrieved May 24, 2008, from http://www.pewInternet.org/reports/toc.asp?Report=19

Fried, C. (1970). Privacy: A rational context. Chap. IX in anatomy of values. New York: Cambridge University Press. (Reprinted from *Computers, Ethics, and* Society, pp. 51-63, M.D. Ermann, M.B. Williams, & C. Gutierrez, Eds., 1990, New York: Oxford University Press.

Fried, C. (1984). Privacy. In F.D. Schoeman (Ed.), *Philosophical dimensions of privacy: An anthology* (pp. 203-222). New York: Cambridge University Press.

Fulda, J. (1997). From data to knowledge: Implications of data mining. *Computers of Society, 27*(4), 28.

Ganesan, S. (1994). Determinants of long-term orientation in buyer-seller relationships. *Journal of Marketing 58*(2), 1-19.

Gotlieb, C.C. (1995). Privacy: A concept whose time has come and gone. In D. Lyon & E. Zureik (Eds.), *Surveillance, Computers and Privacy* (pp. 156-171). Minneapolis: University of Minnesota Press.

Häyry, M., & Takala, T. (2001). Genetic information, rights, and autonomy. *Theoretical Medicine 22*, 403-414.

Jarvenpaa, S.L., Tractinsky, N., & Vitale, M. (2000). Consumer trust in an Internet store. *Information Technology and Management 1*, 45-71.

Järvinen, O.P.(2005). *Privacy management of e-health. Content analysis of 39 U.S. health providers' privacy policies.* PhD Thesis. Turku School of Economics, Turku, Finland. Retrieved May 24, 2008, from http://www.tukkk.fi/tutkimus/Vaitokset/default.asp

Johnson, D.G. (1994). *Computer ethics (second edition).* Englewood Cliffs, NJ: Prentice Hall.

Mason, J.K., McCall, & Smith, R.A. (1999). *Law and medical ethics (fifth edition).* London, England: Butterworths.

Mayer, R.J., Davis, J.H., & Schoorman, F.D. (1995). An integrative model of organizational trust. *Academy of Management Review, 20*, 709-734.

McArthur, R.L. (2001). Reasonable expectation of privacy. *Ethics and Information Technology, 3*, 123-128.

Michelfelder, D.P. (2001). The moral value of informational privacy in cyberspace. *Ethics and Information Technology, 3*, 129-135.

Moor, J.H. (1997). Towards a theory of privacy in the information age. *Computers and Society, 27*(3), 27-32.

Moor, J.H. (1998). Reason, relativity, and responsibility in computer ethics. *Computers and Society, 28*(1), 14-21.

Rachels, J. (1975). Why is privacy important? Philosophy and public affairs, *12*(4). (Reprinted from *Computers, Ethics, & Social Values*, pp. 351-357, D.G. Johnson & H. Nissenbaum, Eds., 1995, Englewood Cliffs, NJ: Prentice Hall.

Regan, P. (1995). *Legislating privacy: Technology, social values, and public policy.* Chapel Hill, NC: University of North Carolina Press.

Sitkin, S., & Roth, N.L. (1993). Explaining the limited effectiveness of legalistic remedies for trust/distrust. *Organization Science, 4*(3), 367-392.

Somerville, A. (1999). English V. Genetic privacy: Orthodoxy or oxymoron? *Journal of Medical Ethics, 25*, 144-150.

Tavani, H.T. (1999a). Informational privacy, data mining, and the Internet. *Ethics and Information Technology, 1*, 137-145.

Tavani, H.T. (1999b). KDD, Data mining, and the challenge for normative privacy. *Ethics and Information Technology, 1*, 265-273.

Thibaut, J.W., & Kelley, H.H. (1959). *The social psychology of groups.* New York: Wiley.

Thompson, P.B. (2001). Privacy, secrecy and security. *Ethics and Information Technology, 3*, 13-19.

Uslaner, E.M. (2000). *Trust, civic engagement, and the Internet.* European Consortium for Political Research. University of Grenoble, April 6-11. Retrieved May 24, 2008, from http://www.bsos.umd.edu/gvpt/uslaner/Internettrust.pdf

Warren, S., & Brandeis, L.D. (1890). The right to privacy. *Harvard Law Review, 4*, 193-220.

ENDNOTES

1 See for example Council of Europe: Convention For the Protection of Individuals with Regard to Automatic Processing of Personal Data. Council of Europe, European Treaty Series No. 108. Signed January 28, 1981 entered in force October 1, 1985; DIRECTIVE 95/46/EC Of the European Parliament

and of the Council of 24 October 1995 on the protection of individuals with regard to the processing of personal data and on the free movement of such data; DIRECTIVE 97/66/EC of the European Parliament and of the Council of 15 December 1997 concerning the processing of personal data and the protection of privacy the telecommunications sector

2 See for example the Fair Information Practices of The Federal Trade Commission (FTC, 1973; FTC, 1998; FTC, 2000), TRUSTe (http://www.truste.com), BBBOnLine (http://www.bbbonline.com), and HONcode (http://www.hon.ch).

3 Health Insurance Portability and Accountability Act of 1996, 42 U.S.C.A. 1320d to d-8 (West Supp., 1998). The Department of Health and Human Services finally issued administrative provisions for this bill in late December 2000. Available at: http://aspe.hhs.gov/admnsimp/index.htm or Federal Register, December 28, 2000, for the implementation details (which go into full effect in 2003).

Chapter VIII
Trust in Patient-Centered E-Health

Richard Klein
Clemson University, USA

Michael Dinger
Clemson University, USA

ABSTRACT

Patient-centered e-health (PCEH) offerings see the emergence of divergent, new third parties, through initiatives, including (a) medical content aggregation, (b) health-based online communities, and (c) patient-physician Internet-based portals. Here, the product is digital and heterogeneous for medical content aggregators; virtual and heterogeneous for online communities; and digital, context-specific, and asynchronous for patient-physician portals. With patients expressing privacy and confidentiality concerns in communicating personal health information electronically, growing numbers of PCEH initiatives give rise to many unique issues with respect to patient trust. Existing electronic commerce research focuses on trust in online vendors, potentially providing an incomplete picture with respect to patient trust in PCEH. An accurate and holistic understanding of patient trust encompasses different combinations of cognitive processes, disposition to trust, and institution-based trust, all shaping trusting

INTRODUCTION

E-health encompasses "the use of emerging information and communication technology, especially the Internet, to improve or enable health and healthcare" (Eng, 2001, pp.20). Surveys estimate that 40% of Internet users go online to obtain medical information (Baker, Wagner, Singer, & Bundorf, 2003). Accordingly, Internet-focused firms, such as WebMD (http://www.WebMD.com/), are among the fastest growing in the healthcare industry (Wareham & Klein, 2003). Vendors have developed and subsequently deployed Internet-based IT innovations increasingly aimed at patients and their caregivers (Eudes, 2006). The growing use of the Internet within this industry gives rise to many unique and emerging issues with respect to patient trust.

Consider that within the United States, the debate over national electronic health records has cited concerns with privacy and confidentiality (Dixon, 2007). Patients have expressed similar privacy and confidentiality concerns in communicating personal health information electronically (Bernhardt, Lariscy, Parrott, Silk, & Felter, 2002; Hassol, Walker, Kidder, Rokita, Young, Pierdon, Deitz, Kuck, & Ortiz, 2004). Accordingly, patient trust emerges as a complex issue with respect to growing uses of the Internet and Internet-based technologies. Furthermore, patient trust constitutes a critical success factor for patient-centered e-health (PCEH) initiatives, including (a) medical content aggregators, (b) health-based online communities, and (c) patient-physician Net-based portals, noted in Figure 1. As more patients turn to the Internet in managing their medical conditions; healthcare providers, medical content aggregators, as well as Internet-based solution vendors must understand the factors that affect patient trust with respect to different trustee constituencies.

In years past, trust has been perceived as a traditional and simple patient-physician dyad. This trust still exists in face-to-face environments such as doctors' offices and hospitals. However, with the addition of multiple third parties in Internet-based environments, the potential exists for divergent levels of trust and for different constituencies to influence actions.

Medical content aggregators, such as Dr. Koop (http://www.drkoop.com/), must garner the trust of patients in order for their services to provide value, promoting use that ultimately translates into greater performance through advertising revenues and/or subscription fees. Additionally, patients must trust the author of the content provided. If patients do not have the requisite trust in the source of the content, it will likely go unused as patients turn to alternate outlets.

Increasingly, patients have the opportunity to participate in a variety of online communities and interact with virtual support groups, such as Caring4Cancer (http://www.caring4cancer.com/). However, patient involvement may be dependent upon trust in the vendor hosting the online community. Moreover, patients would have little impetus to participate in an online forum in which the other group participants are judged untrustworthy.

Finally, patient-physician Internet portals have the capacity to securely manage personal medical information for online access by patients. Medfusion (http://Medfusion.net/) and other such portals, however, must garner a requisite level of trustworthiness in controlling and protecting sensitive data. Given the confidential nature of

Figure 1. Patient-centered e-health initiatives

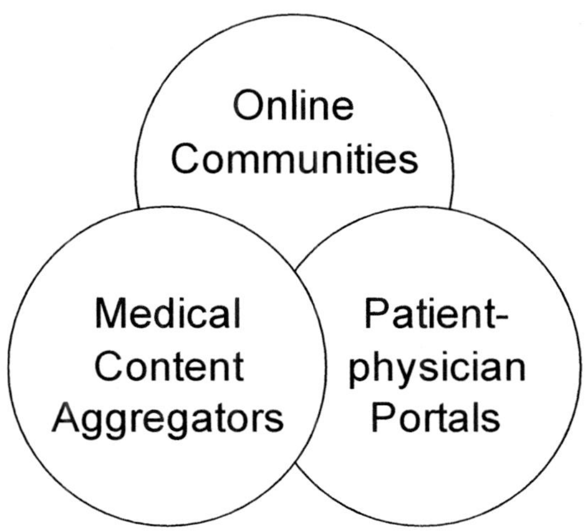

personal medical information, portals perceived as untrustworthy may fail to be adopted, resulting in quick abandonment by patients. Patients must also put a high level of trust in their healthcare provider to update personal health information and respond to communications.

Ultimately, trust has a significant impact on these PCEH initiatives. Particularly, trustworthy environments may realize additional benefits in the form of increased loyalty, yielding subsequent performance benefits for vendors. On the other hand, environments that fail to imbue trust will likely lack sufficient traffic, fewer subscribing healthcare providers, and subsequently lower revenue levels.

This work examines different theoretical perspectives on trust relevant to emerging PCEH initiatives and unique aspects of patient trust in different PCEH contexts. The current work focuses on the role of trust, considering three significant types of initiatives: (a) medical content aggregators, (b) health-based online communities, and (c) patient-physician Internet-based portals. Notably, firms may support multiple initiatives, as is the case with WebMD. The company offers content aggregation in addition to patient-physician portals through its subsidiaries.

The following section provides background specific to patient trust in online environments. The next section integrates specific relevant dimensions of trust with the three major PCEH initiatives considered. The final section highlights future trends and conclusions.

TRUST

In the absence of absolute rules and regulations, trust serves as a primary mechanism for reducing social complexity (Luhmann, 1979). Trust has been defined as "the willingness of a party to be vulnerable to the actions of another party based on the expectation that the other will perform a particular action important to the trustor (i.e., party doing the trusting), irrespective of the ability to monitor or control that other party" (Mayer, Davis, & Schoorman, 1995, pp.712). A variety of disciplines—including information systems (Ba & Pavlou, 2002), marketing (Morgan & Hunt, 1994), economics (Rousseau & Wachtel, 1998), psychology (Ferrin, Dirks, & Shah, 2006), and sociology (Currall & Judge, 1995)—have studied trust extensively. Specifically, prior work investigates the role of trust in relationship commitment (Rousseau & Wachtel, 1998), factors contributing to initial trust formulation (McKnight, Cummings, & Chervany, 1998), the trust an individual has in an organization (Bhattacherjee, 2002), and trust between individuals within organizations (Mayer et al., 1995).

Research investigating the effect of trust on commitment to a relationship finds higher levels of trust in an exchange partner correlated with higher levels of commitment to that partner (Morgan & Hunt, 1994). These findings highlight the importance of trust in fostering recurring use on the part of patients, which is so crucial to the long run success of PCEH initiatives. Since there are issues of risk and vulnerability inherent in such relationships, patients accordingly seek to engage in exchanges with trustworthy parties (Morgan & Hunt, 1994). Here, factors that contribute to trust also positively contribute toward developing some level of commitment.

Within theoretical discussions of trust, a number of concepts informing PCEH initiatives appear regularly. First, in order for trust to be relevant, a given relationship must exhibit some form of risk. The absence of risk in a given situation mitigates the need for trust (Luhmann, 1979). In any given e-health situation, there is risk involved, particularly for the patient. There is the risk that "expert" content could be wrong, that advice or support from peers could be poor or not genuine, or that sensitive personal information could be leaked or otherwise misappropriated through an Internet portal. Such risks necessitate some level of trust on the part of patients. Hence, perceived risk influences trust (Mayer et al., 1995) within this context.

Consistent with the stated definition of trust, patient trusting beliefs; namely, ability, benevolence, and integrity; are considered. The next section outlines the notion of disposition to trust, which serves as the basis for initial formation of trusting beliefs. Trusting beliefs are then discussed. Consistent with an integrated model of organizational trust (Mayer et al., 1995; McKnight et al., 1998), additional factors shaping patient beliefs within the PCEH context include cognitive processes and institution-based trust, as depicted in Figure 2.

DISPOSITION TO TRUST

Disposition, or propensity, to trust encompasses the general willingness to trust others. Such propensity will shape the extent to which the patient puts trust in a given trustee (i.e., party being trusted) absent prior experience with, or information about, the trustee. Trust disposition differs across patients with disparate developmental experiences, personality traits, and/or cultural backgrounds (Hofstede, 1980). Research finds that propensity to trust does not determine trust in a specific situation with a particular set of circumstances (Johnson-George & Swap, 1982). Instead, Mayer et al. (1995) posit that disposition to trust has a significant impact on other aspects of the trust construct, namely trusting beliefs, often called factors of trustworthiness.

Hence, disposition to trust encompasses (a) faith in humanity, or an overall perception of trustworthiness concerning people in general, and (b) trusting stance, or individual beliefs about the relative benefits of trusting another in general (McKnight et al., 1998). Faith in humanity affects initial trusting beliefs drawing upon already developed thought patterns (Kramer, 1994). In the absence of relevant, situation specific information, beliefs, and understanding about human nature shape trust (Wrightsman, 1991). Additionally, trusting stance further influences willingness to trust another, without consideration of beliefs about the party. A high trusting stance finds the

Figure 2. Theoretical trust perspectives (Adaptation of Mayer et al., 1995 and McKnight et al., 1998)

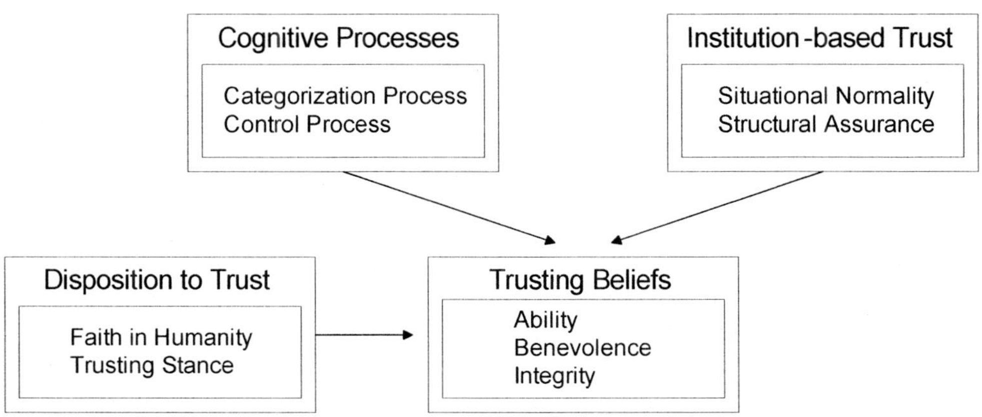

trustor willing to trust others with the expectation that trust breeds positive outcomes (McKnight et al., 1998). Collectively, these two dimensions of disposition to trust play a role in effecting trusting beliefs, or specific factors of trustworthiness, given specific circumstances.

Trusting Beliefs

Mayer et al. (1995) propose an integrated model of trust that is composed of characteristics of the trustor, or person doing the trusting; the trustee, or person being trusted; and the perceived risk inherent in the relationship. The characteristics of the trustor are largely composed of an innate propensity to trust others. As a baseline personality characteristic, one patient might be more apt to place trust in others, whereas a different patient might be naturally more skeptical. Here, the characteristics of perceived trustworthiness of the trustee include (a) ability, (b) benevolence, and (c) integrity.

Ability refers to a more specific brand of trust, in which trust is placed in others with respect to specific tasks. Namely, ability considers the requisite set of skills, competencies, and/or characteristics that enable the trustee to exert influence or hold a position within a specific domain (Mayer et al., 1995). Benevolence refers to the trustee "wanting to do good to the trustor, aside from an egocentric profit motive" (Mayer et al., 1995, pp.718). This trust factor focuses on the intentions and motivations of the trustee (Deutsch, 1958). The final factor, integrity, assesses the extent to which trustee actions are consistent with some set of acceptable trustor standards (McFall, 1987). Moreover, a party is judged to have integrity when the trustor believes the other party to have a strong sense of justice. Integrity, like benevolence, reflects ethical traits (McKnight, Choudhury, & Kacmar, 2002a).

Collectively, these three factors create trust through perceived trustworthiness in the trustee. A trustee might be skillful and benevolent and yet be highly inconsistent concerning moral actions, or even hold a moral code entirely different from the trustor. Moreover, McKnight et al. (2002a) posit that these three factors, or trusting beliefs, play out within Internet-based contexts. Existing empirical research demonstrates that these beliefs shape trust's influence on purchase intentions in electronic commerce environments (McKnight, Choudhury, & Kacmar, 2002b), adoption of advice from online recommendation agents (Wang & Benbasat, 2005), and use of patient-physician electronic communications (Klein, 2007a).

Cognitive Processes

Cognitive processes consist of (a) categorization processes and (b) illusions of control processes (McKnight et al., 1998). Categorization processes are broken into unit grouping, reputation, and stereotyping. Unit grouping occurs when the trustee is perceived to be in the same group as the trustor, subsequently yielding a higher level of trust (Kramer, Brewer, & Hanna, 1996). Reputation categorization focuses on the state of the trustee's reputation, which reflects professional competence (Barber, 1983; Powell, 1996). Finally, stereotyping constitutes general judgments based on occupation, gender, and race (Orbell, Dawes, & Schwartz-Shea, 1994). Illusions of control comprise token control efforts, or the trustor's ability to influence or generate some result from the potential trustee in order to judge trustworthiness (Langer, 1975).

Institution-Based Trust

In considering patient trusting beliefs in organizational entities, factors specific to the trustee also influence patient perceptions. It has been noted that online electronic commerce environments exhibit high degrees of institution-based trust as consumers transact with new and often unfamiliar third-parties (Pavlou & Gefen, 2004). Institution-based trust focuses on beliefs that requisite structures exist, enabling one to act with the expectation of future successful encounters (Zucker, 1986). As such, institution-based effects encompass (a) situational normality, or the relative state of normality in the setting, and (b) structural assurances, or the availability of recourse in the form of guarantees, regulations, and/or legal action.

Situational normality beliefs reflect perceptions of the appearance of a normal or "customary" environment (Baier, 1986). This concept extends to individual comfort levels with socially constructed roles based in a shared understanding among members of a social system (McKnight et al., 1998). Prior work categorizes structural safeguards as institutional "side bets" (Shapiro, 1987). Here, regulations seek to assure expectations about transactions (Sitkin, 1995). Guarantees mitigate trustor perceptions of risk through agreements extended by firms (Zaheer, McEvily, & Perrone, 1998). Finally, legal recourse attaches some level of significance to promises made by firms through potential social disapproval and/or legal action (Sitkin, 1995).

PATIENT-CENTERED E-HEALTH INITIATIVES

In this chapter, we are addressing three common types of PCEH initiatives: (a) medical content aggregation, (b) online communities, and (c) patient-physician portals. Content providers enable patients to search and find medical information via the Internet. Patients are also able to avail themselves of a variety of support groups through online communities. These Internet-based communities enable patients to interact with others who have experienced, or are currently experiencing, similar health issues or concerns ranging from weight management to cancer. Finally, patient-physician portals provide services to patients and physicians by enabling communications as well as storage and access to personal health records (PHR).

While electronic commerce research examining trust informs our understanding of patient trust in PCEH contexts, some distinct circumstances emerge. Existing efforts examining trust within electronic commerce environments focus on the online vendor. However, multiple intermediaries permeate most Net-based environments. Prior work examines the "perceived effectiveness" of feedback mechanisms, escrow services, and credit card guarantees, in the context of studying trust in the online intermediary and community of sellers within online auction markets (Pavlou & Gefen, 2004). Other research operationalizes trust solely with respect to the online intermediary or vendor (Cheung & Lee, 2001; Gefen, Karahanna, & Straub, 2003; Jarvenpaa & Tractinsky, 1999; McKnight et al., 2002b). Clearly, divergent trusting beliefs may exist with respect to organizations other than the primary vendor, including Internet service providers, financial institutions, and product manufacturers. Most efforts to date examine homogeneous products, while assuming service providers and financial institutions are, at best, controls.

The PCEH context cannot assume homogeneity across products. Content aggregators obtain medical information from different sources. Online communities attract different patient participants, potentially structuring and managing communities differently across vendors. Further, patient-physician portals offer divergent functionality and interfaces among competitors, with subscribing healthcare providers often adopting different mixes of functionality from the same intermediary. Additionally, from the patient perspective, PHR access and communications with providers constitute divergent core offerings (Klein, 2007b).

Within PCEH, the "book" purchased from Amazon (http://www.amazon.com/) effectively becomes the medical content, online community, or patient information access/communication offered through PCEH initiatives. Here, the product is digital and heterogeneous for medical content

Figure 3. PCEH initiative trustees

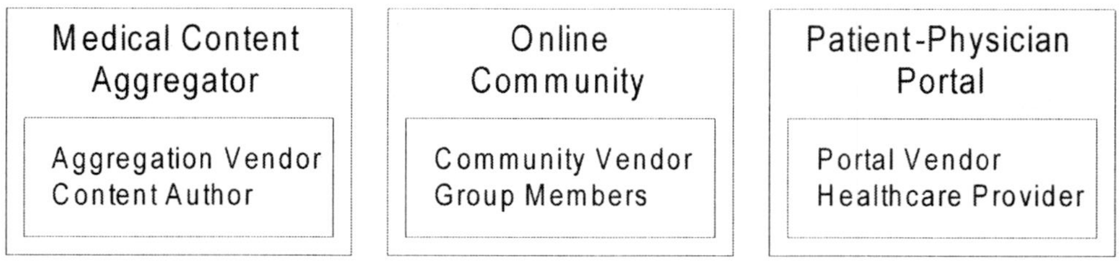

aggregators; virtual and heterogeneous for online communities; and digital, context specific, and asynchronous for patient-physician portals. Each initiative entails multiple trustees (some of whom are vendors) while others encompass partners. Specifically, trust in content author, group members, and healthcare providers constitute partners within each initiative and emerge as relevant in shaping patients' trust in the PCEH initiative. Figure 3 highlights the relevant PCEH trustee constituencies considered in this chapter.

Medical Content Aggregators

Medical content aggregators pursue information management business models by collecting and filtering information-based goods such as data and media products (Wareham & Klein, 2003). Such initiatives depend on patient use as a mechanism for deriving revenue through advertising and, in some cases, subscription fees. Due to risks in following inaccurate or ill-advised health-related information, the number of aggregators available, and ease of switching between firms, the patient has the motivation and option to choose the provider perceived most trustworthy. Patients are more likely to maintain a committed relationship with an organization that is perceived trustworthy (Morgan & Hunt, 1994). Here, patient trust in the aggregation vendor and content author are anticipated to drive use.

Trust in Aggregation Vendors

Among trusting beliefs, ability may shape trust in content aggregators to a greater extent than benevolence and integrity. Patient perception of content aggregator ability is largely shaped by technical aspects of Web site operations in addition to the relevance and quality of available healthcare information. Where patients encounter problems in navigation and/or dead links, the vendor will likely be deemed lacking with respect to requisite technical capabilities. Similarly, where health content is lacking or of a poor quality, the vendor may be judged incapable of successfully facilitating aggregation of quality information. Hence, online content providers can further increase perceptions of ability by sourcing content created by reputable experts in given fields. Arguably, no one expert will have experience in all medical fields; therefore, vendors can maximize perceptions of ability by having many experts create content within their given field.

Formation of trusting beliefs here partially depends on categorization processes and institution-based trust (McKnight et al., 1998). A salient factor in formation of patient trust toward an online vendor engaged in medical information management is often reputation. A positive reputation is perceived as a marker of trustworthiness (Doney & Cannon, 1997). Firms that make a significant investment in reputation development have much to lose, and therefore, can be perceived as more trustworthy. Consider the case of Dr. Koop, which emerged as one of the first Internet startups aggregating and distributing healthcare content to patients. Marketing and branding capitalized on the name and reputation of Dr. C. Everett Koop, the highly regarded former United States Surgeon General.

In electronic commerce environments firm size, in addition to reputation, has been perceived as a primary antecedent of trust (Jarvenpaa & Tractinsky, 1999). Larger organizations have more to lose from untrustworthy behavior. Additionally, reputation and firm size are suggested to positively influence each other (Doney & Cannon, 1997; Ganesan, 1994). As an organization grows larger, it may become more reputable, or at least better known. Similarly, organizations with quality reputations are likely to grow larger. Jarvenpaa & Tractinsky (1999) posit that reputation is partially a function of perceptions of firm size. Therefore, a vendor can enhance initial judgments of trust by managing the firm's reputation and perceptions of its size.

Initial trust formation also depends on institution-based factors, namely situational normality and structural assurance (McKnight et al., 1998). Beliefs about structural assurance are particularly relevant to intermediaries managing healthcare content. If the patient believes that the vendor makes guarantees concerning available content, that regulations monitor provided content, or even that some form of recourse is available, the likelihood of trusting increases. Given risks with respect to disclosure of personal information, vendors often take steps to develop and publish privacy policies as well as terms and conditions of use. Frequently, this information is easily and prominently available through homepages. The MayoClinic.com (http://www.mayoclinic.com/), for example, posts its "Privacy Policy" and "Terms and Conditions of Use," and goes a step further by noting posting dates for each.

Prior work also notes the use of third-party seals by organizations such as Health on the Net Foundation Code of Conduct (http://www.con.ch/), Truste (http://www.truste.org/), and URAC (http://www.urac.org/). These organizations aid in establishing guarantees with respect to firm standards of conduct and practices in addition to providing for limited recourse by consumers (Luo & Najdawi, 2004). Fung and Lee (1999) suggest that reputation for an online organization is based on the existing brand name and such seals of approval.

As noted, many content aggregation business models are predicated on revenue generation through advertising and subscription fees. In the case of advertising, such commercial pursuits on the part of vendors give rise to issues specific to benevolence- and integrity-based trusting beliefs. Specifically, content vendors must take great care in managing advertising initiatives, so that the vendor is not perceived as acting purely in pursuit of profits. While patients may expect, and accept, some level of advertising, vendors engaged in targeted efforts based on profiling of searches might go too far, encroaching on expectations of anonymity. Further, such situations might give rise to integrity issues in addition to benevolence. Not only might such a vendor be viewed as pursuing pure profit motives, but also actions might run counter to patients' expectations of acceptable online privacy.

Trust in Content Authors

The second trustee relevant to patient trust in medical content aggregators focuses on the author of sourced information. In accessing specific healthcare information from an online content aggregator, patients form opinions about the trustworthiness of the content author, with ability anticipated to be the dominant trusting belief. Patients' positive perceptions of the author's medical expertise will, in all likelihood, result in higher perceptions of ability and greater subsequent use of content.

Cognitive processes via reputation and institutional-based trust via situational normality, aid in the formation of trusting beliefs. Author reputation, or even the reputation of affiliated institutions, credentialing boards, and/or medical schools, can aid in enhancing trusting beliefs. Similarly, the reputation of peer reviewers may serve to advance authors' reputations.

For institutional-based trust, situational normality plays a greater role than structural assurance, in contrast to the content vendor. Situational normality serves to inform individual cognitive processes of reputation categorization. Here, the presence or absence of certain information contributes toward perceptions of situational normality, ultimately informing reputation. Consider a search of WebMD for information on a specific disease. Retrieved articles identify the author, date last updated, and professional peers reviewing the content. Patients can obtain additional information regarding both the author and reviewers through hyperlinks to their Web sites. While not providing for guarantees or recourse, this information helps to establish the legitimacy of the authors and their work.

In sum, medical content aggregation initiatives need to acknowledge both the content aggregator and original source of the content as garnering trust of patients. For the vendor and author, ability constitutes the critical factor shaping trustworthiness. For the aggregator, reputation and structural assurance influence trusting beliefs, while content authors rely upon reputation in conjunction with aspects of situational normality in shaping perceptions of trustworthiness.

Online Communities

Online community initiatives give rise to patient trust issues with respect to the vendor sponsoring the community and the support group members. As was the case with content aggregation initiatives, vendors depend on patient use to fuel revenue through advertising and/or subscription fees. Here again, greater perceived trustworthiness increases the likelihood of a committed relationship (Morgan & Hunt, 1994).

Trust in Community Vendor

With respect to trusting beliefs, ability and again integrity may constitute dominant perceptions of trustworthiness. Technical aspects of the operation of Web sites shape patient perceptions of vendor ability. Navigation issues and problems with chat sessions (e.g., Java applet and User Defined Protocol failures) will likely garner negative perceptions with respect to requisite capabilities. Additionally, compared with medical content aggregators, participation in online communities dictates the disclosure of increasing amounts of personal medical information. One can use content aggregator Web sites anonymously. However, in participating in an online community a patient must often disclose substantial personal health information within the context of engaging in a support group. Accordingly, in addition to perceptions of ability, integrity also constitutes a significant patient trusting belief.

For the vendor, cognitive processes in the form of reputation and beliefs about structural assurance are particularly relevant in shaping trusting beliefs. Reputation emerges as a positive influence on patient perceptions. Existing firms with an established brand in the marketplace find themselves at an advantage in regards to engendering perceptions of professional competence among patients (Powell, 1996). Weight Watchers (http://www.weightwatchers.com/) provides an excellent example of an established firm capitalizing on a quality reputation to support use of its online community. Here again, one might expect such online communities and larger organizations to benefit from their reputations (Doney & Cannon, 1997).

From an institutional-based trust perspective, given risks with respect to disclosure of personal information, vendors can take steps to develop and publish privacy policies as well as terms and conditions of use statements. Further, third-party seals may again be important in establishing guarantees with respect to standards of conduct and practices in addition to providing for limited recourse (Luo & Najdawi, 2004).

Trust in Group Members

Online support group members must also garner some level of trust from a patient in order to generate participation. Before a group can become beneficial to the patient, that patient has to make a potentially risky emotional investment in the other members of the group. Moreover, patients who view the group as trustworthy are more likely to stay committed (Morgan & Hunt, 1994). The social identity of de-individuation effects (SIDE) model suggests that computer-mediated anonymity can reinforce adherence to strong group boundaries and social norms (Postmes, Spears, & Lea, 1998), further supporting committed relationships.

With respect to trustworthiness factors, ability may be the least salient. In a support group situation, a patient may not be overly concerned that other participants are highly skillful in treating a specific illness or even highly qualified to offer medical advice. Instead, the patient is likely to be more concerned with the benevolence and integrity of the rest of the support group members. If the patient believes members are involved for reasons of personal gain, the patient will be less inclined to trust. Additionally, if members exhibit characteristics of a moral code distinctly different from the patient, or if the behavior of members is inconsistent or erratic, patients will again be disinclined to trust.

Initial trust formation in support group settings depends to a large extent on individual patient disposition to trust as well as cognitive processes and institution-based trust (McKnight et al., 1998). Notably, patients who are predisposed to trust will exhibit higher levels of faith in humanity, and put more emphasis on the value of trust in a relationship (Wrightsman, 1991). These patients will be more likely to trust others in a support group.

In terms of cognitive processes, patients may categorize the members of a group based on unit grouping and stereotypes. Unit grouping is the process of placing other people in or out of the same group as the trustor (Kramer et al., 1996).. If the patient is looking to join a support group of other people experiencing the same situation, the effect of unit grouping will positively influence intent to trust (Brewer & Silver, 1978; Zucker, Darby, Brewer, & Peng, 1996). Returning to the example of Weight Watchers, everyone is experiencing a related health issue and working a homogeneous treatment plan. Since the patient and members of the support group are "in the same boat," the patient is more inclined to trust.

If the patient has personal stereotypes regarding support groups or members, trusting inclinations could be positively or negatively influenced. Subsequently, patient perceptions of the group as relatively normal may affect trusting beliefs (Garfinkel, 1963). Situational normality dictates that circumstances deemed highly unusual may see patients disinclined to trust. As such, patients with experience specific to online communities, and subsequently some comfort level with the environment, may be more inclined to trust an online support group. Consider patients with prior experience interacting in online communities such as Facebook (http://www.thefacebook.com/) and MySpace (http://www.myspace.com/). Such patients might be naturally inclined to easily assimilate into a health-based online community.

It is further worth noting that firm size may be a significant factor influencing trusting beliefs (Jarvenpaa & Tractinsky, 1999). The size of the organization behind the support group may positively influence willingness to trust the vendor in conjunction with reputation. However, the size of the support group itself may have a different effect. Patients might feel lost in a support group that is too large, or be uncomfortable in a support group that is too small. Depending on patient preferences, some support groups could be considered too large, while too small to another patient. The effect of group size may rest entirely on the preferences of the patient. For example, Caring4Cancer boasts numerous options for cancer patients seeking an online community, allowing patients to find a group conducive to personal preferences.

Within online communities, patients focus on trusting the vendor that manages the community and the members of the support group. With respect to the vendor, ability and integrity emerge as the dominant trusting beliefs with cognitive processes via reputation and structural assurance serving to influence perceptions. By contrast, benevolence and integrity are potentially the key factors when considering trusting beliefs in support group members. Patients draw upon individual cognitive processes, namely unit grouping and situational normality, in forming trusting beliefs.

Patient-Physician Portals

Patient-physician portals enable electronic patient communications with healthcare providers and access PHR. Patients face significant risk through their use of these portals. Namely, patient trust within this context must first consider the online vendor hosting the portal. Additionally, given the asynchronous nature of this PCEH initiative with both patients and providers engaged in two-way communications and interactions with each other (Wilson, 2003), patients must also trust their healthcare provider.

Trust in Portal Vendors

Ability and integrity potentially dominate patient trusting beliefs in portal vendors. As is the case with both aggregation and online community vendors, technical aspects of the Internet-based solution influence perceptions of organizations' ability. A poor interface may predispose patients to question vendors' technical skills. Moreover, given the increased presence of personal health information in these portals, patient perceptions of integrity become critical. Both the information access and communication aspects of these applications necessitate the flow of some level of personal data. Even if a patient never accesses PHR and only uses the system to request a prescription refill, the prescription itself might engender highly confidential information, as would be the case with HIV medications. Patients have consistently expressed privacy and confidentiality concerns in communicating electronically with providers (Bernhardt et al., 2002).

Some patients, however, may be naturally more inclined to trust that personal information is secure, whereas others might be naturally more skeptical of the security of electronic environments. The patient may also categorize the patient-physician portal based on reputation. As noted in discussing aggregation and online community vendors, reputation likely shapes patient perceptions of factors of trustworthiness. Additionally, based on other factors, including firm size (Morgan & Hunt, 1994), the patient may perceive a portal reputable, positively influencing trusting beliefs.

If the patient perceives that institution-based factors offer protections, intentions to trust may increase. The perception of protections in the form of guarantees, regulations, and/or legal recourse will positively influence trust. Structural assurance may play a significant role in shaping patient trusting beliefs. For example, accessing confidential patient information via the Internet through a patient-physician portal requires patient consent under the Health Insurance Portability and Accountability Act (HIPAA, 1996) in the United States. While vendor guarantees may serve to mitigate risk (Zaheer et al., 1998), legal recourse through HIPAA regulations attaches external significance to firm promises (Baier, 1986). Hence, portal vendors must take steps to engender the highest sense of integrity in patients. Here again, privacy policies in addition to terms and conditions of use constitute essential postings on Web sites. Third-party seals like Health on the Net, Truste, and URAC may also serve to instill a sense of integrity (Luo & Najdawi, 2004). Vendors have also sought out the aid of medical professional associations in fostering a positive image. For example, Medfusion prominently notes their partnership with the American Academy of Family Physicians on their Web site, complete with the Academy's logo and a hyperlink to their Web site.

Trust in Healthcare Provider

In considering individual healthcare providers, patients should trust their respective provider to manage healthcare needs. It is important that patients first hold a trusting relationship with their provider before participating in patient-physician portals (Andreassen, Trondsen, Kummervold, Gammon, & Hjortdahl, 2006). Lacking this trusting relationship, patients are unlikely to communicate with their physician in an electronic format. Also, if an existing offline relationship breaks down, the online relationship will break down as well. Assuming this trusting relationship exists, patients need to then trust that their communications are delivered to their physicians and that their personal medical information is indeed private and secure. Whereas trust is transferable to an extent to online contexts (Stewart, 2003), trusting beliefs, cognitive processes, and institutional-based factors may be task specific, warranting consideration of potential distinctions.

Patient perceptions of benevolence and integrity may prove more influential than ability with respect to the trustworthiness of the healthcare provider in interactions through portals. Beliefs specific to provider integrity will in all likelihood fall in line with beliefs established in the context of the physician-patient relationship. Surveys note that patients have confidentiality concerns with respect to online PHR and patient-physician communications (Bernhardt et al., 2002; Hassol et al., 2004). However, findings also suggest that three-quarters of adults desire to communicate with their healthcare provider electronically (Conhaim & Page, 2003). Similarly, the market finds patients demanding ever increasing convenience and access to providers (Ball & Lillis, 2001). Accordingly, healthcare providers that offer portal access to communications may be perceived as more caring or benevolent. Additionally, the office staff, nurse, or physician that initiates the discussion of the patient-physician portal may shape beliefs. Physicians taking an active role in PCEH initiatives may be perceived as more caring.

One cannot, however, ignore the benefits that healthcare providers receive by offering their patients access through Web-based applications. Empirical work has yet to establish the performance impacts of portals on healthcare practice operations. Providers do bear the burden of the costs of making portals available to their patients, although vendors point toward potential efficiency gains in streaming communications and disseminating information. Evidence of the performance benefits of administrative uses of information technology exist in other business settings (Devaraj & Kohli, 2003; Gurbaxani & Whang, 1991). Further, efficiency benefits not only the firm but also clients and customers (Teece, 1980). Hence, healthcare providers offering Internet-based access may be perceived as benevolent, empowering patients through advanced technology.

With respect to the role of institution-based factors in shaping beliefs, structural assurance is important, as healthcare providers will often obtain written consent when establishing patient accounts through vendors. Such procedures serve to reinforce guarantees on the provider side, while also influencing trusting beliefs with respect to the third-party vendor. The extent to which the patient perceives a healthcare provider to be acting in a competent manner with respect to the portal likely also impacts perceptions of integrity. A provider that automatically establishes patient accounts through the portal absent formal, informed consent consistent with HIPAA regulations may be deemed to lack integrity. By contrast, where one observes providers executing formalized procedures aimed at ensuring confidentiality, patients will likely judge the provider to have greater integrity.

Patient trusting beliefs in both the portal vendor and their healthcare provide may contribute toward use and ultimate success of the PCEH initiative. The relevant factors of trustworthiness and antecedents do differ however. For vendors, ability and integrity may contribute more to overall trusting beliefs, with reputation-based cognitive processes and structural assurance shaping beliefs. By contrast, healthcare providers must be perceived as benevolent and have a high degree of integrity. Here again, institution-based structural assurance initiatives potentially drive perceptions of beliefs, particularly integrity.

FUTURE TRENDS

Future trends specific to PCEH initiatives might be embedded in consolidation trends among firms within the healthcare sector. Firms like WebMD have begun pursuit of diversification strategies, consolidating product and service offerings to the market. These firms may bring together multiple PCEH initiatives under a single organizational umbrella. Such endeavors can leverage efficiencies, in the form of combined professional expertise, content, reputation, and information systems/technology infrastructure. Furthermore, by making use of such synergies, firms may be able to offer unique combinations of value to patients. For example, in time, one might find that the patient-physician portal vendor also facilitates content aggregation and maintains online communities. Such evolutions might serve to make our understanding of patient trust substantially more complex.

Even in the absence of outright consolidation of vendors; one should expect growing integration of PCEH initiatives where the healthcare provider serves as the nexus of PCEH offerings available to patients. Consider the case of Kaiser Permanente (http://www.kaiserpermanente.org/). As a full-service managed care provider, Kaiser oversees all aspects of patient care through outright ownership of provider practices, pharmacies, and medical facilities. Kaiser's HealthConnect system facilitates all three PCEH initiatives to varying degrees (Goedert, 2005), complicating the trust issue. Moreover, managed care plans create additional unique considerations, including to what extent, does the "plan" become a trustee.

CONCLUSION

This work posits that in PCEH initiatives, patients form trusting beliefs in multiple constituencies when utilizing PCEH applications. In considering trusting beliefs with respect to PCEH initiatives, different beliefs potentially prevail across different constituencies for each initiative. Even in considering the vendor across all three initiatives, given the nature of each, the requisite level of integrity might vary while ability persists at a high level. Consider that anonymous searches for information through a content aggregator does not give rise to significant integrity concerns, while participation in an online health-based support group might as confidential information might be discussed, even semi-anonymously. Further, use of a patient-physician portal bears the exchange of personal medical data. Here, the presence of confidentiality and privacy concerns yield greater attention with respect to trustee integrity.

It is also proposed that while empirical electronic commerce research informs our understanding of PCEH initiatives, it provides for a misleading and incomplete picture with respect to patient trust. Existing efforts have focused the trust construct on the online vendor, where the product is to a great extent independent of the firm. Within the PCEH context the product is digital and heterogeneous in the case of medical content aggregators; virtual and heterogeneous for online communities; and digital, context specific, and asynchronous for patient-physician portals. An accurate and holistic understanding of trust within this context can only be achieved by considering the broader population of trustee constituencies.

REFERENCES

Andreassen, H.K., Trondsen, M., Kummervold, P.E., Gammon, D., & Hjortdahl, P. (2006). Patients who use e-mediated communication with their doctor: New constructions of trust in the patient-doctor relationship. *Qualitative Health Research, 16*(2), 238-248.

Ba, S., & Pavlou, P.A. (2002). Evidence of the effect of trust building technology in electronic markets: Price premiums and buyer behavior. *MIS Quarterly, 26*(3), 243-268.

Baier, A. (1986). Trust and antitrust. *Ethics, 96*(2), 231-260.

Baker, L., Wagner, T.H., Singer, S., & Bundorf, M.K. (2003). Use of the internet and e-mail for healthcare information. *Journal of the American Medical Association, 289*, 2400-2406.

Ball, M.J., & Lillis, J. (2001). E-health: Transforming the physician/patient relationship. *International Journal of Medical Informatics, 61*(1), 1-10.

Barber, B. (1983). *The logic and limits of trust.* New Brunswick, NJ: Rutgers University Press.

Bernhardt, J.M., Lariscy, R.A.W., Parrott, R.L., Silk, K.J., & Felter, E.M. (2002). Perceived barriers to internet-based health communication on human genetics. *Journal of Health Communication, 7*(4), 325-340.

Bhattacherjee, A. (2002). Individual trust in online firms: Scale development and initial test. *Journal of Management Information Systems, 19*(1), 211-241.

Brewer, M.B., & Silver, M. (1978). Ingroup bias a function of task characteristics. *European Journal of Social Psychology, 8*(3), 393-400.

Cheung, C.M.K., & Lee, M.K.O. (2001). Trust in Internet shopping: Instrument development and validation through classical and modern approaches. *Journal of Global Information Management, 9*(3), 23-35.

Conhaim, W.W., & Page, L. (2003). Is the doctor online? *Information Today, 20*(2), 29-31.

Currall, S.C., & Judge, T.A. (1995). Measuring trust between organizational boundary role persons. *Organizational Behavior and Human Decision Processes, 64*(2), 151-170.

Deutsch, M. (1958). Trust and suspicion. *Journal of Conflict Resolution, 2*(4), 265-279.

Devaraj, S., & Kohli, R. (2003). Performance impacts of information technology: Is actual usage the missing link? *Management Science, 49*(3), 273-289.

Dixon, P. (2007). *World privacy forum comments about the ethical, legal, and social implications of using genetic healthcare data in electronic health records.* U.S. Department of Health and Human Services (Ed.). Washington, D.C.: World Privacy Forum.

Doney, P.M., & Cannon, J.P. (1997). An examination of the nature of trust in buyer-seller relationships. *Journal of Marketing, 61*(2), 35-51.

Eng, T.R. (2001). *The eHealth landscape: A terrain map of emerging information and communication technologies in health and healthcare.* Princeton, NJ: The Robert Wood Johnson Foundation.

Eudes, J.A. (2006). Gateway to the Web. *Marketing Health Services, 25*(4), 38-39.

Ferrin, D.L., Dirks, K.T., & Shah, P.P. (2006). Direct and indirect effects of third-party relationships on interpersonal trust. *Journal of Applied Psychology, 91*(4), 870-883.

Fung, R., & Lee, M. (1999). EC-trust (trust in electronic commerce): Exploring the antecedent factors. In W. Haseman & D. Nazareth (Eds.), *Proceedings of the Americas Conference on Information Systems* (pp. 517-519). Charlotte, NC: Association for Information Systems.

Ganesan, S. (1994). Determinants of long-term orientation in buyer seller relationships. *Journal of Marketing, 58*(2), 50-69.

Garfinkel, H. (1963). A conception of, and experiments with, "trust" as a condition of stable concerted actions. In O.J. Harvey (Ed.), *Motivation and social interaction: Cognitive determinants* (pp. 187-238). New York: The Ronald Press Company.

Gefen, D., Karahanna, E., & Straub, D.W. (2003). Trust and TAM in online shopping: An integrated model. *MIS Quarterly, 27*(1), 51-91.

Goedert, J. (2005, July 1). Kaiser readies new Web portal tools. Health Data Management. Retrieved May 26, 2008, from http://www.healthdatamanagement.com/

Gurbaxani, V., & Whang, S. (1991). The impact of information systems on organizations and markets. *Communications of the Association for Computing Machinery, 34*(1), 59-73.

Hassol, A., Walker, J. M., Kidder, D., Rokita, K., Young, D., Pierdon, S., Deitz, D., Kuck, S., & Ortiz, E. (2004). Patient experiences and attitudes about access to a patient electronic healthcare record and linked Web messaging. *Journal of the American Medical Informatics Association, 11*(6), 505-513.

HIPAA. (1996). *Public law no. 104-191, section 1173, U.S.C. 201 C.F.R.* Health Insurance Portability and Accountability Act.

Hofstede, G. (1980). Motivation, leadership, and organization: Do American theories apply abroad? *Organizational Dynamics, 9*(1), 42-63.

Jarvenpaa, S.L., & Tractinsky, N. (1999). Consumer trust in an internet store: A cross cultural validation. *Journal of Computer-Mediated Communication, 5*(2), 1-33.

Johnson-George, C., & Swap, W.C. (1982). Measurement of specific interpersonal trust: Construction and validation of a scale to assess trust in a specific other. *Journal of Personality and Social Psychology, 43*(6), 1306-1317.

Klein, R. (2007a). Internet-based patient-physician electronic communication applications: Patient acceptance and trust. *e-Service Journal, 5*(2), 27-51.

Klein, R. (2007b). Patient portal acceptance: An empirical examination of individual and technology based factors. *European Journal of Information Systems, 16*(6), 751-760.

Kramer, R.M. (1994). The sinister attribution error: Paranoid cognition and collective distrust in organizations. *Motivation and Emotion, 18*(3), 199-230.

Kramer, R.M., Brewer, M.B., & Hanna, B.A. (1996). Collective trust and collective actions. In R.M. Kramer & T.R. Tyler (Eds.), *Trust in organizations: Frontiers of theory and research* (pp. 357-389). Thousand Oaks, CA: Sage, Inc.

Langer, E.J. (1975). The illusion of control. *Journal of Personality and Social Psychology, 32*(2), 311-328.

Luhmann, N. (1979). *Power and trust.* New York: John Wiley.

Luo, W., & Najdawi, M. (2004). Trust-building measures: A review of consumer health portals. *Communications of the Association for Computing Machinery, 47*(1), 108-113.

Mayer, R.C., Davis, J.H., & Schoorman, F.D. (1995). An integrative model of organizational trust. *Academy of Management Review, 20*(3), 709-734.

McFall, L. (1987). Integrity. *Ethics, 9*(1), 5-20.

McKnight, D.H., Choudhury, V., & Kacmar, C. (2002a). Developing and validating trust measures for e-commerce: An integrative typology. *Information Systems Research, 13*(3), 334-359.

McKnight, D.H., Choudhury, V., & Kacmar, C. (2002b). The impact of initial consumer trust on intentions to transact with a Web site: A trust building model. *Journal of Strategic Information Systems, 11*(3-4), 297-323.

McKnight, D.H., Cummings, L.L., & Chervany, N.L. (1998). Initial trust formation in new organizational relationships. *Academy of Management Review, 23*(3), 473-490.

Morgan, R.M., & Hunt, S.D. (1994). The commitment-trust theory of relationship marketing. *Journal of Marketing, 58*(3), 20-38.

Orbell, J., Dawes, R., & Schwartz-Shea, P. (1994). Trust, social categories, and individuals: The case of gender. *Motivation and Emotion, 18*(2), 109-128.

Pavlou, P.A., & Gefen, D. (2004). Building effective online marketplaces with institution-based trust. *Information Systems Research, 15*(1), 37-59.

Postmes, T., Spears, R., & Lea, M. (1998). Breaching or building social boundaries? SIDE effects of computer-mediated communication. *Communication Research, 25*(6), 689-715.

Powell, W.W. (1996). Trust-based forms of governance. In R.M. Kramer & T.R. Tyler (Eds.), *Trust in organizations: Frontiers of theory and research* (pp. 51-67). Thousand Oaks, CA: Sage, Inc.

Rousseau, P.L., & Wachtel, P. (1998). Financial intermediation and economic performance: Historical evidence from five industrialized countries. *Journal of Money, Credit and Banking, 30*(4), 657-678.

Shapiro, S.P. (1987). Policing trust. In C.D. Shearing & P.C. Stenning (Eds.), *Private policing* (pp. 194-220). Newbury Park, CA: Sage Publications, Inc.

Sitkin, S.B. (1995). On the positive effect of legalization on trust. In R.J. Bies, B.H. Sheppard & R.J. Lewicki (Eds.), *Research on negotiation in organizations* (pp. 185-217). Greenwich, CT: JAI Press.

Stewart, K.J. (2003). Trust transfer on the World Wide Web. *Organization Science, 14*(1), 5-17.

Teece, D.J. (1980). Economies of scope and the scope of the enterprise. *Journal of Economic Behavior and Organization, 1*(3), 223-247.

Wang, W., & Benbasat, I. (2005). Trust in and adoption of online recommendation agents. *Journal of the Association for Information Systems, 6*(3), 72-101.

Wareham, J., & Klein, R. (2003). Intermediation structures in electronic healthcare portals. In A. Armoni (Ed.), *Effective healthcare information systems* (pp. 237-248). Hersey, PA: IRM Press.

Wilson, E.V. (2003). Asynchronous healthcare communication. *Communications of the Association of Computing Machinery, 46*(6), 79-84.

Wrightsman, L.S. (1991). Interpersonal trust and attitudes toward human nature. In J.P. Robinson, P.R. Shaver & L.S. Wrightsman (Eds.), *Measures of personality and social psychological attitudes: Volume 1: Measures of social psychological attitudes* (pp. 373-412). San Diego, CA: Academic Press, Inc.

Zaheer, A., McEvily, B., & Perrone, V. (1998). Does trust matter: Exploring the effects of interorganizational and interpersonal trust on performance. *Organization Science, 9*(2), 141-159.

Zucker, L.G. (1986). Production of trust: Institutional sources of economic structure 1840-1920. In B.M. Straw & L.L. Cummings (Eds.), *Research in organizational behavior* (pp. 53-111). Greenwich, CT: JAI Press.

Zucker, L.G., Darby, M.R., Brewer, M.B., & Peng, Y. (1996). Collaborative structure and information dilemmas in biotechnology: Organizational boundaries as trust production. In R.M. Kramer & T.R. Tyler (Eds.), *Trust in organizations: Frontiers of theory and research* (pp. 90-113). Thousand Oaks, CA: Sage, Inc.

Chapter IX
Involving Patients and the Public in E-Health Research

John Powell
Warwick Medical School, University of Warwick, UK

Natalie Armstrong
Social Science Group, Department of Health Sciences, University of Leicester, UK

ABSTRACT

This chapter deals with the principles and practice of patient and public involvement in e-health research, and discusses some of the issues raised. In the first part of this chapter, we discuss the problems of defining an "e-health consumer," and discuss why, how and when to involve consumers in e-health research. We also set out principles to guide effective consumer involvement, and the benefits that this can bring in the e-health arena. In the second part of this chapter, we describe how consumers were successfully involved, through a variety of methods, in the development and evaluation of an Internet-based intervention to aid diabetes self-management. Patient and public involvement in research is not the same as undertaking research on patients or the public. It is about understanding, incorporating and benefiting from the relevant consumer perspective, at various levels, throughout the stages of a project.

INTRODUCTION

Consumer involvement in research is not the same as undertaking research on consumers. It is about understanding and incorporating the consumer perspective into the project, often from the very initial stages. Effective consumer involvement can bring many benefits to e-health research projects—from identifying the most relevant outcome measures, to aiding recruitment of research participants, to assisting the dissemination of findings. We are indebted to staff at the UK consumer involvement charity INVOLVE for their assistance with our consumer involvement strategy at Warwick Medical School, and for the materials on consumer involvement available at www.invo.org.uk.

The achievement of meaningful and useful involvement of consumers in research is a challenge for all health services researchers. It is of particular interest to those working in the field of e-health for several specific reasons which themselves create further challenges. First, e-health is a new field with an emerging research agenda, and is therefore well placed to benefit from the different insights that consumers can bring. But equally, as a new area do consumers have sufficient knowledge to give informed comment? Second, while it is relatively straightforward to identify (for example) people with diabetes to help with diabetes research, e-health consumers do not in general define themselves as such. This creates challenges of definition, and challenges for recruiting consumers. Third, e-health researchers will naturally look to methods of e-involvement to achieve consumer participation in research, but these have their own problems. Not least among these is the exclusion of certain consumers who may not be e-health literate (Norman & Skinner, 2006), but who may still have important contributions to make.

In this chapter, we will establish the principles and conceptual basis for involving patients and the public in the development and evaluation of e-health applications. We will also review and discuss current approaches to consumer involvement in the development of e-health applications. Finally, we will demonstrate how consumers were successfully involved in the development and evaluation of an Internet-based intervention to aid diabetes self-management.

BACKGROUND

The terminology in this area can be problematic (Herxheimer & Goodare, 1999). Health consumers have been defined, in a rather all encompassing fashion, as "patients, past patients, prospective patients, long-term users of health services, relatives caring for patients or users, and people who speak for these primary consumers through local and national support and activist groups, community organizations such as community health councils, local and national coalitions of such groups, and international networks" (Williamson, 2001, p. 661). None of the alternative terms used to describe people who interact with health services and whose views we wish to capture (consumers, users, patients, clients, lay individuals, and so on) is value-free (Coulter, 2002). These terms are often

Box 1. Ten reasons for involving consumers in e-health research (Incorporating findings from Hanley et al., 2004)

1. To ensure that research topics which are relevant to real people get priority
2. To bring a different perspective to help shape an emerging field of research
3. To capture first hand experience of a health condition
4. To improve methods
5. To improve results
6. To facilitate the adoption of research findings
7. To involve the people whose taxes fund public research programmes
8. To involve the people who will be most affected by the research findings
9. To build capacity of consumers with e-health research skills
10. To empower the consumers of e-health services

specific to certain disciplines or locations. This chapter takes a pragmatic approach, discussing consumer involvement, but acknowledging that others may prefer alternate terms.

Ten reasons for involving consumers in e-health research are listed in Box 1. This list draws on work in the United Kingdom by the charity INVOLVE, as well as our own experience. The first of these reasons is to ensure that the topics that are researched in the first place are those which have some relevance to the consumers of health services. Researchers can sometimes pursue esoteric lines of enquiry and it is possible to lose touch with the bigger picture. Consumers may also have valuable local knowledge which cannot be captured in other ways. If consumers are involved in research departments and in grant funding bodies, they can help to ensure that topics of relevance to patients and the public get chosen in the first place. The second reason for consumer involvement is linked to the first: that consumers will bring a different, lay perspective to research. Researchers, policy-makers and practitioners who have traditionally set the research agenda bring their own disciplinary perspectives and the views of lay representatives can be a constructive challenge to these. For example fresh ideas from a lay person may ensure that alternative research approaches are considered. This is particularly important in an emerging research area such as e-health where new ideas and techniques are being developed all the time.

The third reason is concerned with capturing first hand experience of a health condition. The last few years have witnessed the rise of the informed, expert patient (Gray, 2002). It is now widely accepted that those with first hand experience of a health condition have acquired valuable expertise which was previously unrecognised by many in the health professions. Research can benefit from capturing and harnessing this expertise. For example, expert patients may be able to give researchers an insight into day-to-day living with a health condition, which will allow researchers to design their study to minimise disruption to patients and maximise concordance. Consumer involvement can bring further significant improvement to both the methods and the results of a research project. For example, the selection of the most appropriate, consumer-relevant outcome measures for an intervention study will improve the methods. Results can be improved by maximising recruitment to a study, and consumer involvement can achieve this through identifying the optimal situations for recruitment, such as time and location, and by facilitating access to otherwise hard to reach groups.

A further reason concerns the adoption of research findings. If consumers are involved in a research project, it can increase the face validity of that project for other consumers and for professionals. Improved face validity will mean that findings are more likely to be seen as valid and to be adopted. Furthermore, consumers can advise on the best routes for disseminating findings to the public, and the appropriate vocabulary to use. The next two reasons are both moral issues. There is a strong moral argument that members of the public should be involved in publicly funded research which they have contributed to through taxation. There is a further moral argument that the people whose lives are ultimately going to be most affected by the research findings should have a prior influence on the research. These moral considerations are gaining prominence with publicly funded research programmes.

The penultimate reason concerns the need to build capacity of consumers with the knowledge and experience to influence e-health research. One of the main barriers to meaningful consumer involvement at present is the availability of consumers with the requisite skills. A sustainable programme of consumer involvement in e-health research needs to build this capacity in order to help future research.

Finally, e-health and in particular the emergence of the Internet as a healthcare tool has been seen as part of the wider movement of increasing consumerism in healthcare and the rise of an informed and empowered healthcare consumer (Henwood, Wyatt, Hart, & Smith, 2003). The easy access to expert information on the Internet, and to personal accounts of illness, poses challenges to professionals (Hardey, 2001). Consumer involvement in research can be seen as a further erosion of professional dominance, and a further contributor to service user empowerment.

HOW TO INVOLVE CONSUMERS IN E-HEALTH RESEARCH

The three levels of consumer involvement have been categorised as consultation, collaboration (also described as active involvement), and user-controlled (also described as user-owned) (Clayton, Oakley, & Pratt, 1997; Hanley, Bradburn, Barnes, Evans, Goodare, Kelson, Kent, Oliver, Thomas, & Wallcraft, 2004). Below these three levels any contribution is considered to be passive (Clayton et al., 1997), where consumers may be supportive but are not truly involved.

The consultative approach is one in which lay people are canvassed for their views on specific issues by the researchers. The commonest method is some form of cross-sectional approach such as a questionnaire survey. This is a relatively simple and straightforward process, and provides a method of identifying lay opinions without making any commitment to act on them (Hanley et al., 2004). Service users were consulted as part of the national listening exercise (postal and e-mail questionnaire) conducted by the UK National Health Service Service Delivery and Organisation research programme in 2002 (Cherry & Anderson, 2002), which identified e-health as one of its research priorities. Other methods of consultation include public meetings, focus groups, and interviews. If consultation is limited to structured questions then responses may fail to address issues which were not previously identified by the researchers. For this reason it can be important for methods of consultation to be flexible in allowing the collection of free-text data. Consultation methods can also be frustrating for those taking part as they may never see what effect their contribution has had. Others go further in criticising the consultative approach as being a form of tokenism whereby the powerless can hear and may have their voices heard but have no influence and no idea as to whether their views are having an effect (Arnstein, 1969).

Collaboration describes the situation of consumers being active partners with professionals in the research process. The benefits of this approach are that consumers can have a more direct influence on the research process, including shaping design aspects such as recruitment and consent procedures, and being involved in the interpretation and dissemination of findings (Hanley et al., 2004). By being active collaborators who can see what effect their influence is having, consumers have a vested interest in delivering successful research. Disadvantages for consumers include the time, skills, and resources required to contribute at a level equal to their researcher colleagues. The perceived power difference between consumer and researcher can be an inhibitory factor. Methods of collaboration generally involve consumers joining the project team and/or the steering group and contributing as equal colleagues at the relevant meetings and discussions. For example, at Warwick University, in an ongoing study of carers' use of information and communication technology, we have involved carers as equal colleagues on the steering group to advise on project progress, and in particular, helping with methods of recruitment and dissemination of results.

User-controlled research is where lay people take the lead role in the research. The benefits are the possibility of addressing issues that professional researchers would miss or disregard, the development of research capacity among consumers, and the empowerment of consumers (Hanley et al., 2004). Problems occur when the research is no longer perceived as being independent, and the reduced role of the professional researcher may threaten the rigour of the methods. Handing over the control of some element of a research project to a lay person may cause difficulties for a professional researcher. To combat this issue, consumers taking a lead role in research need adequate training and support. This emerging area has recently been reviewed by a team at Brunel University in the UK (Turner & Beresford, 2005). They see user-controlled research as a response to feelings of disempowerment and discontent with traditional approaches. There are currently very few published examples in the e-health arena, although one of the issues with user-controlled research is that it does not always get published in scientific journals.

WHEN TO INVOLVE CONSUMERS IN E-HEALTH RESEARCH

Box 2 shows that consumers can be usefully involved, whether using consultative, collaborative or user-controlled perspectives, at any stage of the research process. That is not to say that they should always be involved at all stages, or always from the same perspective. Consumer involvement should be undertaken with a specific project aim in mind, and in the stage of the process and nature of involvement should be determined by this aim. Involvement without thoughtful planning as to what it might achieve, even if it occurs throughout the research process, can be as tokenistic and valueless as the handpicked inclusion of an acquiescent consumer on a researcher dominated committee.

It is tempting for e-health researchers to harness e-methods to involve consumers. These methods (such as e-mail or Web-based surveys, e-mail consensus gathering, Internet discussion boards) certainly have cost advantages. They also access a population likely to have high levels of e-health literacy, and who may be hard to identify using traditional methods. In establishing an e-health User Group at the University of Warwick, we initially wrote to local patient and carer groups seeking volunteers but had a poor response, we suspect because people do not generally define themselves as e-health consumers in the same way that they may well define themselves as being (for example) diabetic and belonging to a wider community of diabetics. E-methods are, therefore, valuable in capturing the views of the e-health consumer population. However e-health

Box 2. Ten stages in the research process at which consumers can be involved (adapted from Hanley et al., 2004)

1. Identifying topics for research
2. Prioritising research proposals
3. Commissioning specific projects
4. Designing methods
5. Undertaking research
6. Analysing data
7. Interpreting results
8. Disseminating findings
9. Evaluating the research process
10. Managing research

researchers must not neglect the views of those who are not regular Internet users. These views can be of equal value, as one of the challenges for e-health is to identify barriers to uptake.

There are other pitfalls for the e-health researcher to avoid. The first of these is tokenism. Consumer involvement is now widely regarded by research funding bodies as an essential component of research. It is also perceived as being time consuming and problematic. There is a danger that projects will pay lip-service to the concept by the tokenistic inclusion of perhaps one lay person in a peripheral role. Such an approach would ignore the added value that consumers can bring to research. E-health researchers are in a position to combat tokenism by harnessing new methods of e-involvement of large numbers of consumers, for example through e-mail and discussion board consultation.

A further, related pitfall is that of representativeness. It is not possible for all lay representatives to be elected unanimously by their peers, share all the characteristics of those peers, and be able to convey the accurate, current views of their peers. Compromises have to be made. Researchers must be aware that the views and characteristics of some consumers will not be shared by others and should strive to capture all diverse opinions within their chosen method of consumer involvement. With a small selection of consumers the required technique is therefore more akin to purposive sampling in qualitative research than a large random sample.

PRINCIPLES TO GUIDE CONSUMER INVOLVEMENT

Certain principles can be used to guide effective consumer involvement (Baxter, Thorne, & Mitchell, 2001; Faulkner, 2005).

- **Clarity.** There needs to be clear identification of the roles and responsibilities of all involved with a project, including consumers. The use of a job description for consumers contributing to a project can be very valuable in providing this clarity.
- **Openness.** The whole process of consumer involvement must be transparent. This includes full details of the research, how consumers' views will be taken into account alongside other influences, and the required commitment from consumers (including information on the duration of the process).
- **Respect.** The involvement of consumers must be nonexploitative. Their views should be taken into account as originally stated to them and they should be kept informed of the consequences. There should be recompense for any out of pocket expenses such as travel costs.
- **Accessibility.** The processes put in place to involve consumers should maximise accessibility. Attention, therefore, needs to be paid to terminology used in documents (avoiding jargon), to the times and locations of meetings, and to any special needs that the relevant user group may have. Linked to accessibility is the notion of inclusiveness. Consumer involvement should not present any barriers to participation due to disability, language, or other characteristics such as age, gender, ethnicity or religious beliefs. Involved consumers should reflect the diversity of the consumer population.
- **Support.** Consumers need to be properly prepared and receive training to undertake their tasks if necessary. This should be provided by the research project. Financial support should be provided if consumers have to forego their usual employment in order to participate. Researchers may also choose to make honoraria payments to reflect the contribution of consumers. Other forms of support may also be necessary—for example, in an upcoming study of the use of information and communication technolo-

gies by carers of people with dementia, we will be providing respite care to allow us to involve carers.

CONSUMER INVOLVEMENT IN THE DESIGN AND EVALUATION OF AN INTERNET-BASED TOOL FOR DIABETES SELF-MANAGEMENT

At the University of Warwick, we have been undertaking a project to design and evaluate a tool for Internet-based self-management and support of people with diabetes (Armstrong, Hearnshaw, Powell & Dale, 2007; Armstrong, Powell, Hearnshaw & Dale, 2007). This "Virtual Clinic" allows a person with diabetes to communicate with his or her health professionals via a messaging system, find information on diabetes, and participate in both asynchronous peer-to-peer discussion boards and real-time chat sessions. This project aims to evaluate the feasibility, acceptability, and effectiveness of such a system through a programme of research comprised of three stages: first, a stakeholder consultation with consumers; second, a pretesting session to trial the intervention developed; and third, a six month pilot study with patients and health professionals. Throughout this project, we have strived to bring meaningful public and patient involvement to our work. In this section we describe these activities to illustrate how consumer views have been captured and incorporated in a real example.

We involved consumers in the following ways:

1. Use of a consumer panel to shape the study;
2. Membership of the project steering group;
3. Interviews and focus group discussion to shape the design of the intervention;
4. E-mail consensus gathering to refine the intervention;
5. A workshop bringing together consumers, practitioners and researchers;
6. A computer-lab based intervention pretest and focus group discussion.

The methods and results of these activities are described, together with an assessment of their strengths and weaknesses.

1. Use of a consumer panel to shape the study. For several years, Warwick Medical School's "Warwick Diabetes Care" has supported a user group of lay people with diabetes whose purpose is to support researchers in all areas of diabetes research. The Warwick Diabetes Care Research User Group (WDCRUG) meets bi-monthly, and one of its main roles is to examine developing research projects and provide input and feedback from a consumer perspective. It is typical for WDCRUG to be involved from an early stage in a project's development, for example to help with defining a research question/topic or to suggest the best ways to recruit participants. With regard to our work on developing the "Virtual Clinic" tool, the WDCRUG was consulted throughout development of the study and made comments on early draft proposals. Their early positive feedback on the "Virtual Clinic" concept provided encouragement that this was a project worth pursuing and they have been kept up to date with developments and study progress since then.

In terms of assessing the strengths and weaknesses of this particular form of consumer involvement, it is interesting to contrast our experience of consulting the well-established, disease-specific, WDCRUG with the first author's attempts to establish an e-health user group at Warwick Medical School. This aims to be a virtual network of individuals who have an interest in using the Internet to support their healthcare or the healthcare of someone they care for. The network will primarily run by e-mail and bulletin board, with occasional face-to-face meetings. However, while WDCRUG found that it was relatively easy to identify individuals who define themselves as "diabetes users," it has been extremely difficult to find volunteers who perceive themselves as "e-health users" and wish to take such a role on this advisory panel. We wrote to all consumer and carer organisations in the local health community requesting volunteers to form this group, but recruited less than ten volunteers. Interestingly, several of these volunteers had a health problem that severely restricted their mobility and would restrict attendance at face-to-face meetings. The establishment of the e-health user group continues, with attempts to "snowball" sample from a few initial volunteers. We also hope to involve some of the diabetes service users engaged in the "Virtual Clinic" work, to help build "e-health user" capacity.

2. Membership of the project steering group. From the outset, the direction of the research has been guided by a project steering group with members from a diverse range of backgrounds, including lay and health professional representation. Having lay and professional involvement on an equal basis in the project steering group has been of great importance to the study. In particular, the lay member has helped to ensure that both the research protocol and the intervention under development have incorporated the consumer perspective. For example, the sampling strategy for our focus groups was guided by advice from the lay representative. It has been our experience that finding representatives to sit on this steering group was relatively straightforward, using existing links with diabetes user groups to request volunteers. The on-going commitment to attend meetings on a regular basis has been slightly more problematic, with the need for a flexible approach to the timetabling of meetings, to avoid clashes with work commitments. This will be a particular issue for any study with lay representatives in full time employment. To reduce the amount of face to face contact time required, and the hassle this can cause, we also encouraged e-mail comments on documents, from all representatives on the steering group, and we consulted specific members (including lay representative) by telephone and e-mail on issues which required their expertise.

3. Interviews and focus group discussion to shape the design of the intervention. When developing the "Virtual Clinic" tool, we wanted to ensure that it was able to meet the needs of consumers as closely as possible. To this end, we carried out a detailed consultation with patients receiving their care in a local diabetes clinic, as well as with the health professionals working there. In order to gather detailed and consumer-led data, a qualitative approach was taken. Three focus groups with patients were held, each containing between three and five participants (twelve in total: two male and ten female). Additionally, five interviews were carried out with health professionals. Both the focus groups and the interviews were similar in format. First, a demonstration was given in order to familiarise participants with the concepts we were developing and the features the "Virtual Clinic" may contain. Following this, the discussion was opened up for participants to give their input. The topic guide in both cases focused upon: participants' initial reactions to the idea, the most and least important/useful elements, whether they would be likely to use such a system, factors that may facilitate or hinder use, what the benefits may be, and any concerns they may have. Interviews and focus groups were audio-recorded and transcribed, and transcripts analysed thematically.

This method of involving consumers in our work was very successful and provided valuable insights into how participants saw the new tool fitting in with, and improving, their current experience of receiving diabetes care. It was important for us as researchers to receive feedback about which elements patients felt would be most useful. This enhanced our understanding of how the intervention could best help patients. For example, participants focused heavily on how they would value the peer-to-peer support available through asynchronous discussion boards and real-time chat. This feature was not well developed in the prototype version that was used for the focus group demonstrations, and we were, therefore, alerted to the need to develop this aspect more fully. In contrast, an element of the intervention that had previously been felt to be important to patients, the facility to upload blood glucose readings from their meter and display them graphically on screen, received only a lukewarm reception. It was also useful to capture patients' views on the usability of the "Virtual Clinic." It was clear that their preference was for an intervention that was straightforward and easy to use, rather than a more complex intervention with many features, but which they would be unlikely to use. This important feedback highlighted the value of practical usability over "flashiness," and gave us the confidence to go ahead with later stages of the work with a more basic version of the "Virtual Clinic" than originally planned.

We found that the organisation and recruitment for this stage of the work was relatively straightforward. The work was approved by the relevant NHS Research Ethics Committee and the NHS Trust in which the diabetes clinic was based, and all participants gave written consent to take part. Patients were largely happy to take part and "give something back" to the health service that they felt had helped them.

4. E-mail consensus gathering to refine the intervention. Following the interviews and focus groups discussed above, a process of e-mail consensus gathering was used to collect the views and experiences of those using Internet-based systems for other long-term conditions and to continue refinement of the "Virtual Clinic." A message was posted on discussion boards for conditions including asthma, epilepsy, mental health, and diabetes, and consumers were invited to e-mail their comments on our system (described in detail in the posting) and the positive elements of other systems they had used. This approach worked less well than the interviews and focus groups, and had a limited response. We found that the majority of responses were received from people who had seen the posting on diabetes boards, with very limited input was received from those with other conditions. This again raises the issue discussed above of the need to carefully define what is meant by a consumer in particular cases, and that perhaps people see their experience of a particular health condition as more salient to giving advice than any shared experience as an "e-health consumer." Certainly, it seems likely that people with long-term conditions other than diabetes either did not see the relevance, or did not feel that they could make a meaningful contribution to an intervention for another health condition of which they had no experience.

5. A workshop to bring together consumers, practitioners and researchers. A more successful method of consumer involvement was a one-day workshop organised to bring together a wider group of stakeholders with expertise in the area of the use of information technology (IT) in the care of people with diabetes. Participants came from a range of backgrounds, including patients, health professionals, and researchers in the area of diabetes care and the use of IT in healthcare. The workshop facilitated discussion and debate on the potential role that IT can have in the care of people with diabetes in general, and considered specific aspects of the "Virtual Clinic" research project. The format included large group plenary sessions and small group discussions. This workshop helped to locate the study within wider debates and developments about the increasing role of e-health in diabetes care, both nationally and internationally, and to explore some of the emerging challenges of the research project.

6. A computer-lab based intervention pre-test and focus group discussion. Following development of an intervention that we felt could meet the needs of consumers as identified through the previous work, a pretest of the intervention was undertaken with consumers. These volunteer patients were recruited from three local hospitals. The session took the form of a computer-lab based session, in which consumers were introduced to the system, logged on and asked to experiment with using it, followed by a focus group in which they gave us their feedback. In preparation for this pretest, the "Virtual Clinic" was set up with some introductory messages posted on the discussion board and example material in other sections, such as links to information on diabetes, dates in the calendar section, and messages from the research team about forthcoming data collection points. Consumers tested the system for approximately thirty minutes and were encouraged to use it interactively (for example by replying to the pre-posted messages and starting new threads), in addition to simply exploring what features it offered. Following this hands-on session, the consumers took part in a discussion that focused on: their general experience of using the system, the features they liked or disliked, the positive and any negative aspects of using the system, and whether they thought using the "Virtual Clinic" would be beneficial. We were very pleased that consumers reported the "Virtual Clinic" as being easy and straightforward to use; with all the features they could envisage needing. We feel the development of a system that so comprehensively meets consumers' needs is a direct result of our commitment to involving consumers in the development of the project from the outset.

The "Virtual Clinic" study is still ongoing, and we aim to achieve further consumer involvement at the next stages of interpretation of findings, dissemination, and developing protocols for further research.

CONCLUSION

In this chapter, we have discussed the involvement of patients and the public in e-health research. We have established the principles and conceptual basis for involving patients and the public in the development and evaluation of e-health applications. We have described the reasons for such engagement, and the levels and stages at which this can take place. We have also used our experience in one research project to illustrate some of the methods of involvement and demonstrate how consumers were successfully involved in the development and evaluation of an Internet-based intervention to aid diabetes self-management.

The widespread acceptance of the value of involving consumers in research is a relatively recent phenomenon, going hand-in-hand with the recognition of the role of the informed, expert patient. As an emerging area for research, e-health is well placed to be at the forefront of effective consumer involvement. E-methods can and should support public and patient involvement. The use of such methods to effectively harness consumer views represents an exciting area for future research. However, given the existence of the digital divide, care must also be taken to include the views of the digitally excluded, as well as the digitally included—to involve the have-nots as well as the have-Nets. Those with low levels of e-health literacy may be exactly the people to provide insights into the facilitators and barriers in the adoption of e-health technologies.

ACKNOWLEDGMENT

The authors gratefully acknowledge receiving advice from staff at the UK consumer involvement charity INVOLVE (http://www.invo.org.uk), and the use of materials produced by INVOLVE as referenced in the text. This chapter is based on a talk given at the MedNet 2006 conference, held in Toronto, Canada.

REFERENCES

Armstrong, N., Hearnshaw, H., Powell, J., & Dale, J. (2007). Stakeholder perspectives on the development of a virtual clinic for diabetes care: Qualitative study. *Journal of Medical Internet Research, 9*(3), e23. Retrieved May 26, 2008, from http://www.jmir.org/20073/e23

Armstrong, N., Powell, J., Hearnshaw, H., & Dale, J. (2007). Design of a trial of internet-based self-management for diabetes. *Journal of Telemedicine and Telecare, 13*(Supplement 1), 1-2.

Arnstein, S.R. (1969). A ladder of citizen participation in the USA. *Journal of the American Institute of Planners, 35*(4), 216-224.

Baxter, L., Thorne, L., & Mitchell, A. (2001). *Small voices, big noises. Lay involvement in health research: Lessons from other fields.* Exeter, UK: Washington Singer Press.

Cherry, C., & Anderson, S. (2002). *Refreshing the national listening exercise: Report of the findings.* London, UK: National Co-ordinating Centre for NHS Service Delivery and Organisation.

Clayton, A., Oakley, P., & Pratt, B. (1997). *Empowering people: A guide to participation.* Oxford, UK: INTRAC.

Coulter, A. (2002). *The autonomous patient: Ending paternalism in medical care.* London, UK: The Stationery Office.

Faulkner, A. (2005). *Service user involvement in the UK Mental Health Research Network. Guidance for good practice.* London, UK: UK Mental Health Research Network Service User Research Group England (SURGE).

Gray, J.A.M. (2002). *The resourceful patient.* Oxford, UK: eRosetta Press.

Hanley, B., Bradburn, J., Barnes, M., Evans, C., Goodare, H., Kelson, M., Kent, A., Oliver, S., Thomas, S. & Wallcraft, J. (2004). *Involving the public in NHS, public health, and social care research: Briefing notes for researchers (second edition).* Hampshire, UK: INVOLVE.

Hardey, M. (2001). E-health: The Internet and transformation of patients into consumers and producers of health knowledge. *Information, Communication and Society, 4*(3), 388-405.

Henwood, F., Wyatt, S., Hart, A., & Smith, J. (2003). Ignorance is bliss sometimes: Constraints on the emergence of the 'informed patient' in the changing landscapes of health information. *Sociology of Health and Illness, 25*(6), 589-607.

Herxheimer, A., & Goodare, H. (1999). Who are you, and who are we? Looking through some key words. *Health Expectations, 2*(1), 3-6.

Norman, C.D., & Skinner, H.A. (2006). E-health literacy: Essential skills for consumer health in a networked world. *Journal of Medical Internet Research, 8*(2), e9. Retrieved May 26, 2008, from at http://www.jmir.org/2006/2/e9/

Turner M., & Beresford, P. (2005). *User controlled research. Its meanings and potential. Final report.* Hampshire, UK: INVOLVE.

Williamson, C. (2001). What does involving consumers in research mean? *QJM: An International Journal of Medicine, 94*(12), 661-664.

Section II
Applications

Chapter X
Using Interaction Design to Improve Usability of a PHR User Interface Based on Visual Elements

Stefano Forti
e-Health Applied Research Unit, FBK-Fondazione Bruno Kessler, Italy

Barbara Purin
e-Health Applied Research Unit, FBK-Fondazione Bruno Kessler, Italy

Claudio Eccher
e-Health Applied Research Unit, FBK-Fondazione Bruno Kessler, Italy

Nicolò Luppino
Faculty of Art & Design, University of Venezia, Italy

Carlo Busolin
Faculty of Art & Design, University of Venezia, Italy

Diego Conforti
Department of Health, Autonomous Province of Trento, Italy

Gianni Martini
Freelance Social Researcher, Trento, Italy

ABSTRACT

This chapter presents a case study of using interaction design methods for exploring and testing usability and user experience of a Personal Health Record (PHR) user interface based on visual and graphical elements. To identify problems and improve the design of PHR user interface we conducted two task-oriented usability testing based on the think-aloud technique for observing users during their interaction with a high-fidelity PHR prototype, and questionnaires and semistructured interviews for measuring user satisfaction. Our study demonstrates that a user-centered approach to interaction design involving the final users in an iterative design-evaluation process is important for exploring innovative user interfaces and for identification of problems in the early stages of the development cycle of a PHR.

INTRODUCTION

The Markle Foundation's Connecting for Health working group in its report "Connecting Americans to their healthcare" (Markle Foundation, 2004) defines Personal Health Record (PHR) as: "an electronic application through which individuals can access, manage and share their health information in a secure and confidential manner" (pp. 13). In the last years, PHR has been gaining great attention from healthcare institutions and organizations, due to its potential for a more active involvement of citizens in their care and improvement of relationships and communication between patients and their healthcare providers (Brailer, 2004; Cohn, 2007). Recently, in its report on the prevention of medication errors (IOM, 2007), the Institute of Medicine has identified PHR systems as a viable technology to support consumers' self-management.

Worldwide research institutions, government and healthcare authorities have identified PHR as a top priority, established broad areas for research and evaluation of PHR systems, and acknowledged the necessity of demonstration and pilot projects as a critical next step to address and exploit the full potential of PHR-based systems and services (Brailer, 2004; Cohn, 2007; Markle Foundation, 2004; Tang, Joan, Ash, Bates, Overhage, & Sands, 2006).

In order to design a working system, the involvement of final users is a crucial phase, even though it is often undervalued (Nielsen, 1993). For example, in healthcare settings, it has been demonstrated that the most innovative project could fail because of a rushed interface design (i.e., an interface limited to a subjective taste) that can compromise the user's acceptability, strongly influencing the use of a system (Bates, Kuperman, Wang, Gandhi, Kittler, Volk, Spurr, Khorasani, Tanasijevic, & Middleton, 2003). This seems to be particularly true in the context of development of a PHR-based system, since we are dealing with citizens, a deeply nonhomogeneous group, due to the disparity of age, cultural level, living context, healthcare and computer literacy.

Interaction design emphasizes the importance of involving final users throughout the whole process of design of the product or system within an iterative design-evaluation process. Preece, Rogers, and Sharp (2002, pp. 170, 285) state that a user-centered approach to development "forms a central plank" of interaction design process and "the real user and their goals, not just technology, should be the driving force behind development of a product."

In the last years, several groups have applied user-centered approaches and usability testing in healthcare settings for the design and implementation of clinical information systems (Coble, Karat, Orland, & Kahn, 1997; Kushniruk & Patel, 2004; Kushniruk, Patel, Cimino, & Barrows, 1996; Zhang, Johnson, Patel, Paige, & Kubose, 2003). To our knowledge, only few studies have applied a user-centered approach to design and development of a PHR system (Tran, Zhang, Stolyar, & Lober, 2005).

During the last year, the Department of Health of the Autonomous Province of Trento (NE Italy) has promoted a feasibility study on the design of a PHR-based system. One of the preliminary research questions of the study was to explore whether and how visual design solutions can promote user's usability and acceptance of a PHR-based system. A first requirement for using a visual approach in the design of the PHR system was to create a clean nonredundant interface that would reassure and communicate calm and serenity to users and guide them through a user-friendly navigation throughout the PHR. A second, but not less important, requirement is that a user interface based on visual elements would be portable and usable in a touch-screen paradigm on mobile devices (i.e., palm top) with minor modifications.

This chapter describes the use of interaction methods, particularly usability testing, for exploring and testing usability and user experience of a

PHR user interface based on visual elements.

This chapter is organized as follows: The first section introduces basic concepts on interaction design. The second section briefly illustrates visual design, and the third section describes how we take into account visual design recommendations, in order to create an innovative PHR user interface. The fourth section presents the usability testing for evaluating the PHR user interface prototype. The fifth section reports conclusions and briefly outlines future activities.

Interaction Design

Interaction design can be described as a user-centered approach to design that involves four basic activities (Preece, Rogers, & Sharp, 2002). These activities regard the identification of needs and requirements, the development of alternative designs, the creation of interactive version of the design, and the evaluation of the usability and acceptability of the interactive version. Interaction design emphasizes the importance of involving final users throughout the whole process of design of the product or system within an iterative design-evaluation process.

There are two important aspects that characterize the interaction design process. The first aspect regards the evaluation phase, in particular the usability testing methods, through which "specific usability and user experience goals should be identified[...] at the beginning of the project" with the aim of helping designers and developers "to choose between alternative designs and to check on progress as the product is developed" (Preece, Rogers, & Sharp, 2002, pp. 170). The second concerns the concept of iterative design in which cycles of design-test-measure-and-redesign are repeated several times as often as necessary. Preece et al. (2002, pp. 170) state that iteration is "inevitable because designers never get the solution right the first time," particularly "if you are trying to innovate."

Interaction design consists of several techniques and approaches to perform an iterative user-centered evaluation of the system under construction. The evaluation design phase identifies four different evaluation paradigms: "quick and dirty" evaluation, usability testing, field studies, and predictive evaluation (Preece et al., 2002). We opted for the usability testing since it has been demonstrated to be an effective methodology for user interface design (Dumas & Redish, 1999; Rubin, 1994), and fits well a user-centered approach to the iterative development of applications.

Usability testing provides for several techniques, which can be categorized in user observation, asking users' opinion, and testing user performance (Preece, Rogers, & Sharp, 2002). In particular, the think-aloud technique (Erikson & Simon, 1985) is a powerful tool for observing users while using the system, since it allows the externalizing users' thought processes. For this reason, it is increasingly being used for the practical evaluation of human-computer interfaces, also in the medical informatics domain (Kushniruk & Patel, 2004). This technique, combined with the analysis of video recorded user interactions, has been reported to represent a valuable tool for building electronic medical record interfaces (Jaspers, Steen, van den Bos, & Geenen, 2004; Johnson & Johnson, 2006; Sharda, Cohen, & Patel, 2006; Waller, Franklin, Pagliari, & Greene, 2007).

The goal of evaluation is not only to design efficient systems (usability goals), but also to develop systems capable of eliciting positive responses from users motivating them to use the systems and increasing the likelihood of future use (user's experience goals). Recently, user-centered design has received major attention in the healthcare domain (Zhang, 2005) as it has been considered necessary for the successful development of health information systems (Johnson, Johnson, & Zhang, 2005; Rose, Schnipper, Park, Poon, Li, & Middleton, 2005).

Visual Design

Visual design (or visual communication) is composed of two intertwined parts: visual organization, and personality. Visual organization deals with the creation of informative layouts through the principles of perception and visual weight, while personality (or "look and feel") is mainly concerned with the use of fonts, colours, shapes, textures, and images to elicit a positive emotional response by the user (Wroblewski, 2002). Using techniques of graphical design for developing alternative designs has been demonstrated that stimulates innovative interactive system design (Danis & Boies, 2000).

Visual design may play an important role in user's acceptance and usability of PHR. In fact, when citizens cope with the use of a PHR for the management of their clinical data, they should experience this moment not as a heavy work task but rather as a voluntary and quiet activity, useful for their own health. Although it has been demonstrated that visual design can positively contribute to usability of Web applications and support or impair different aspects of user's behaviour (Wroblewski, 2002), unfortunately it is often underused in design and implementation of healthcare information systems.

A PHR User Interface Based on Visual Elements

At a first step, starting from a defined PHR data model, we adopted the visual design approach to design the pages constituting the PHR interface making broadly use of visual elements. The key-element is a circle connected to similar circles in an organic shape that evokes water drop's molecular structure. Such element characterizes all pages and was chosen as vital elements for mankind. Each element has proper dimension, colour, and spatial positioning depending on its function and importance, as well as a label identifying the subject.

Designing an effective home page is a crucial task. An improper home page can seriously jeopardize the PHR objectives. In fact, the home page is the one page that all citizen-visitors will view. It is the blueprint for the success of PHR since it produces the first impression of the overall System. It should clearly show what the system is about.

Our PHR (Figure 1) is organized around a "menu-home page" that acts as a gateway to the system and provides the map to guide users in the navigation throughout the PHR. Commonly, the content-navigation menu of a Web site is an interactive list that usually appears on the left or right side of the screen. In the home page of our PHR, we have substituted it by a graphical menu making use of organic shapes and pictograms. The clinical information organization is displayed in a geographic-like map: relative relationships are represented by using connections, and the content hierarchy was realized by using different colours, drops' dimensions, and spatial distribution. For example, the "emergency" drop has been positioned on the top left portion of the screen and filled in red in order that, according to the western world of reading, it stands out as the most important element. Also, we used the position of the elements to communicate a temporal pattern. For example, the "biological testament" drop has been positioned on the bottom right, because it regards the last part of the lifetime. By moving the mouse pointer over a shape, a tooltip box appears showing user the information content.

Cyan was chosen as the basic color for the PHR because it is relaxing. In combination with the light-gray background and a rational amount of empty space, this makes the home page minimal, so as not to look too cluttered and confusing. Important items were placed consistently toward the top and center of the page. All items were appropriately vertically and/or horizontally aligned on the pages. A common visual organization has been consistently applied in each page of the PHR. Important clickable items giving access to the PHR services (e.g., vocabularies, help online, print utilities) were placed in a menu bar in the same location, and closer to the top of the page. In this way, they can be immediately found. Under the menu bar on the left side of the page, a rectangular frame shows icon-based elements acting both as the page location path and as a navigation toolbar. The page central area is used for the management of specific services or clinical data (e.g., Web messaging between citizens and health operators).

Considerable effort was dedicated to guide and support the management of clinical information. Clicking over a drop in the home page menu, an organized information subsection is displayed (Figure 2), which on the left side presents a non-clickable image of the previously selected drop. The latter provides location information at a glance and to reassure the user.

After selecting one of the available information-items, the user accesses information-management pages through the forward button (Figure 2, bottom right). A summary page displays a table with the most meaningful data, which are an extract of the whole information recorded in the PHR. The selection of a record allows users to view, modify, or delete the related data. For some clinical information, helpful graphs are also available (see Figure 3).

A button to insert new data is always displayed on the bottom right of the summary page. Pages for data entry have a wizard step-by-step structure to help users fill in the forms. This also allowed us to avoid the use of scroll bars and to have all information always visible in the frame. Most of fields have icon-buttons for specific support services (e.g., vocabularies, calendar, and lists of possible values).

INTERACTION DESIGN APPROACH TO THE DEVELOPMENT OF A VISUAL-BASED PHR: A CASE STUDY

Methods

There are several types of usability tests that can be performed at different moments of a system's life cycle (Kushniruk & Patel, 2004). For example, exploratory tests aim to explore preliminary user interfaces for examining if users are able to navigate from screen to screen and/or within a screen. Exploratory tests can be very useful at the early stage of the development of a system when critical design decisions are to be taken, because wrong assumptions could cause usability problems later (Rubin, 2004).

After having designed the first prototype of the PHR, we performed an early exploratory usability test to explore the effectiveness of our user interface and to gather information on problems that user may encounter when interacting with the PHR specifically related to our design choices.

Study Design

To identify problems and solutions and further refine the prototype we adopted a usability testing based on the think-aloud technique for observing users (Kushniruk & Patel, 2004), and questionnaires and semi-structured interviews for measuring user satisfaction.

The study was divided in two phases with eight participants in each phase (Phase I and Phase II). In fact, according to Nielsen (1993), a number of 5-12 participants is considered adequate to elicit the major issues that would arise in a usability testing. Phase I was carried out on the first prototype of the system. After that, the problems highlighted by the analysis of gathered data served as a guideline to refine the prototype interface. Phase II was carried out on the refined version of the PHR prototype.

In this phase users were asked to carry on the same tasks performed in Phase I. The first eight participants were selected among the patients of a primary healthcare practitioner working in Trento. The second group of participants was recruited among the administrative and technical personnel of our Institution (the Bruno Kessler Foundation of Trento). We enrolled two different groups of citizens because people participating in a usability test phase may get experienced with the system and are no longer novice users seeing the design for the first time (Nielsen, 1993). If the user population is large, as it is the case of PHR users, it is more convenient to conduct usability tests involving groups of users with homogeneous characteristics (Nielsen, 2000). For this first study, we have focused our attention on users with previous experience with Internet as they are the most probable early adopter of PHR systems (Markle Foundation, 2004). Hence, the inclusion criterion was skill in using the Web: namely, use of Internet from more than one year and for more than one hour per week.

The tests were conducted at the General Practitioners' School in Trento and at the Bruno Kessler Foundation building in order to make it convenient for the participants. The test rooms were quiet and pleasant so as to avoid external distraction. Each test session lasted 90 minutes and was managed by the same examiner whose role was to collect data without influencing test's participants.

Data gathering was accomplished in the following ways:

Table 1. Usability test participants' characteristics

Characteristics	Phase I n	Phase II n
Age range (years)		
18-29	0	2
30-39	3	2
40-49	4	4
50-59	1	0
Sex		
Female	6	4
Male	2	4
Education		
High school	6	8
University	2	0
Internet experience		
Less than one year	0	0
More than one year	8	8
Time spent using the Internet		
1 to 3 hours per week	3	2
More than 3 hours per week	5	6
Reason for using the Internet		
At home	0	0
At work	1	1
Both	7	7

Table 2. Usability testing tasks

TASK 1 You decide to record some clinical information about your birth family. Your grandmother on your mother's side died of breast cancer at the age of 80. She had been diagnosed with an ischemic disease since she was 71. She had Alzheimer and cat allergy.
TASK 2 You decide to record some information about your health condition. Last year you were discovered to be allergic to wasp stings that cause you asthma attacks. You treat your allergy with Sandimmum in 50 mg pill form.
TASK 3 You decide to record some information about your health condition. Your family doctor has prescribed Nimesulide for you. You started the drug therapy in May 28. You had taken pills on a full stomach at dinner and before going to bed. But after 10 days you decided to stop therapy because of a bed heartburn.

Table 3. Coded problems in phase I usability testing

Coded categories	Description	Think-aloud (13 comments)	Semi-structured interview (9 comments)
Layout/screen organization	The subject comments on the layout or screen organization.	38.4%	77.8%
Navigation	Subject comments on basic navigation, or indicates he/she can't move through interface etc.	23.1%	0%
Resolution	The subject mentions the resolution of information presented.	15.4%	11.1%
Meaning of labels	The subject comments on the meaning of labels in the interface itself.	15.4%	0%
Color	The subject mentions the use of colors.	7.7%	11.1%
Graphics	The subject explicitly mentions graphics.	0%	0%
Overall ease of use	The subject comments on the overall ease of use.	0%	0%

- A background questionnaire to address possible sources of variation among users: age, gender, educational qualification, and experience with Internet (Table 1);
- The observation of the participants while surfing the PHR pages. During this phase, users were encouraged to "think-aloud" commenting on any difficulties they encountered while performing three data input tasks regarding family's health history, personal health history, and drug treatment (Table 2). These scenarios reflected realistic situations that a PHR user could actually experience. Video and audio were captured by using the Camtasia Studio© Software. By analyzing the content of the recordings, we determined the task completion times and the success of each, as well as a list of problems encountered.
- Two post-task questionnaires for assessing user satisfaction, which users were asked to fill after the completion of the tasks. The first one was mainly focused on usability aspects of the user interface (Table 4) while the second aimed to investigate emotional reactions (Table 5).
- A post-task semi-structured interview, which aimed to explore subjective user

Table 4. Usability questionnaire results

Questions (note 1)	**Phase I**	**Phase II**	**P (Mann Whitney U test)**
Q1: This PHR is visually appealing	0.88	1.25	NS
Q2: It was easy to move from one page to another	-0.25	0.75	0.015
Q3: The overall organization of PHR is easy to understand	-0.25	1.13	0.001
Q4: Individual pages are well designed	0.38	0.63	NS
Q5: Terminology used in PHR is clear	1.00	1.13	NS
Q6: The content of PHR met my expectations	0.25	1.00	NS
Q7: I would be likely to use this PHR in the future	0.63	1.50	0.05
Q8: I was able to complete my tasks in a reasonable amount of time	0.25	1.00	NS
Q9: Overall, this PHR is easy to use	0.00	1.13	0.028

Notes
1. five-point Likert scale(-2=strongly disagree; -1=disagree; 0=neutral; +1=agree; +2=strongly agree)

Table 5. User experience questionnaire results

Questions (note 1)	**Phase I**	**Phase II**	**P (Mann Whitney U test)**
Q1: Intuitive/Not-intuitive	1.00	2.00	NS
Q2: Interesting/Boring	1.38	2.75	0.015
Q3: Clear/Confusing	-0.25	2.13	0.007
Q4: Comfortable/Uncomfortable	0.38	1.50	NS
Q5: Engaging/Unattractive	1.25	1.38	NS
Q7: Satisfying/Displeasing	0.50	1.25	NS
Q8: I like/I dislike	0.38	2.25	0.021

Notes
1. Seven-point semantic scale.Each response was converted to a numerical value in the range [-3, 3].

experiences beyond what was previously observed. Information was gathered starting from a set of summative exit questions about issues that we wished to explore. Such themes regarded troubles found during the previous tasks and what the user like/dislike most about the PHR interface (Table 3).

- A final post-test questionnaire, which asked participants their general opinion about the personal health record.

Statistical Analysis

The first user questionnaire concerning overall usability issues was based on a five-point Likert-type scale ranging form -2 to 2, with 0 as neutral point. User experience was measured through a seven-point differential scale, because it has been demonstrated that this tool is appropriate for registering the aesthetic preferences and gathering information from the participants on their feeling and emotional reaction about the system use. We quantified each judgment of the semantic scale by assigning a score ranging from -3 to +3. For the presentation of the results of both questionnaires, we adopted the more intuitive approach to represent the desirable traits of the system with the higher numbers. Because no assumption can be made on the normality of the rating distributions, the nonparametric Mann-Whitney U test for two independent samples was used to test the null hypothesis that the probability distributions of the scores of the two groups are equal. The conventional level of significance $p = 0.05$ was chosen to reject the null hypothesis.

RESULTS

Participants' Background

The characteristics of the two groups of users are outlined in Table 1. All participants had an Internet experience of more than one year; 62% in the Group I, and 75% in the Group II used Internet more than three hours per week. In both groups, 87% of the participants used Internet both at work and at home.

User Performance

The time for each task completion was recorded. Users performed better using the second version of PHR prototype in terms of user success (100% vs. 91%) and the lesser amount of time to complete each task. The average times to complete the Task 1 in Phase I and Phase II were 4.22 minutes and 3.18 minutes, respectively. The average times to complete the Tasks 2 and 3 were 4.15 minutes and 5.16 minutes in Phase I and 2.52 minutes and 4.23 minutes in Phase II. The average time to complete the scenario (all the three tasks) was 12.41 minutes in Phase I and 10.34 minutes in Phase II. This difference, however, was not statistically significant.

Analysis of the Process Data

Think-aloud reports transcribed in a word processing file were analyzed to identify problems users experienced when interacting with the prototype system. These data were transformed as recommendations to developers to improve and refine the system. A content analysis (Preece, Rogers, & Sharp, 2002) was performed using coding categories described in previous literatures about human-computer interaction (Kushrinuk & Patel, 2004). Such coding categories include *information content, comprehensiveness of graphics and text, problems in navigation* and *overall system understandability*. The same content analysis was made on the data gathered through the semistructured interviews conducted after task completion.

We analyzed all comments (13 coming from the think-aloud reports, and nine from the semistructured interviews), and found that we could categorize the problems into the seven groups shown in Table 3. Specific Kushrinuk's subitems such as *understanding of system instruction/error messages*, *consistency of operations*, *response time* and *visibility of system status* did not apply to our analysis since the prototype did not allow to save/retrieve input data.

The most frequent problems were related to the *layout and screen organization* (Figure 1). First of all, the drop-menu did not visualize the whole information organization, so the user had to surf several pages before finding the desired information; in this context, drop-associated tooltips did not help the user. Second, since the family health history records belonged to the personal profile information group, the user inferred that also the sibling subitems (e.g., *personal data, life, psycho-social profile*) were related to user's family rather than to him/her. Third, many users did not understand that a different color for the *clinical history* drop was used as a signal that this element served only to explore the information rather than allowing data input. In our opinion, this misunderstanding was also due to the label "clinical history" we used.

Even though only the kind of problems discussed above emerged during the semistructured interviews (probably because these problems were perceived as overwhelming), navigation problems also impaired the interaction of the users with the interface. In particular, problems related to both the navigation buttons and navigation toolbar. Moreover, these submenu-like lists in information subsections (see Figure 2) were difficult to use, because they required users to select an item, and then click the forward button to go on, instead of just double clicking the item to open the related page.

Users had difficulties also with input data forms either containing poorly organized fields or with insufficient information about the use of the fields.

Finally, some subjects mentioned the use of colors and suggested to change the color of some elements according to their taste.

The video recordings confirmed all these results and gave us valuable suggestions about how to modify the system interface to reflect those comments.

Figure 1. The home page of our PHR before usability testing. All elements were disposed from left to right according to a temporal ordering on the horizontal axis reflecting the ordering of the events in a person's lifetime. The "emergency drop" (in red) and the "clinical history drop" (in yellow) are tools for the exploration of the recorded data. Clinical information that does not change frequently is represented in blue while information often updated is in cyan. Drops are logical groups of clinical data. The connection between them represents relative relationships while content hierarchy is represented thought drops' dimension and spatial distribution. When the mouse pointer is over a shape, a tooltip box shows user all the content information in that drop.

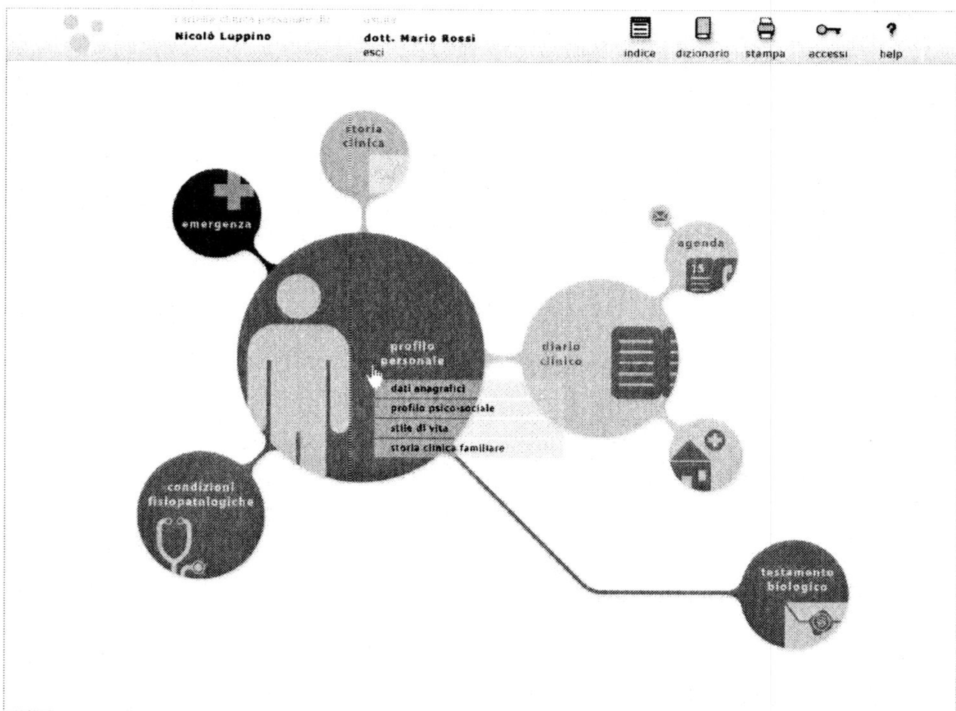

Design Recommendations

In the refinement phase, the major changes were made on the menu-home page. Drops were added so that the whole information organization was displayed. To this end, small nonclickable drops were added to provide tooltips briefly explaining the content. To access this information, the larger connected drop must be selected. The *family health history* was associated with a new drop separated from the *personal profile* one, as shown in Figure 4. The new location was chosen in consideration of the temporal ordering on the horizontal axis. We decided also to decrease the dimensions of the *personal profile* drop and to increase the dimensions of the *clinical diary* one. This is because the former organizes quasistatic information while the latter, allows users to manage data that change frequently, and is of more frequent use. To point out that the *emergency* and *clinical history* drops do not support data input, they were cut off from the main menu. The color of the *clinical history* drop was changed to green in order to not divert user attention away from the other drops on the page.

Detailed one-click, drop-like submenus substituted for submenu-like lists in the information subsections. In this way, menu and submenu have the same aesthetic and the forward button is not necessary.

In all internal pages (Figure 5), a common text page location path works as the main navigation toolbar. Near it, a small nonclickable image of the main menu represents the position of the current page in order to provide this information at a glance. On the top of the opposite page side, two small *emergency* and *family health history* drops are always available for the exploration of the recorded information.

Finally, the forms have been updated by adding instructions for filling in the forms and by fixing errors in labels.

Figure 2. The personal profile subsection before the usability testing. A nonclickable image on the left side of the page represents the drop previously selected. On the right side of the page there is a list of all information available. By selecting an item and clicking the forward button (bottom right of the page) the user accesses to the relative information-management page.

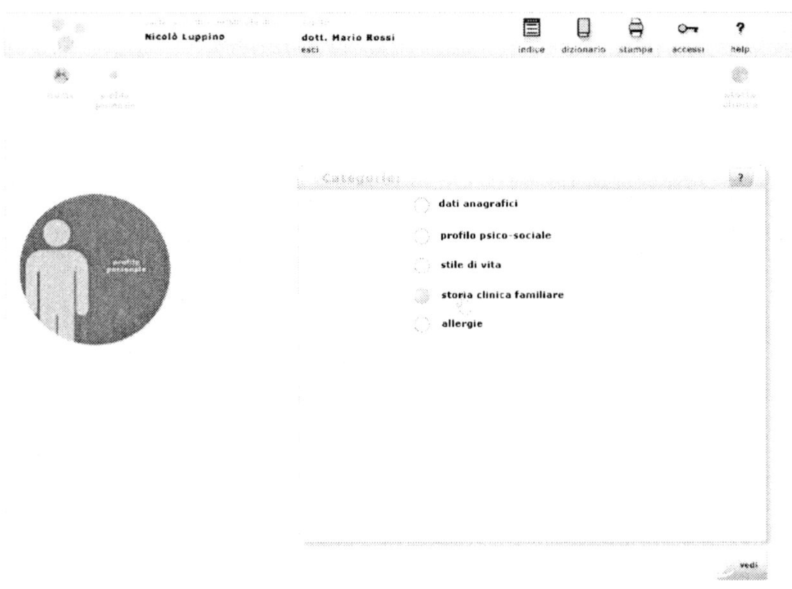

Figure 3. The drugs treatment subsection. The figure A on the top displays a summary page for drug treatments. By clicking on a column's header data are sorted accordingly. The selection of a record allows users to view, modify or delete data by using the buttons below the table. A helpful graph about the drug prescription is also available (figure B). The button on the bottom right of the summary page displays the wizard for input data forms (figure C).

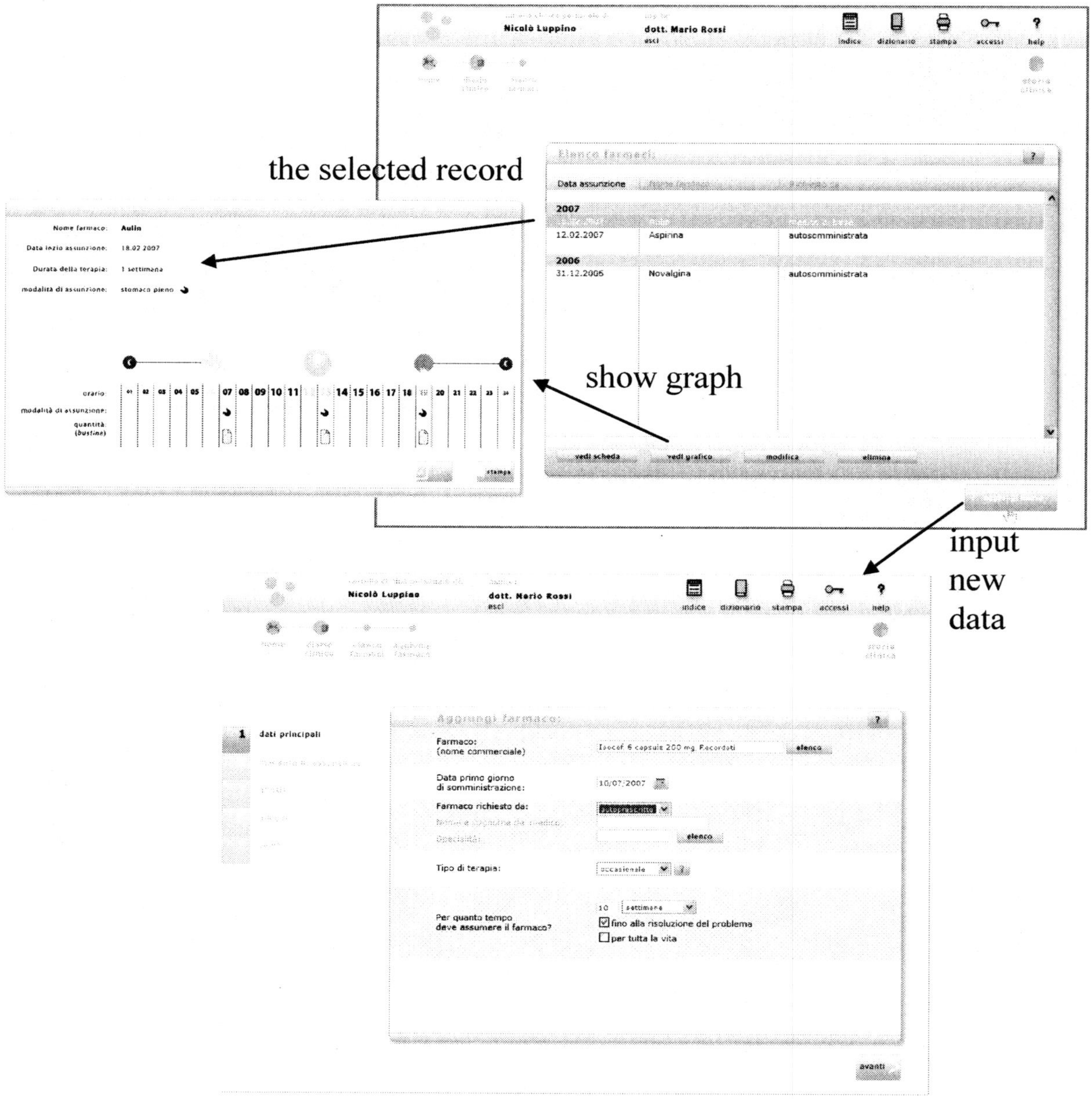

Figure 4. The home page of our PHR after usability testing. The smallest non-clickable drops are added so that to display the whole information organization. The user must select the connected bigger drop to access the information. The "family history drop" is now set apart from the "personal profile" one. Its new location is based on the temporal ordering on the horizontal axis. The "clinical diary drop" is bigger than the "personal profile" one because it gathers information that changes frequently. The "emergency drop" (in red) and the "clinical history drop" (in green) are cut off from the clinical information menu since they are tools for exploring recorded data.

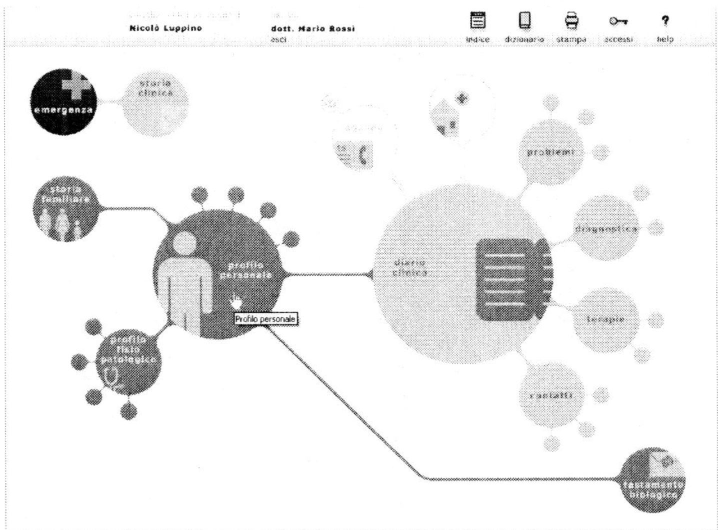

Figure 5. The "user profile" information subsection after usability testing. A drop-like submenu substitutes the menu-like list. Now menu and sub-menu have the same aesthetic. One click on a smallest drop is enough to open the relative page. The selected drop is highlighted in colored in the small non-clickable image on the top left of the page. Near this image there is a common textual page location path that works as a navigation toolbar.

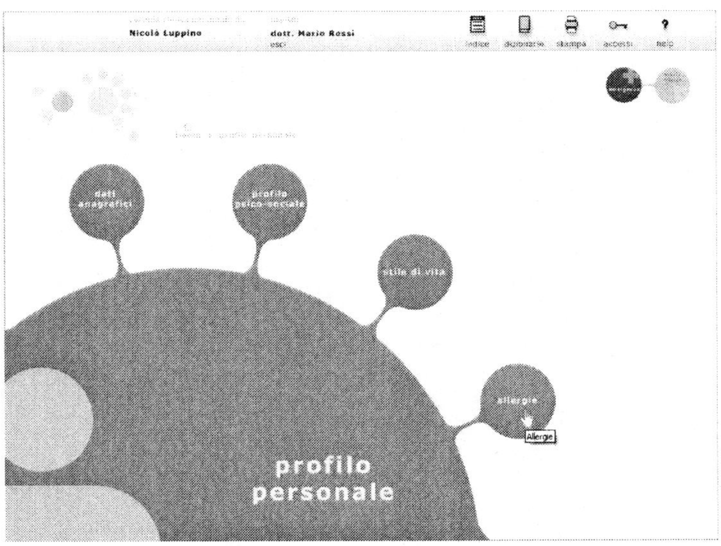

User Satisfaction

The results of the interface usability survey are reported in Table 4. For each question, the table shows the average scores of the questions for Phase I and Phase II, along with the level of significance of the difference. The negative score of questions Q2 and Q3 after Phase I reveals that users encountered serious problems when navigating through the pages and in understanding the overall organization of the information. These results were confirmed by the content analysis of audio-video recording and semi-structured interview. A qualitative comparison of the two phases shows an increase of the average ratings for all questions, indicating a general improvement of the usability after the refinement of the user interface. In particular, for four questions the difference was statistically significant indicating that the interaction design solved some of the problems encountered by the users in the first phase: namely, those related to the easiness of navigation, information organization, and the positive attitude toward use of the system. It is worthy to note that in the refined prototype not all the navigation problems were solved, as indicated by the relatively low score of 0.75 of question Q2.

The results of feeling and emotional reaction questionnaires about the system use are shown in Table 5. As for the preceding table, the average scores for Phase I and Phase II and the level of significance of the difference are reported. As before, the qualitative comparison of the results of the two questionnaires revealed that the users of refined version of the PHR interface experienced a more positive emotional reaction compared to the users of the first version. In particular, the first version of the interface was clearly perceived by the users as confusing (question Q3, average score -0.25), whereas the user judgment of the refined version was reversed (av. score 2.13). The difference of scoring of question Q3 between the two phases was statistically significant. Moreover, changes introduced after the interaction design phase made the PHR interface significantly more interesting (question Q2) and more pleasant (question Q8).

At the end of the usability test, we gathered users' opinions and beliefs about the usefulness of the PHR and their attitude toward using it in real situations. Users were asked to rank their opinion on a seven-point Likert scale from one (not much) to seven (very). All the answers received a very high score. In response to the question, "Do you think that a PHR can be relevant for your health?" the average score was 6.7. The questions, "Do you think that PHR is important for improving the relationship with your general practitioner?" and "Do you think that PHR is beneficial in case of emergency?" were ranked 6.6 and 6.9, respectively. The relevance of PHR in the context of paediatric care was ranked 6.8. All the participants stated that they would like to use the system in the future and would recommend the system to a friend.

CONCLUSION

This chapter demonstrates, through a case study, that interaction design methods incorporating user-centered principles in an iterative design-evaluation process can contribute to improve the design of the user interface of a PHR. One of the key characteristics of the user-centered approach of interaction design is to involve users not only towards the end of system development (e.g., in a summative evaluation), but to involve them throughout the entire development cycle, starting from very early exploratory phases. This work demonstrates that the involvement of representative users at the early stages of the development cycle is fundamental not only for exploring innovative user interfaces, but also for early identification of problems in the user interface that could create more serious usability issues at later stages of the system development.

This study represents an exploratory test to examine the usability and acceptability of an innovative interface based on visual elements and provides evidence that the use of visual and graphical elements in the user interface of PHR elicits positive response from users. Particular attention, however, must be paid to the early identification of usability problems that may impair the use of such kinds of PHR. The involvement of citizens for carrying out iterative usability testing on refined versions of PHR represents an effective way for achieving this.

The work we have described in this chapter is part of a longer-term iterative cycle of PHR evaluation and redesign. In fact, design-evaluation and redesign cycles on different modules of prototyping versions will be applied through the whole development life cycle of the PHR system that we are implementing in the Province of Trento (NE Italy). Currently, our work has been focused on Internet experienced people. Future usability testing will regard the use of the system by people with less computer experience, different health literacy, chronic conditions, more varied ages, etc.

A comparison test to compare this innovative user interface with a more conventional user interface is currently undergoing. We intend to apply iterative usability testing on all the modules and functions that will constitute our PHR system. For example, the graphical representation of the personal clinical history will be designed and tested involving both health operators, the primary users of this PHR functionality, and citizens.

ACKNOWLEDGMENT

This work was supported by the Department of Health and the Department of Research and Innovation of the Autonomous Province of Trento.

REFERENCES

Bates, D.W., Kuperman, G.J., Wang, S., Gandhi, T., Kittler, A.,Volk, L., Spurr, C., Khorasani, R., Tanasijevic, M., & Middleton, B. (2003). Ten commandments for effective clinical decision support: Making the practice of evidence-based medicine a realty. *Journal of the American Medical Informatics Association, 10*, 523–530.

Brailer, D.J. (2004). *The decade of health information technology: Delivering consumer-centric and information-rich healthcare*. National Coordinator for Health Information Technology. Retrieved May 26, 2008, from, from http://www.hhs.gov/healthit/documents/hitframework.pdf

Coble, J.M., Karat, J., Orland, M., & Kahn, M. (1997). Iterative usability testing: Ensuring a usable clinical workstation. In *Proceedings of AMIA Annual Symposiu* (pp. 744–748).

Cohn, S.P. (2006, February). *Personal health records and personal health record systems*. Chairman National Committee on Vital and Health Statistics. Retrieved May 26, 2008, from, from http://www.ncvhs.hhs.gov/0602nhiirpt.pdf

Danis, C., & Boies, S. (2000). Using a technique from graphic designers to develop innovative system design. In *Proceedings of DIS 2000* (pp. 20–26).

Dumas, J.S., & Redish J.C. (1999) *A practical guide to usability testing*. Portland, OR: Intellect Books.

Ericsson, K.A., & Simon, H.A. (1984). *Protocol analysis: Verbal reports as data*. Cambridge, MA: The MIT Press.

Institute of Medicine (IOM). (2007). *Preventing medication errors*. Washington, D.C.: National Academies Press.

Jaspers, M.W., Steen, T., van den Bos, C., & Geenen, M. (2004). The think-aloud method: A guide to user interface design. *International Journal of Medical Informatics, 73*(11-12) 781–795.

Johnson, C.M. & Johnson, T.R. (2006). The significance of cognitive modelling in building healthcare interfaces. *International Journal of Medical Informatics, 75*(2) 163–172.

Johnson, C.M., Johnson, T.R., & Zhang, J. (2005). A user-centered framework for redesigning healthcare interfaces. *Journal of Biomedical Informatics, 38*(1) 75–87.

Kushniruk, A.W., & Patel, V.L. (2004). Cognitive and usability engineering methods for the evaluation of clinical information systems. *Journal of Biomedical Informatics, 37*(1), 56–76.

Kushniruk, A.W., Patel, V.L, Cimino, J.J., & Barrows, R.A. (1996). Cognitive evaluation of the user interface and vocabulary of an outpatient information system. In *Proceedings of AMIA Annual Symposium* (pp. 22–26).

Markle Foundation. (2004). *Connecting Americans to their healthcare, final report.* The Robert Wood Johnson Foundation. Retrieved May 26, 2008, from http://www.connectingforhealth.org/resources/wg_eis_final_report_0704.pdf

Nielsen, J. (1993) *Usability engineering.* San Diego, CA: Academic Press.

Nielsen, J. (2000). *Jakob Nielsen's alertbox, March 19, 2000: Why you only need to test with 5 users.* Retrieved May 26, 2008, from http://www.useit.com/alertbox/20000319.html

Preece, J., Rogers, Y., & Sharp, H. (2002). *Interaction design: Beyond human-computer interaction.* New York: John Wiley & Sons, Inc.

Rose, A.F., Schnipper, J.L., Park, E.R., Poon, E.G., Li, Q., & Middleton, B. (2005). Using qualitative studies to improve the usability of an EMR. *Journal of Biomedical Informatics, 38*(1), 51–60.

Rubin, J. (1994) *Handbook of usability testing: How to plan, design, and conduct effective tests.* New York: John Wiley and Sons.

Sharda, P., Das, A. L., Cohen, T.A., & Patel, V. (2006). Customizing clinical narratives for the electronic medical record interface using cognitive methods. *International Journal of Medical Informatics, 75*(5), 346–368.

Tang, P.C., Joan, S., Ash, J.S., Bates, D.W., Overhage, J.M., & Sands, D.Z. (2006). Personal health record: Definition, benefits, and strategies for overcoming barriers to adoption. *Journal of the American Medical Informatics Association, 13*(2), 121–126.

Tran, D.T., Zhang, X., Stolyar, A., & Lober, W.B. (2005) Patient-centered design for a personal health record system. In *Proceedings of AMIA Annual Symposium* (pp. 1140).

Waller, A., Franklin, V., Pagliari, C., & Greene, S. (2007) Participatory design of a text message scheduling system to support young people with diabetes. *Health Informatics Journal, 12*(4), 307–321.

Wroblewski, L. (2002). *Site-seeing: A visual approach to Web usability.* New York: Hungry Minds, Inc.

Wroblewski, L. (2006). *Where visual design meets usability.* Retrieved May 26, 2008, from http://www.lukew.com/ff/entry.asp?363

Zhang, J. (2005). Guest editorial: Human-centered computing in health information systems. *Journal of Biomedical Informatics, 38*(1), 1–3.

Zhang, J., Johnson, T.R., Patel, V.L., Paige, D.L., & Kubose, T. (2003). Using usability heuristics to evaluate patient safety of medical devices. *Journal of Biomedical Informatics, 36*(1–2), 23–30.

Chapter XI
Healthcare Quality and Cost Transparency Using Web-Based Tools

Jiao Ma
Saint Louis University, USA

Cynthia LeRouge
Saint Louis University, USA

ABSTRACT

This chapter explores the use of Web sites to provide patients with understandable information about the quality and price of healthcare (healthcare transparency). Our first objective is to discuss patients' perceptions of empowerment and need for quality and cost information when choosing medical providers and facilities for healthcare procedures. To meet this objective, we address issues of patient awareness of sources of healthcare quality and cost information, perceived responsibility for managing healthcare costs, and knowledge of appropriate actions to exercise choice of providers. Our second objective is to investigate the potential of Web-based tools, which provide healthcare quality and cost information, to facilitate patients' decision-making processes regarding choice of provider for healthcare services, particularly common outpatient procedures. To meet this second objective, we use insights from user-centered design procedures (e.g., focus groups and in-depth interviews) associated with the development of a healthcare transparency Web-based tool.

INTRODUCTION

On May 10, 2006, Carolyn Clancy, M.D., Director of the Agency for Healthcare Research and Quality, testified before the Joint Economic Committee of the U.S. Congress outlining the commitment of the Department of Health and Human Services (HHS) to provide Americans with understandable information about the quality and price of healthcare. This vision has four objectives:

- Promote quality transparency;
- Promote price transparency;
- Facilitate the greater use of health information technology; and
- Transform healthcare so its incentives support a consumer-oriented healthcare system.

The synergy of these objectives is an informed and empowered healthcare consumer with a panoramic view of his/her healthcare situation.

The Internet has done much to facilitate this view by providing an ever-expanding bounty of information about health prevention and maintenance; however issues such as the general understandability and accuracy of this information still remain. Interactive tools and features that provide communication channels (e.g., peer support groups) and personalized information are increasingly common supplements to content pages. Monitoring devices have also been an area of great advancement and promise.

It is evident that patients have an appetite for prescriptive and preventative healthcare information and tools. However, does this need also exist for healthcare cost and quality transparency? The first objective of this chapter is to better understand patients' perceptions of empowerment and need for procedure quality and cost information when choosing medical providers and facilities. The second objective of the chapter is to address the potential of Web-based tools to facilitate and enable the patients' decision-making processes. To meet these goals, questions of interest include:

- Do patients perceive quality and cost information as important to their choice of healthcare provider?
- Do patients feel empowered with quality and cost information to make decisions about where to have medical procedures (e.g., mammogram and bone density tests) or tests (e.g., spinal tap or allergy testing) performed?
- Would a Web-based tool that provides quality and/or cost information be compatible with the patients' decision-making processes?
- What factors should be considered in designing a useful and usable Web-based tool to provide quality and/or cost information for patients?

We review existing literature, assessment of existing healthcare transparency Web applications, and insights from user-centered design techniques from an on-going study involving developing such a tool to reveal issues, controversies, and problems associated with healthcare quality and cost Web-based tools, and discuss solutions. We adapt the constructs from a Theoretical Compatibility Model (Karahanna, Agarwal, & Angst, 2006) to use as thematic dimensions to organize our presentation of Web-based quality and cost tool compatibility, as well as provide insight within the landscape of existing information systems research.

BACKGROUND

In America's democratic consumer culture, consumers can easily obtain information about price and quality for most purchases using existing resources (e.g., mass media such as TV, print publications, Web sites) to assist with purchase decisions. A noted exception is healthcare where cost and quality information is still limited

(Greenberg, 2006). In a consumer-driven system, healthcare buyers with financial incentives will demand quantitative and qualitative information on competing health plans, facility options, providers, and specific healthcare treatment. Plans and providers will be motivated to supply this information in order to manage cost and utilization as necessary to stay competitive.

Healthcare transparency is about disseminating information (quality and cost) in a patient-friendly manner to allow patients to make informed healthcare decisions based on value. Ideally, transparency creates incentives at all levels and motivates the entire system to provide better care for less money (HHS, 2007). Providers will improve when they see how their practices compare to others, and consumers benefit from making informed decisions. Additionally, it is theorized that healthcare transparency will encourage patients to become better healthcare shoppers by factoring quality and price into decisions about care, which will lead to a positive impact on management of healthcare costs at both individual and industry levels (Openshaw, 2006). It is through these ideals that some embrace healthcare transparency as an element in change and reform in America's healthcare system (Greenberg, 2006). A modern healthcare system and a democratic consumer culture demand a modern information strategy (Lansky, 2003).

The Internet plays and will continue to play a key role in consumer research, plan enrollment, ongoing administration, and customer service (Beauregard, 2006). According to Coulter (2005), alternative ways of accessing health advice are becoming more popular. For instance, a recent UK survey of people aged 45 and older found over 30% of respondents had searched for health information on the Web. In addition, the Agency for Healthcare Research Quality (AHRQ) recommends a wealth of Web-based resources for healthcare quality information and tips, as well as print resources (AHRQ, 2007) to assist consumers in making more informed healthcare decisions. As such, emerging Web-based tools and resources are a logical choice for providing patients with healthcare quality and cost information—for example, CompareYourCare hosts 22 tools (including three English/Spanish bilingual tools) that compare and rate the quality of healthcare, according to national treatment guidelines, and assist self-care by providing up-to-date information and skills to better manage an illness or maintain good health (http://www.compareyourcare.org/). This site was developed by the Foundation for Accountability (FACCT), and is owned by HealthGrades Inc. Among the efforts of making healthcare more "transparent," a handful of states like New York, Florida, Maryland, and Texas provide state-sponsored Web sites (e.g., New York State Healthcare Report Card at http://www.abouthealthquality.org/index/about) which enable patients to compare hospital and, physician prices (a range of charges or average prices) and performance.

The aforementioned states are using this type of "transparency" to force poorly performing providers out of business and push providers at the high end of the spectrum to voluntarily lower their fees (Lemov, 2006). Hospitals were found to respond positively to public reporting by immediately improving their quality scores during the preparation of disclosing quality data. Most of the hospitals were able to spot their failings from site information and changed policies as appropriate to meet the standards.

The objectives of these sites are not only to prompt organizational action, but also to influence patients' decision-making behavior. Site information about the cost and quality of care is offered to patients to accommodate their higher responsibilities in paying and managing healthcare costs. However, despite the free and easily accessible data, little empirical evidence has shown that patients have altered their behaviors in response to publicly reported quality or cost measures (Lemov, 2006). In fact, there is little elaboration on patient issues related to cost and quality transparency. Furthermore, there is no clear indication that patient input was considered in creating the design and content of these sites. Hence, this chapter focuses on trends, issues, controversies, and solutions for using Web-based tools to provide healthcare transparency from the patient perspective.

TRENDS, ISSUES, AND CONTROVERSIES

Quality and Cost in the Healthcare Decision Process

Do patients perceive quality and cost information as important to their healthcare provider decision-making process?

Service marketing literature indicates that customers attempt to evaluate both functional quality (i.e., delivery quality, which includes an assessment of reliability, responsiveness, assurance, empathy, and tangibles) as well as technical performance quality in deriving quality judgments. However, the entire quality judgment will be made on delivery quality elements, if someone lacks the ability to assess technical quality (Gronroos, 1984). In reference to healthcare, Bowers and Keife (2002) pointed out that functional quality traditionally has received more weight, because patients often lack the technological sophistication to understand details of their diagnoses and treatment and place paternalistic trust in their physicians to make the right decisions.

However, times are changing. The 1996-2000 FACCT study on patients and healthcare quality found that patients are beginning to seek outside information and use it to ask questions of their healthcare providers and participate in healthcare decisions (FACCT, 2000). About one-third of the patients in the FACCT study used the Internet for seeking health information. When selecting a physician, the FACCT study found that patients were interested in factual information, such as years in practice, malpractice record, hospital affiliation, and so on. About 28% of those studied accessed Web sites to read and post messages about a physician. Segmentation of the adult population in the FACCT study suggests that the most passive healthcare participants are older men with lower than average incomes with at least one chronic condition, while the most aggressive information seekers are women with higher-than-average incomes.

Recent trends also show a shift related to healthcare costs. American healthcare is moving toward consumer-driven health plans, which require significant copays or deductibles and/or utilize personal flex spending accounts (these accounts allow participants to allocate limited amounts of pre-tax dollars to cover healthcare costs). As early as 1986, Rosenstein (1986) called attention to the trend in making patients more financially responsible for medical care services by increasing their out-of-pocket costs. For patients with consumer-driven plans, cost is an important factor. In fact, Rosenstein predicted that cost will eventually become one of the major criteria used in healthcare selection. In response to patients' increased concerns regarding costs, changes in healthcare are under way. For instance, walk-in retail clinics, which target providing convenient access/limited service at a competitive price, are spreading nationwide. More than a dozen clinic operators plan to open thousands of clinics in stores such as Wal-Mart, CVS, Walgreen's, and Kerr Drug. Prices at these walk-in clinics are posted on an electronic sign as in a fast-food restaurant (Schmit, 2006).

Cost and quality information are not separate issues, but are intertwined in making an assessment of healthcare value. In a national survey of healthcare consumers in Taiwan on patient perceived quality and expensiveness, Cheng, Wei, and Chang (2006) found that patients indicating higher perceived quality (i.e., physician technical or functional interpersonal skill ratings) were less likely to report that charges were expensive. Using consumer cost theory, this study concluded that perceived value rather than the price or quality alone is the essence of competition in the healthcare market. Hence, when the quality of the healthcare services meets a consumer's expectation and the consumer considers the price to be worth the anticipated quality, then consumer satisfaction emerges and consumption of those services continues.

Consumer Empowerment

Do patients feel empowered with cost and quality information to make decisions about where to have medical procedures performed?

The traditional paternalistic approach of decision-making in healthcare assumed that (1) doctors and patients shared the same goals; (2) only the doctors were sufficiently informed and experienced to decide what should be done; and (3) patient involvement would be limited to giving or withholding consent to treatment. Evidence shows that higher engagement of patients in decision-making and active involvement in managing their healthcare leads to more appropriate and cost-effective use of health services and better health outcomes (Coulter, 2005). Consumer empowerment includes consumer activation and public disclosure of performance information (Bethell, 2000). Consumer activism refers to patients proactively seeking information about healthcare, health, quality, and cost (e.g., looking up information about a new prescription such as precautions and side-effects). Public disclosure refers to a critical mass of patients having timely access to relevant and understandable information about healthcare performance (e.g., obtaining information on healthcare professionals' backgrounds before agreeing to see them).

When it comes to quality and cost information, the healthcare industry has been described as an imperfect competitive market of uncertainty and information asymmetry (Cheng et al., 2006). This asymmetry impairs patient empowerment in the decision-making process. Healthcare might be the only industry where a consumer can walk through the door, obtain a service not knowing how much it costs, and walk out without paying. This point is highlighted by a recent study, which found patients were able to guess the price of a Honda Accord within $300 and estimate the tab for a coast-to-coast round-trip airline ticket within $37, but were off by $8,100 for a four-day hospital stay (Howley, 2006). Hence, public disclosure of healthcare quality and cost information provide information that is not presently known. This additional information may empower consumers to exercise judicious choices in healthcare decisions, such as where to have medical procedures performed.

Web-Based Quality and Cost Tool Compatibility

Would a Web-based tool that provides quality and/or cost information be compatible with the patient's decision-making process?

While the trend is toward patient empowerment and healthcare information seeking, the question of compatibility between a Web-based tool and the patient's decision-making process is not yet sufficiently answered. Compatibility is a multifaceted issue. Two general aspects of compatibility are normative/cognitive compatibility (referring to feelings or thoughts) and operational compatibility (referring to the compatibility of an innovation to what people do) (Rogers, 1995; Tornatzky & Klein, 1982). With respect to cognitive compatibility, patients' thoughts and feelings on how cost information factors into their healthcare decision model need to be considered. If cost information is not currently a major factor, a key challenge in controlling costs through cost transparency will be how to best reframe patients' thinking about cost as a decision factor. With respect to operational compatibility, the propriety of a Web tool used for this purpose and its design need to be further considered. Recent work in the information systems domain further breaks down operational compatibility into compatibility with preferred work style, existing work practices, and prior experience, as well as elements of technology acceptance (Karahanna et al., 2006).

There is little evidence in research, and to some degree in practice, to determine whether providing healthcare quality and cost transparency via the Internet is compatible with patients' existing needs and preferences. Compatibility in this context is complicated by the issues that what is deemed as relevant information is situational to patients (e.g., specific insurance coverage or health condition). The information infrastructure needs to offer information that people want, and distribute it when and where they need it. In addition, the information delivered by a Web-based tool needs to be personalized to meet each patient's and family members' specific needs (e.g., health needs, language, culture, information seeking behavior) (Lansky, 2002).

To begin to explore the compatibility issue, we adapt the compatibility antecedent constructs from the Theoretical Compatibility Model (Karahanna et al., 2006) to use as a dimensional (thematic) framework to disclose potential compatibility issues. Figure 1 shows the model from the Karahanna et al. study; the model exhibits some statistically significant relationships, along with theoretical relationships proposed for "compatibility with existing practices" that could not be tested. We use the adapted model as a priori prescriptive framework, as opposed to an assessment of a completed innovation in the previous research.

Table 1 provides a comparison of compatibility construct definitions used in the previous study with those used in this study. Some adaptation of construct definition is needed to suit the context of patients' volitional use of a Web-based tool. In the forthcoming section, we propose this model

Figure 1. Theoretical compatibility model (from Karahanna et al., 2006, pp. 789)

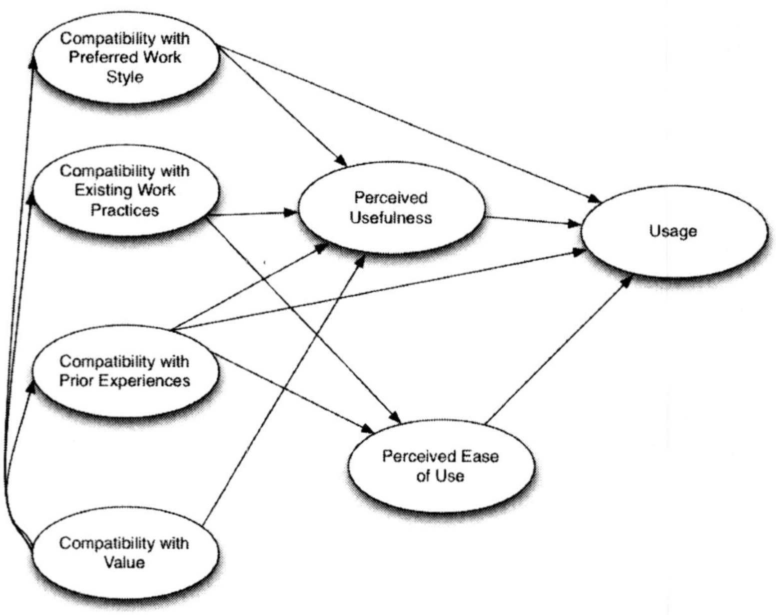

Table 1. Comparison of construction definitions between Karahanna et al. (2006) and current study constructs

Karahanna et al. (2006) Construct	Karahanna et al. (2006, pp. 787) Definition	Current Study Construct	Current Study Definition
Compatibility with Preferred Work Style	Captures the possibility offered by the technology of being consistent with a desired work style	Compatibility with Preferred Task Style	Patient's self-concept regarding the functionality (way) they would like to explore healthcare cost and quality information; cost and quality functional requirements
Compatibility with Existing Work Practices	Measures the extent to which a technology "fits" with a user's current work process	Compatibility with Existing Task Practices	Current practices patients use to find cost information or information seeking strategies used to find health information on the Internet.
Compatibility with Prior Experience	Reflects a fit between the target technology and a variety of users' past encounters with technology	Compatibility with Prior Experience	Existing knowledge or perceptions of fact regarding cost/quality information and experience in using healthcare cost comparison sites.
Compatibility with Value	Epitomizes the match between the possibilities offered by the technology and the user's dominant value system	Compatibility with Healthcare Cost and Values	Patient's dominant value system that affects factoring of healthcare cost and quality into healthcare decisions.

as a way to inform future design and acceptance of an innovation.

PATIENT COMPATILITY: CONSIDERATIONS TO ENHANCE EASE-OF-USE AND VALUE

What factors should be considered in designing a useful and usable Web-based tool for providing quality and/or cost information to patients?

To address the final question of interest, we continue the discussion using insights from user-centered design procedures associated with the development of a particular healthcare transparency Web-based tool (sponsored by a healthcare insurer). We provide insights regarding patients' preferred task styles, existing task practices, prior experiences, and values to use as considerations in developing a transparency tool compatible with the patient perspectives. Insights from these procedures are not intended to draw final conclusions, but to inspire further work in research and practice in meeting patient healthcare quality and cost transparency needs through the use of Web-based tools.

User-Centered Design Methods

The user-centered design (UCD) methods that were used include focus groups and in-depth interviews (IDIs) with primary target users. Participants for both the focus groups and IDIs were randomly selected from a consumer sample provided by a professional marketing firm. The following selection criteria were used to define the sample:

- A variety of group and individual health insurance plans were represented
- A mix of males/females
- Variety in the age range between 18–55 years
- Participants were involved in, or responsible for, household healthcare decisions

- Insurance customers with an annual deductible under $500 and those with an annual deductible in excess of $500
- Participants were computer and Internet users

Members of the pool were assigned to either a focus group or an IDI. Two focus groups were conducted with the potential users of a Web-based tool. Each focus group consisted of eight-to-ten participants and lasted approximately one and one half hours. One focus group included insurance customers with an annual deductible under $500, and one group with an annual deductible in excess of $500. An experienced moderator and a panel of analysts conducted and analyzed the focus groups, respectively. Appendix A provides a general outline of the protocol used to explore beliefs and attitude structures related to healthcare transparency and the use of a Web site to provide this transparency. Exact questions and the flow of conversation evolved around the topics to best suit the characteristics and flow of the groups.

Twelve people participated in IDIs individually. IDIs are a nondirective, qualitative type of interview with an emphasis on listening to people talk in response to a minimal number of specific questions, which are primarily open-ended (Miller & Crabtree, 1999). This research technique provides value through qualitative insight into the belief and attitude structures, which may be used, particularly in business contexts, for strategy development. The IDIs were conducted by a professional interviewer and each lasted approximately 45 minutes. The objectives of these interviews that guided the discussion were: (1) to examine reactions to the concept and design of the Web-based tool, and (2) to extend exploration of focus group topics regarding healthcare transparency beliefs and attitudes. The IDIs began with a discussion of beliefs particularly related to cost transparency and migrated to concept evaluation. Projective techniques were used during the IDIs to allow respondents to engage in free-flowing and creative descriptions of their healthcare cost and quality information needs and how to meet these needs using the prototyped Web-based tool. The concept discussion was followed by a prototype review. The prototypes used in the IDIs were high-fidelity mockups of screen designs, which were a lifelike simulation of the final product with a refined graphic design. However, the back end of the product was simulated rather than real (Isensee & Rudd, 1996).

The Theoretical Compatibility Model in Figure 1 was used as a coding scheme for organizing insights from the investigation using the UCD techniques into compatibility dimensions. Two researchers participated in the coding process and worked together to reach final coding consensus.

Preferred Task Style

To make a decision on the choice of a provider or facility, the UCD data indicated that patients need quality information to accompany cost information, which aligns with the previous discussion of value. When it comes to quality information, participants stated they wanted performance metrics for the healthcare facilities. For cost information to be useful, it must be specific. In other words, participants indicated that patients need explicit and accurate cost information for obtaining the procedure of interest at specific facilities, instead of an average or a range of costs. Hence, the ability to specify parameters within the Web-based tool to customize information to individual situations is important. For example, some participants indicated they liked to be able to calculate their "out-of-pocket" costs based on their individual plan benefits. To meet this need, a calculator to determine "out-of-pocket" cost is an appropriate feature. As another example, some patients want to limit their search to facilities within a specific driving distance.

Multiple sources of data enhance usefulness, particularly regarding quality. To illustrate, some participants expressed an interest for a health transparency Web tool to include links to facility Web sites for further research regarding quality. In addition, people who have undergone similar procedures were considered as a valuable source of information. This was expressed by the desire for online discussion groups and other forums to communicate with other patients. As another alternative, a simple star ratings system was recommended to provide patient feedback for each facility that offers a specified procedure.

However, the UCD data recommended avoiding situations in which patients drown in data and cannot make use of the information. Healthcare cost information must address specific information needs, in order to be useful and meaningful to the patients. Participants mentioned the following factors, which need to be considered in specifying meaningful data regarding healthcare quality and cost transparency:

- Type of service anticipated by the patients
- Specific hospital/clinic providing the service
- Insurance carrier or coverage medium of the patient
- Benefit plan of the patient (deductible, co-insurance, out of pocket limit)
- Procedural information about procedures (such as side-effects and recovery time) is desirable and should be presented with intuitive graphics and imagery where possible.

In seeking to affect patient behavior, entities offering such tools should consider that the Web tool alone might not be enough for a patient to finalize a decision. Participants indicated a Web-based tool should afford users the opportunity to have personal contact via telephone with a "live person," either during or after using the site for questions, or to call a facility for confirmation once they have narrowed down their choices.

Compatibility with Existing Task Practices

The Web-based tool should function in a way that matches patients' natural information seeking behavior. This corresponds to the fact that the user interface needs to be intuitive, informative, and visually appealing, as expressed in various ways by participants. In reviewing UCD data to affirm these generalizations with specific examples, search, sequencing, and support considerations were mentioned.

A desirable search function should generate only effective and "on target" returns. In inquiring what patients may search for, the indication was that patients would seek information to better understand a specific procedure or learn more about a facility beyond the cost information for a procedure of interest. The name of a facility or procedure would be a common search parameter. Regarding the sequencing of information, proxies for quality or general descriptive information (e.g., bed counts, nursing care information) about a facility must be provided before patients can utilize the cost information in their decision-making processes, again aligning with concepts of value using consumer cost theory.

Support services in various forms are an existing practice with many technological tools. Like most users of complex information technology, healthcare patients feel most comfortable knowing a support person is available to help them, in case they encounter problems with the Web tool or have additional questions.

Compatibility with Prior Experience

Utilization of health transparency Web-based tools is a new experience. In recognizing this, participants indicated that public relations and marketing efforts are a must to promote awareness and, most importantly, the value of a health transparency Web-based tool.

Earlier in this chapter, we discussed the general information asymmetry that currently exists, that patients are not well informed regarding healthcare costs, and generally do not know where to look to find this information. Given this asymmetry, patients have little to no experience in accurately estimating healthcare costs and tend to make inaccurate estimates of the costs (Howley, 2006). The UCD data indicates patients may not only be unaware of a specific price or range for a procedure, but that patients may also be unaware that different facilities can have different costs for the same medical procedures or treatments (e.g., colonoscopy). In addition, even if armed with information regarding cost differences, participants doubted that they were empowered to select a facility for medical procedures. Many believed this decision was completely under the control of the physicians. If health transparency tools are to affect behaviors, the lack of knowledge regarding the patient's role in the decision process needs to be remedied through patient education. As such, health transparency Web tools may include such content as "next steps," "how to compare," or "discussing costs with your doctor."

Compatibility with Values

Consumer attitudes and expectations about healthcare are shifting toward increased clinical performance and public accountability. Some patients have become activists who demand and use information about medical treatments, healthcare products, and healthcare standards (Kizer, 2001).

On the subject of healthcare standards for a Web tool, participants indicated concern about the source of the information. Patients demand impartial and credible sources to help with their decisions. The Web tool prototype that participants reviewed during the IDIs was sponsored by a health insurance carrier. Remarks regarding the sponsorship indicated that trust in insurance carriers was generally low among the participants. Many participants believed that carriers bear the responsibility for healthcare costs, and hence, are driven by a "profit motive." Consequently, concerned participants suspected that data provided by the carrier might be biased toward increasing a carrier's profit. To offset perceptions of biased data, there were recommendations to add information provided by credible sources, such as independent ratings of facilities and providers. Examples given included performance metrics, backgrounds, customer evaluations, and activity information (e.g., annual numbers of services performed) for both physicians and facilities.

Regarding the decision process, the UCD data revealed that patients predominantly based their choice of care decisions on the quality of the physician performing the procedure, which is measured using three criteria: (1) past experience with that physician, (2) the physician's reputation and specialization in that procedure, and (3) recommendations of others (e.g., family and friends). The obvious caveat relative to this chapter is that the cost of a medical procedure is not currently a primary factor that patients consider when making decisions regarding personal or family medical procedures.

Part of the emphasis on quality is attributable to minimizing health risks. Participants pointed out that healthcare service was viewed differently from other professional services. Specifically, they indicated some healthcare procedures (e.g., a life-threatening surgery) could not be viewed as commodities. It was also expressed that when it came to a loved-one, particularly a child, even if a procedure was "simple," the focus was quality. Consequently, patients do not view these types of healthcare decisions as potential "shopping" experiences. Also, participants expressed that they had less desire to control costs than with other types of purchases. One focus group participant stated, "Healthcare is perceived [as] too important to be considered as a shopping experience." Participants indicated that they are more likely to research cost information on the Internet for autos, electronic products, and other types of professional services (e.g., funeral, legal service) than they would be for healthcare cost information.

The other reason for concentrating on quality in the healthcare decision process is attributed to the fact that most consumers are not paying directly for medical procedures, whereas they are for other products. Furthermore, patients often feel entitled to insurance coverage or some other form of cost coverage. Participants disclosed a long-standing perception that healthcare costs are someone else's problem. Consequently, UCD participants expressed no need to take responsibility in controlling overall healthcare costs. Underscoring this general position, participants overwhelmingly defined their costs of interest as "out-of-pocket" costs for a medical event, which resulted from copay or coinsurance. Hence, the only time the cost of the procedure may change patient behaviors is when patient out-of-pocket cost is impacted. When patients are not concerned about the cost of procedures until it hits their pocketbook, the potential of the Web tool to change behavior may be restricted. We make the prior statement with caution, because even in cases where out-of-pocket costs exist, UCD data does not reveal any clear indication that patients would use cost information from Web tool on a voluntary basis to change any care decisions.

Earlier in this chapter, we discussed recent trends that show a shift to a greater consumer burden regarding healthcare costs. Some participants in both the IDIs and focus groups showed some variance in their concerns about costs given the nature of the procedures and who were receiving the procedures (less concern with a child or loved-one). Based upon patients' existing values regarding healthcare cost responsibility and defining costs as their out-of-pocket expenses, could movement toward a greater consumer burden shift healthcare transaction processes toward "more of a shopping model?" Cosmetic surgery typically involves out-of-pocket costs and may provide a useful perspective in contemplating this question. Lee and Hoo (2006) argue that most physicians are compensated differently from the way the other professionals were. They further state that physicians would handle medical transactions differently, depending on how they were paid. For instance, a cosmetic surgery transaction has all the characteristics of a normal market transaction in which the seller has a financial interest in how all aspects of the transaction affect the buyer. The cost information of the typical cosmetic surgery is often readily available in three ways: (1) a package price in advance covering all services and facilities; (2) price comparison/shop-around prior to the surgery; and (3) a price that is lower in real terms than the price charged a decade ago for comparable procedures despite considerable technological innovations in the interim. Advertisements may even indicate a price range. There is ample evidence to suggest that consumers consider costs and "shop around" and that cosmetic surgeons compete with at least some consideration to costs. In contrast, in more typical physician-patient interactions, physicians are not paid to be concerned about all aspects of the transaction and therefore typically ignore the effects on the patients of a variety of costs, including cost of time, the cost of drugs, and other additional costs. In summary, differences exist in decision-making for elective medical procedures (e.g., cosmetic surgeries), as opposed to necessary ones (e.g., life-saving surgeries). According to information retrieval studies (Taylor, Cool, Belkin, & Amadio, 2007; Xu & Chen, 2006), costs constitute a relevant factor in information seeking process of elective "less threatening" medical procedures, however, they may not be as relevant or important in selecting essential procedures.

CONCLUSION

Although trends are moving toward patient empowerment and considerations of healthcare quality and cost, patients are not currently empowered when it comes to healthcare quality and cost information. In addition, patients perceived that they had limited responsibility for healthcare costs. The ultimate reason to look at compatibility issues early in the design process is to have some foresight to determine and enhance the potential for technology acceptance and outcomes. In aggregating literature and insights from the UCD data, what healthcare transparency Web tools have to offer may become more compatible with the patients' decision-making process as the healthcare industry continues with emerging trends toward patient information empowerment and increasing patient healthcare cost burden.

Currently, providing health transparency through a Web-based tool will likely influence the consumer healthcare decision processes the most in situations not involving extremely serious healthcare conditions and when the consumer bears the greatest cost burden. Web-based tools that provide understandable comparative cost information and quality indicators may best enable healthcare patients in the decision processes. Furthermore, such tools may also best serve their purposes by providing features that help the consumer deliberate (e.g., forums with peers, calculator, and further contact information).

The Theoretical Compatibility Model (Karahanna et al., 2006) proved to be a viable framework for analyzing the patient perspective and may be well suited to further explore and test consumer health informatics issues related to quality and cost transparency (e.g., acceptance of such Web sites and actual changes of behaviors resulting from using the Web site), as well as other consumer health issues (e.g., adoption of various forms of patient health records). Future work will include assessing existing and forthcoming healthcare transparency Web tools' ability to raise cost and quality awareness and encouraging the use of this information as a change agent for decision-making.

REFERENCES

Agency for Healthcare Research and Quality (AHRQ). (2007). *Improving healthcare quality: A guide for patients and families*. Retrieved May 26, 2008, from http://www.ahrq.gov/consumer/qntlite/

Beauregard, T.R. (2006). *Large employer views of consumer-driven healthcare: Current interest, barriers, and potential solutions*. Manhattan Institute. Retrieved May 26, 2008, from http://www.manhattan-institute.org/consumerdrivenhealthcare/pdfs/Beauregard.pdf

Bethell, C. (2000). *Patient-centered care measures for the national healthcare quality report (defining patient-centered care)*. Retrieved May 26, 2008, from http://www.markle.org/resources/facct/doclibFiles/documentFile_168.pdf

Bowers, M.R., & Kiefe, C.I. (2002). Measuring healthcare quality: Comparing and contrasting the medical and the marketing approaches. *American Journal of Medical Quality, 17*(4), 136-143.

Cheng, S.-H., Wei, Y.-J., & Chang, H.-J. (2006). Quality competition among hospitals: The effects of perceived quality and perceived expensiveness on healthcare patients. *American Journal of Medical Quality, 21* (1), 68-75.

Coulter, A. (2005). What do patients and the public want from primary care? *British Medical Journal, 331*(7526), 1199-1201.

The Foundation for Accountability (FACCT). (2000). *Patients and quality: What do they know? What do they want? Results from FACCT consumer research 1996-2000*. Retrieved May 26, 2008, from http://www.markle.org/resources/facct/doclibFiles/documentFile_196.pdf

Greenberg, J. (2006, July 18). *Will consumer driven healthcare put the brakes on rising costs?* New Hampshire Public Radio. Retrieved May 26, 2008, from http://www.nhpr.org/node/11210

Gronroos, C.A. (1984). A service quality model and its marketing implications. *Europe Journal of Marketing, 18*, 36-44.

Health and Human Services (HHS). (2007). *Value-driven healthcare—transparency: Better care lower cost.* Retrieved May 26, 2008, from http://www.hhs.gov/transparency/

Howley, K. (2006, April). "I can't afford to get sick"—Think your insurance has you covered? Just wait till you need it most. *Reader's Digest.* Retrieved May 26, 2008, from http://www.rd.com/content/the-cost-of-health-care-in-america/

Isensee, S., & Rudd, J. (1996). *The art of rapid prototyping.* MA: International Thompson Computer Press.

Karahanna, E., Agarwal, R., & Angst, C.M. (2006). Reconceptualizing compatibility beliefs in technology acceptance research. *MIS Quarterly, 30*(4), 781-804.

Kizer, K.W. (2001). Establishing healthcare performance standards in an era of consumerism. *Journal of the American Medical Association, 286* (10), 1213-1217.

Lansky, D. (2002). *Information for better quality care—the patients' perspective.* Foundation for Accountability. Retrieved May 26, 2008, from http://www.markle.org/resources/facct/doclibFiles/documentFile_526.ppt

Lansky, D. (2003). *A person-centered view of consumer information in the healthcare marketplace.* Federal Trade Commission/U.S. Department of Justice Joint Hearings on Healthcare and Competition Law and Policy. Retrieved May 26, 2008, from http://www.markle.org/resources/facct/doclibFiles/documentFile_595.ppt

Lee, P.V., & Hoo, E. (2006). Beyond consumer-driven healthcare: Purchasers' expectations of all plans. *Health Affairs 25*(6), w544-w548. Retrieved May 26, 2008, from http://content.healthaffairs.org/cgi/content/abstract/25/6/w544

Lemov, P. (2006, September). Healthcare: A dose of transparency. *Governing Magazine.* Kaiser Family Foundation. Retrieved May 26, 2008, from http://www.governing.com/articles/9hcare.htm

Miller, W.L., & Crabtree, B.F. (1999). Depth interviewing. In W.L. Miller, & B.F. Crabtree (Eds.), *Doing Qualitative Research* (pp. 89-108). Thousand Oaks CA: Sage Publications.

Openshaw, J. (2006, October 31). Checkup lines: Americans need to learn to shop for healthcare. *Market watch.* Retrieved May 26, 2008, from http://www.marketwatch.com/News/Story/consumers-need-become-better-health-care/story.aspx?guid=%7B09F2F091-A840-4D08-AAE3-C4CDD9A8C02C%7D

Rogers, E.M. (1995). *Diffusion of innovations.* New York: The Free Press.

Rosenstein, A.H. (1986). Applications of consumer behavior in medical care. *Journal of Professional Services Marketing, 1*(4), 31-37.

Schmit, J. (2006, August 28). Could walk-in retail clinics help slow rising health costs? *USA Today.* Retrieved May 26, 2008, from http://www.usatoday.com/money/industries/health/2006-08-24-walk-in-clinic-usat_x.htm

Taylor, A.R., Cool, C., Belkin, N.J., & Amadio, W.J. (2007). Relationships between categories of relevance criteria and stage in task completion. *Information Processing & Management, 43*(4), 1071-1084.

Tornatzky, L.G., & Klein, K.J. (1982). Innovation characteristics and innovation adoption-implementation: A meta-analysis of findings. *IEEE Transactions on Engineering Management, 29*(1), 28-45.

Xu, Y., & Chen, Z. (2006). Relevance judgment: What do information consumers consider beyond topicality? *Journal of the American Society for Information Science and Technology, 57*(7), 961-973.

APPENDIX A: FOCUS GROUP PROTOCOL OUTLINE

- To discover the current state of cost information –
  - Do patients have an awareness of costs – if so, sources?
  - How/if patients currently use cost information?
- To discuss the future state of cost transparency –
  - Relevancy of information – what do they need to know, when?
  - Information access – how do they want to get the information?
  - Credibility of information – what makes it trusted?
  - What other factors must play in with cost – i.e. quality?
  - At what point in time does the shopping process start? Proactive, Reactive, not Active?
  - Roles of decision makers/influencers – family members, friends, third party sources, physicians, etc.?
  - Which care situations are open to choice/cost considerations, and which ones aren't?
  - What features are most important when a procedure needs to be done? How does this vary by situation?
- To explore how to encourage use of cost information as a change agent -
  - Discussion about plan designs – current vs. prototypes – what would encourage cost research/ factoring into decision-making?
  - Incentives to factor price into decision-making?
- To determine what patients mean by quality of care.

Chapter XII
Perceptions of E-Health in Rural Communities

Ann L. Fruhling
University of Nebraska at Omaha, Peter Kiewit Institute, USA

ABSTRACT

This chapter is drawn from a comprehensive study that examined the effect Human-Computer Interaction usability factors had on rural residents' perception of trust in e-health services. Written comments provided by participants were examined to develop a qualitative assessment of dimensions that are important to rural residents' perceptions of e-health. Identification of these dimensions will aid e-health system designers and administrators in creating better e-health applications.

INTRODUCTION

Recently, Dr. Patricia Grady, Director National Institute of Nursing Research, reported to Congress that "the healthcare of rural populations is a concern because of poverty, lack of services, and/or health vulnerability of the population" (Grady, 2005). Rural residents typically have limited access to healthcare services, such as specialty physicians, conventional healthcare sites, community-based clinics, and homes (Grady, 2005). The Internet can provide access to a variety of e-health services, such as computer-based healthcare communication intervention programs that provide customized information and social support for rural families. General-purpose e-health applications may also help improve the healthcare delivery to rural areas. These applications include purely clinical applications (e.g., physicians consulting on a diagnosis), emergency health communication applications (e.g., distributing information about Severe Acute Respiratory Syndrome), disease-focused applications (e.g., diabetes self-management support), Internet communication between patients and physicians, and commercial applications that have no association with a patient's own healthcare provider (e.g., WebMD) (Wilson, 2008).

This chapter is drawn from responses to a comprehensive study that analyzed the effect that human-computer interaction (HCI) usability factors have on rural residents' perception of trust when using e-health services. Primary results are reported by Fruhling and Lee (2006). The study also solicited comments from the participants regarding their perceptions of a sample e-health Web site and the likelihood of using such services. Further, the study included a feedback mechanism to gather data from rural residents who did not wish to participate in the overall study. Demographic responses and feedback provide the basis to describe the relevant characteristics of rural residents. Participants' written comments are analyzed to identify qualitative dimensions that are important to rural residents in determining whether to accept and use e-health services.

RELEVANT CHARACTERISTICS OF RURAL RESIDENTS

Participants for this study were selected based on the location where they live. According to experts at the Nebraska Rural Health Research Center, Nebraska communities that have a population between 2,500 and 5,000 are referred to as "rural." A list was developed of six Nebraska communities that meet these criteria and are located at least 25 miles from a similar or larger-size community (see Figure 1). The two communities selected for the study, Broken Bow and Ogallala, are located further than 25 miles from a Critical Access Hospital in addition to the above criteria.

Letters inviting participation in this study were mailed to people living outside the town boundaries of Ogallala and Broken Bow. There were 3,992 rural resident mailing addresses eli-

Figure 1. State of Nebraska showing candidate study communities

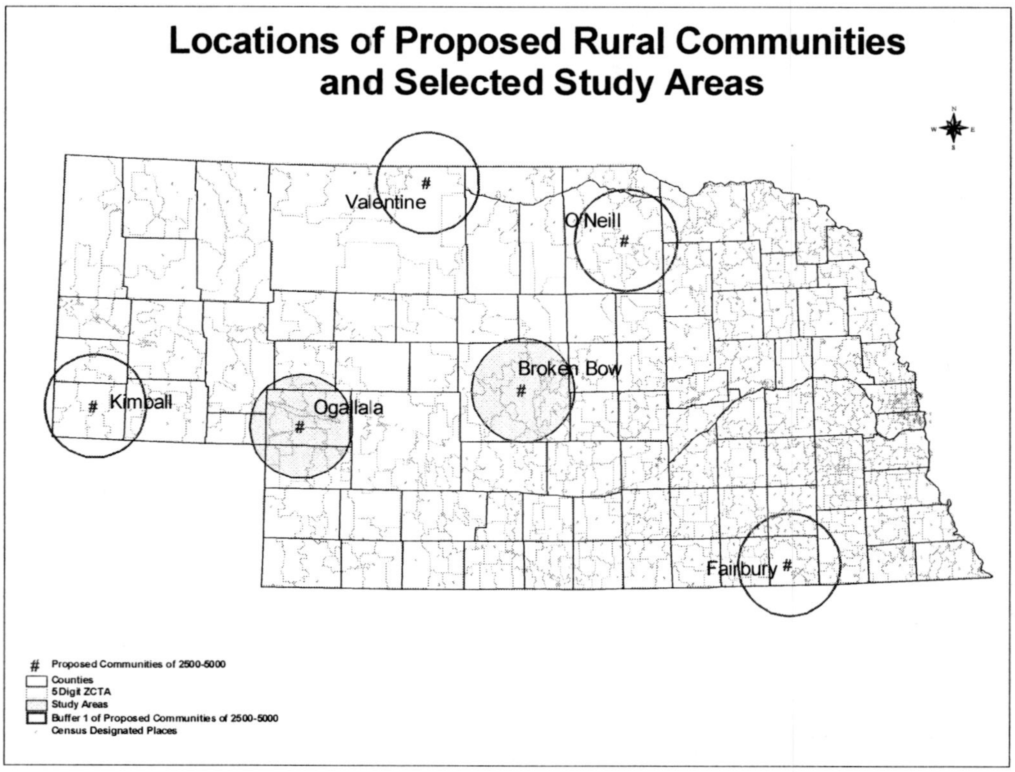

Figure 2. Alegent Health homepage

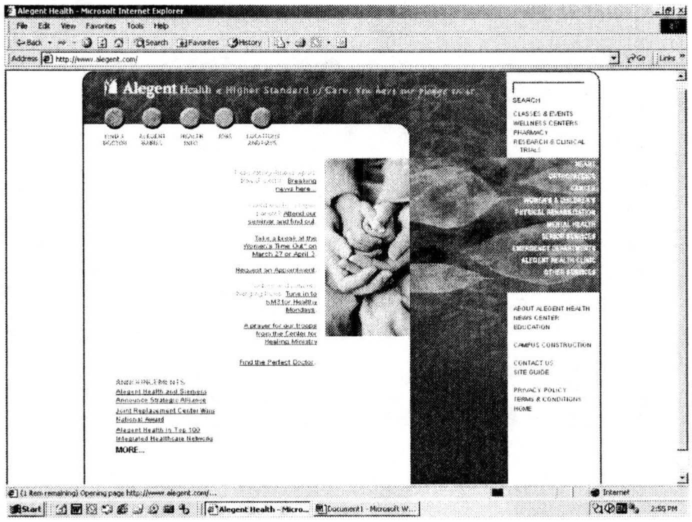

gible for simplified bulk mailing in the Broken Bow area, and 4,758 eligible in the Ogallala area. Because bulk mailing was used, this eliminated the need for individual addressing; however, it did not provide for random sampling.

Participation was voluntary. Each participant was asked to browse the sample e-health Web site to become familiar with its contents and capabilities, and was directed to view various pages on the Web site. Participants were then asked to complete one of four health risk assessments and complete a Web site usability questionnaire survey. Each health risk assessment asked a series of questions about the individual's personal health and then provided a risk assessment analyzing the individual's health condition, based on the participant's responses. If the results of the health risk assessment suggested a serious health problem, the participant was directed to follow up with his or her personal physician. Figure 2 displays the introductory page of the sample e-health Web site.

It is important to recognize that there are additional ethical considerations when dealing with medical and health advice. It was paramount that correct and accurate health information was disseminated. Alegent Health agreed to collaborate in the research. Alegent Health is a recognized and well-respected medical center in the Midwest that has won several national awards relating to the presentation and content of its Web site. Alegent Health allowed its Web site to be altered to include several Web pages directed toward participants in this study.

Out of the 7,850 invitation letters, 276 respondents voluntarily participated in the online e-health study. Of those 276 participants, 260 responses provided data that were complete and matched the generalizing population. More females (64%) participated in the study than males (36%). This was not surprising given that often women are the ones who oversee the healthcare of the members in a family. Over 80% of the participants were married, 7% were single, 8% were divorced, and 4% were widowed.

The respondents' age ranged from 19 years to over 90 years old. 60% of the respondents reported they were 40–59 years of age, and 30% of the respondents were over 65, a figure roughly 10% higher than is represented in the general population. This suggests that as people get older they have more health concerns and, thus, they were

Table 1. Rural residents' Internet connections

Internet Connection Type	Number of Responses	Percentage
Modem/Phone Line	193	74
Cable Modem	24	9
T1 or Faster	23	9
Satellite	9	4
Unknown	11	4

more interested in responding to this particular study.

Participants were asked about their level of education. The results indicated that 85% of the participants had some post-high school education. A majority of the participants (81%) worked outside the home, 7% were at-home spouses, 11% were retired, and 1% were unemployed. As one might expect, many of the participants working outside the home were employed in the agriculture industry (17%). The remaining participants were a cross-section of the professions that serve a community such as bankers, attorneys, physicians, teachers, nurses, clergy, and accountants.

Most of the participants connected to the Internet from home (76%) or from work (21%). The study found that 74% of the participants access the Internet via dial-up connection and only 9% of the participants have high-speed Internet access (see Table 1).

Over 40% of participants reported they use a computer 1–10 hours a week, 27% use a computer 11–20 hours a week, and 33% use a computer more than 21 hours a week. Internet usage was somewhat less. The majority (76%) uses the Internet 1–10 hours a week, 17% use the Internet 11-20 hours a week, and 7% use the Internet more than 21 hours a week.

Based on the responses, one may conclude that many rural residents are experienced and knowledgeable computer and Internet users. It is likely that they are interested in improving their quality of life by having better access to health-care services, and, therefore, have a legitimate interest in e-health. Next, we discuss the health issues that the participants were asked to respond to in the study.

Health Risk Assessments

The participants were asked to select one or more four health risk assessments to complete in the study. These assessments evaluated individual risk relating to:

- Flu and Cold
- Allergies
- Lung Cancer
- Heart Disease

The heart disease health risk assessment was the most popular, and the lung cancer assessment was the least popular. Ten participants answered all four assessments and three subjects did not participate in this portion of the study. For further analysis, the health assessments were grouped according to the seriousness of the illness. Flu and cold and allergies assessments were grouped as low risk assessments, and lung cancer and heart disease were grouped as high risk assessments. The low risk assessment group had 106 responses, and the high risk assessment had 141 responses.

Table 2. Reasons for nonparticipation in the study

Reasons for Nonparticipation	Responses	Percentage
Does not have access to the Internet	334	61%
Does not use a computer	324	59%
Does not have access to a computer	273	50%
Not interested in the Study	128	23%
Concerned with Privacy	125	23%
Other Concerns (with option to write comments)	63	12%

Table 3. Regression analysis

Dependent Variable	Independent Variable(s)	R^2	Adjusted R^2	Std. Error of the Estimate	F	Significance
Age	Does not have access to the Internet	0.889	0.870	0.0813	48.034	.000
Age	Does not use a computer	0.926	0.914	0.0935	75.561	.000
Age	Does not have access to a computer	0.855	0.831	0.1282	35.424	.001

Feedback from Nonparticipants

Included with the invitation letter was a postage-paid return post card that asked rural residents to indicate whether they intended to participate in the study. If the rural resident indicated s/he did not intend to participate in the study, then s/he was asked to choose among six options explaining this decision. Table 2 summarizes reasons given for nonparticipation.

As the respondents' age increased, so did the response percentage for (1) does not have access to the Internet, (2) does not use a computer, and (3) does not have access to a computer as indicated in the regression analysis results presented in Table 3. Male and female responses had minimal differences in the response percentages on reasons for not participating.

IMPORTANT DIMENSIONS IN RURAL RESIDENTS' PERCEPTIONS OF E-HEALTH

As the final stage of participation, a questionnaire survey was administered to participants which included these two open-ended questions:

- What do you look for in a healthcare Web site that would increase your opinion of its trustworthiness?

- Please type any other comments you wish to make.

Most participants responded to both questions. This section examines dimensions that emerged from participants' comments as being important to their perceptions—and potential acceptance and use—of e-health.

Prior Experience with E-Health Web Sites

The participants had varying prior experience using an e-health Web site. Some had never accessed an e-health Web site and some had used them on a routine basis.

For example, an experienced e-health user responds:

I have used several different health Web sites for medical information so I think this is a valuable service. When distance is involved it's great when you can actually call a doctor for his/her opinion on a particular disease or illness and can actually talk to them!

Other participants were just being introduced to e-health:

This is the first time I have connected with a health Web site. We received a letter in the mail, and that is how I discovered this. I'm not real sure of what this Web site entails, but [I] would like some more information on it. I was rather impressed by the information it contained. I do believe that its trustworthiness is [with]in my scope. Thank you.

This diversity of experience suggests it will be necessary for e-health application designers to support novices as well as sophisticated users in order for successful diffusion among rural residents.

E-Health Value

A fundamental value of an e-health Web site for rural residents is that it can be used as the first decision point to determine if an individual has a serious health problem, and if a physician's advice should be sought. Several comments related to this issue:

This could be very useful, as time is very limited for me to see a doctor and [it] could help to make a person decide if they need to see a doctor.

At one time my blood pressure was high, but I am on Toprel and I feel much better. This Web site is a wonderful invention to anyone who visits that has health concerns and doesn't want to stand in line waiting for a doctor to answer questions, [and to bother a doctor] who is too busy to answer those questions.

I did see how this Web site was more or less helpful to a person in a rural area. I had no idea where it was until I called up a map, though I imagined it to be in Omaha. How is this site and this medical group going to help rural people? Wellness check-ups would be good. It is too far for many rural people to use the facilities weekly, but a check-up and follow up may work.

Understanding the Unique Needs of Rural Residents

Although there was considerable positive feedback from most participants, a few expressed skepticism as to whether urban organizations that provided e-health services really understood the unique needs of rural people. One person wrote:

I believe it is unlikely that most rural consumers would find a lot of use for a Web site that originates from an urban/suburban area unless you can make it very applicable to their daily lives - I don't see this site doing a lot of that. It appears more as a commercial for Alegent (which means nothing to me). I also appreciate the attempt and find the fact that you are willing to try to increase this area to be very encouraging. Any connection to "known" providers and services will create a much more trusting environment.

Communicating E-Health Web Site Purpose and Services

Participants suggested that the e-health Web site should provide information, such as whether they are available to answer questions, if they provide information on insurance plans and supplementary Medicare programs, and whether they will refer users to specialists and also to doctors in general. Participants were particularly concerned about how information on the Web site is communicated:

The Web site should provide information that is consistent with other information on the same subject. [The Web site should be a place where] second opinions are not discouraged and excepting questions and receiving courteous replies and true concern for the individual.

Many participants appeared to be well-informed on health matters, and they carefully evaluated the quality, validity, and depth of the health risk assessment questionnaire survey. They communicated a high expectation on the depth and breadth of the information that was offered. This was especially evident in the evaluation of the health risk assessments. The health risk assessments were designed to be simple and quick for the purposes of the usability study. However, this decision may have negatively impacted some of the results. Some of the participants were expecting a more in-depth assessment and response:

I took this survey to find some information on health risk factors. It gave none. I am very disappointed, and this survey hurt your credibility as a health entity in my opinion.

I was disappointed in the basic level of assessment questions asked. Seeing my physician is an assumed response if I am not feeling well. No specific information on allergy management resulted from the answers in my survey response. I did not take an extended time [to browse] the site, however, and so [I] may have missed information that was available. I do appreciate the Internet's ability to connect rural areas to information and services!

These responses suggest that rural residents are interested in knowing the value and purpose of the e-health Web site, and therefore it is important that the Web site clearly communicates its purpose and services in a manner that is convincing to knowledgeable consumers.

E-Health and Healthcare Advertising Do Not Mix

Rural residents are sensitive to e-health Web sites that advertise organizations, products, or services. They are especially concerned that these sites may be biased:

The Web site should have the correct information without the influence of drug companies, helpful resources, and non-biased consideration of both traditional and non-traditional medicine and healthcare ideas.

The Web site should not be trying to sell anything and not trying to get you to switch to another healthcare provider.

Web Site Content and Language is Important

The Web site must contain accurate and verifiable information that is written so that it is complete, yet understandable. Two participants explained this point as follows:

The Web site should have easy access to the term I am trying to find [that is a] current issue to me and the wording used to explain things [should be understandable to me], if it is all medical terms that only a medical student would totally understand, then it is of little use to me.

I would like to see information that is not in doctor's terms to locate a doctor, but state the area [illness, disease or human body part] of reach it covers. Such as Cardiologist - heart doctor. People in rural areas do not understand the [professional medical terminology] terms and names given to what a doctor does for a living.

Reputation of Sponsoring Organization is Important

The participants in this study were looking for a "Seal of Approval" from a physician or a recognized hospital. Several commented that it was important to them for the e-health Web site to have a partnership with a known healthcare provider, a recognized expert in the field, or a health organization with name recognition. They also suggested that their likelihood of using the e-health Web site would increase if it was endorsed by their own family physician. Many stated that the reputation of the organization sponsoring the e-health Web site was very important, and they would evaluate the credentials of the sponsors:

A health Web site should enlist the advice of a licensed medical doctor/physician assistant/registered nurse or a doctor/pa-c/rn who is currently practicing or recently trained and who is up on current health issues.

I prefer the health Web pages that come from medical associations (i.e. AMA). I find their information to be reliable and useful. I do use the Mayo Clinic Web site sometimes, so I might use a Web site from a local hospital.

I usually use Mayo's site because of my confidence in Mayo. A Web site backed by the University, a reputable clinic or known group of MD's would interest me. As you know there are less than reputable medical Web sites on the Internet. We need to know who we are dealing with to trust the medical information received.

I would trust a Web site more if it was endorsed by my family physician.

Security and Privacy Issues

Both security and privacy issues were raised. In this study, no personal contact information was requested (e.g. phone number or address), and no self-identifying information was requested that would link the response to a specific individual. However, it is likely that concern regarding security and privacy issues would increase if more self-identifying information and data were requested. Security and privacy are especially important when there is interaction between a physician and a patient. One participant summed up it as follows:

[My] biggest fear would be the possibility of hackers looking for specifics. At this point in time we really don't feel we have information/details of any interest to whatever a hacker might be looking for; consequently, for this survey there is no [credit] card numbers or social security information that you are asking for. Once that information is requested, our trust in a Web site is diminished.

E-Health Web Site Trustworthiness and Confidentiality

Potential users of e-health services are concerned about trust and confidentiality. They want to know who will have access to their health information and how it will be used:

The Web site should provide a list of contacts of everyone who handles or has access to information provided by [the] Web site user.

If I had questions about my health or my family's health that backed up or built on our family physician's diagnosis, it would increase my opinion of the Web site's trustworthiness. The same would be true if the Web site's information was similar to other medical reading.

Usability of the E-Health User Interface

Some participants had problems navigating the e-health Web site:

It is harder for some[one] with less than the best eyesight anymore, to read words on some colored backgrounds. Also, getting from step 1 to step 2 of the survey took me too long because I forgot I had to close the box I was in - I would have liked to [have] seen a prompt at the end of the survey to get me right to the next step.

It was very difficult to find the buttons to move around. The fonts are too small. There is too much reading on a page. Simplify your home page.

These comments suggest that special support for visual impairment in order for some rural residents to use e-health effectively, especially aging individuals.

Technological Infrastructure Issues and Constraints

Many rural citizens do not have access to a high bandwidth Internet connection. Because of this barrier, Internet connection speed is more of an issue than in urban communities. Some of the problems the participants expressed were:

My Internet server [provider] doesn't always allow me to see all of a Web site; this was true for the Alegent Web site. A lot of the links and various buttons were unreadable to me.

My only hesitation in completing this survey is that our Internet connections are SO slow here that it takes longer to do something on the computer on Internet, so it is usually things of importance.

These comments suggest the amount of graphics and images used to convey health information needs to be minimized or the e-health site will be of limited use to many rural residents.

Appreciation of Interest in Rural Communities

There were many comments expressing appreciation for the concern and interest in expanding healthcare delivery options to rural citizens. Those engaged in farming, ranching, and agriculture find it is often difficult to take off time to travel the long distance that is necessary to see to a doctor. These jobs require daily physical attention, and finding substitutes when someone is not available to work is a challenge as most people in rural communities are already employed:

When you live 85 miles from Kearney, 100[miles] from Grand Island, 3 1/2 hours' drive from Lincoln & 4 hours from Omaha, people that live where I do just accept that some healthcare is not available close. Sometimes I feel that the "big cities" think that the state revolves around them.

Anytime someone is interested in helping the rural community, I appreciate it. We fight to keep our schools, hospitals, etc. We have the best life possible in the rural areas; trust among neighbors and an interest in each other.

E-health needs to apply to rural situations. The Web site needs to communicate an understanding of rural residents, appreciation of their daily life challenges and constraints, and clearly explain how it can improve the quality of healthcare for rural residents. Providing general health information is not enough. Rural residents have well-developed expectations on what e-health Web sites and services can do for them. They are expecting answers for specific problems, actionable advice, and interaction with e-health service providers.

Summary

Both e-health designers and administrators can benefit from this analysis. Several key implications emerged:

- Potential rural users of e-health vary greatly in prior experience with e-health.
- The value and purpose of e-health needs to be emphasized and presented clearly.
- E-health needs to clearly identify what health services are provided.
- E-health is valuable primarily in addressing health issues that are specific to users rather than general health information.
- E-health should avoid advertising organizations, products, or services.
- E-health content and language must be understandable.
- E-health should be endorsed by recognized and respected institutions and/or medical experts.
- E-health needs to convey to rural residents an understanding of their unique needs.
- E-health security and privacy concerns are high among rural residents.
- The Web site graphics may need to be limited due to lack of available high bandwidth connectivity.
- The main reason most rural residents did not participate was due to not having to access to a computer or the Internet. Over time, this problem will likely diminish.

DISCUSSION

The scope of this research was analyzing perceptions of an e-health Web site, which in many cases, is the entry point to many other more sophisticated and expansive health services such as video conferencing among physicians and patients. It is speculated that e-health services will continue to proliferate throughout the healthcare community and in time will become a frequent part of routine patient-physician healthcare relationships and communications. In the future, it is expected that it will be common for a patient to have Web-based online nonurgent consultations with his or her physician. The advantage of this type of e-health service is that physicians can handle less-critical problems in a lower-cost "virtual" office visit that eliminates the need for patients to travel and wait for appointments (Edlin, 2002). Other opportunities for e-health services include patients making appointments with their physicians, requesting prescription renewals online, e-mailing their physicians, and reserving various medical apparatus (e.g., crutches or walkers). It is likely that e-health users in both rural and urban settings will embrace e-health services as the technology continues to mature and becomes more affordable. However, the findings in this study suggest numerous steps that can be taken to improve perceptions of e-health in the short-term.

Limitations

The results of the study may have been impacted because of limited Internet access and bandwidth. The Alegent Health Web site is a highly graphical Web site which requires substantial telecommunications bandwidth for fast performance. Participants using dial-up Internet connections to access the Alegent Health Web site may have experienced slow response when navigating through the Web site. This, in turn, may have affected their perspective towards using e-health options for healthcare delivery.

CONCLUSION

If e-health services are to reach their potential, there still are barriers that need to be overcome. For example, reimbursement to providers of e-health services needs to be addressed. Also, licensure of physicians will have to be adjusted to reflect that e-health crosses state lines, as it is the states' responsibility to license physicians (Krizner, 2002). Having an adequate technology infrastructure available can be difficult to achieve, particularly for rural communities. This issue is partially being addressed by the U.S. Congress, which has begun to provide grant funding through a variety of agencies, including the FCC and the Agriculture Department to improve rural technology infrastructures.

E-health provides many opportunities to improve access to healthcare for both rural and urban communities. This chapter presented an in-depth analysis of potential rural e-health users' needs and expectations of e-health Web site services. Further research is needed to know how these results compare to potential users in urban communities.

REFERENCES

Edlin, M. (2002). Embracing e-health simplifies transactions, improves patient relations. *Managed Healthcare Executive, 12*(8), 30-32.

Fruhling, A., & Lee, S. (2006). The influence of user interface usability on rural consumers' trust of e-health services. *International Journal of Electronic Healthcare*, *2*(4), 305-321.

Grady, P.A. (2005). *Fiscal year 2006 budget request.* Witness appearing before the House Subcommittee on Labor-HHS-Education Appropriations. Retrieved May 26, 2008, from http://www.ninr.nih.gov/NR/rdonlyres/BF2F5680-88F0-4CBF-B86D-E12AE6101246/0/FY2006BudgetRequest.pdf

Krizner, K. (2002). Telemedicine still looks for inroad to total acceptability. *Managed Healthcare Executive*, *12*(5), 44-47.

Wilson, E.V. (2008). Creating patient-centered e-health. In N. Wickramasinghe, & E. Geisler (Eds.), *Encyclopedia of Healthcare Information Systems*, (pp. 318-324). Hershey, PA: IGI Publishing.

Chapter XIII
Assessing a Patient-Centered E-Health Approach to Chronic Disease Self-Management

Elizabeth Cummings
University of Tasmania and Smart Internet Technology Co-operative Research Centre, Australia

Stephen Chau
University of Tasmania and Verdant Health, Australia

Paul Turner
University of Tasmania and Smart Internet Technology Co-operative Research Centre, Australia

ABSTRACT

This chapter explores how in developing patient-centred e-health systems it is possible to accommodate heterogeneous characteristics of end-users and their diverse health and care contexts. It concurs with conventional sociotechnical design paradigms that argue systems must be easy to use, fulfill a perceived need, and present a clear value proposition to ensure successful adoption and utilisation by patients. The chapter also highlights the need for awareness of a number of key challenges relating to emerging discourses on 'empowering patients' and 'e-health'. The implications of these challenges for the development of a truly patient-centred e-health approach are explored in a detailed case study. This chapter contributes to research focused on supporting patients to become genuine co-participants in their own care, health and well-being. However, it also acknowledges that part of the challenge of achieving this goal requires a focus on assisting clinicians to learn to respond to this shift in the autonomy of decision-making.

BACKGROUND

Health reform has been a major item on political and policy agendas across the developed world. Alongside changes to health system funding arrangements, medical insurances and the legal and regulatory environments, e-health initiatives have been identified as major drivers for stimulating the changes necessary to address the crisis. By opening up opportunities for increased information access, cost effectiveness, improved information delivery, update and evaluation the economic case for more information and communication technology (ICT) is strong. However, this deployment also raises a number of sociotechnical, clinical, and legal challenges that have become increasingly evident as the implementations of more sophisticated ICT solutions have met with mixed success or failed to generate their forecast benefits. E-health innovations do have huge potential to support a "better connected health system" that is more efficient, safer, and knowledge-based and provides universal, accessible, and affordable care. However, many approaches to e-health continue to downplay high levels of complexity and uncertainty that exist in the delivery of healthcare services and make problematic assumptions about how ICTs will benefit patients, health professionals, and the healthcare system as a whole (Cummings & Turner, 2007).

The growing crisis in healthcare delivery is also at least partly attributable to the increasing incidence of chronic illness and complex medical conditions associated with the rapidly ageing populations of most 'first world' countries. The focus on chronic illness is directly related to the fact that up to 75% of patients presenting for healthcare have chronic conditions (Epping-Jordan, Bengoa, Kawar, & Sabate, 2001; Fries, Friday, Gira, Cooper, England, Graves, Sokolov, & Wright, 1993). There have been numerous responses to chronic illness, including one set of approaches that emphasize the importance of enfranchising and empowering the patients and/or their carers to become co-participants in their own care. At the most basic level, these approaches are premised on assumptions that patients are both able and willing to participate, that their involvement will improve disease treatment, management, and education, and the net result will be positive results in terms of health outcomes. To date, the wide range of methodologies and assessment procedures used by those implementing these approaches has made comparisons difficult. Although most evaluations have reported some benefits, it is evident that considerable complexity and uncertainty remains regarding how best to support self-management of chronic illness (Warsi, Wang, LaValley, & Avorn, 2004).

INTRODUCTION

This chapter examines a number of key challenges related to the emerging discourses on "empowering patients" and "e-health." The implications of these challenges are explored in a detailed case study. The case study presented in the second part of this book chapter highlights the inherent challenges of moving towards a patient-centred model of healthcare. The case study focuses on a controlled trial that aims to assist people with chronic respiratory conditions, including chronic obstructive pulmonary disease (COPD) and cystic fibrosis (CF), to achieve increased levels of self-efficacy for self-management through interactions with case mentors (community health nurses), and the adoption and use of Web and mobile information systems.

This chapter promotes a patient-centred e-health approach. It is argued that benefits from such an approach can only be realised if systems are specifically designed and implemented on the basis of a detailed understanding of end-users, their needs and complex interactions with one another, the health system, and the wider environment. Without such a holistic approach, there is a concern that the existing inequities of access to quality healthcare faced by many patients will be further compounded by an emerging e-health divide. We must avoid widening this divide to allow the existing inequalities between information "haves" and "have-nots" to be compounded by presenting additional financial, technological, and skill barriers to chronically ill patients (many of the poorest, oldest, and most vulnerable members of our societies) as more health information and services come to be provided primarily online.

Various forms of ICT are increasingly being deployed to allow patients to monitor their health conditions within the comfort of their homes. However, the emergence of these types of systems presumes that patients are both willing and able to adopt and utilise these systems, and that doing so will be beneficial in terms of health and other outcomes. Clearly, from a patient-centred perspective it is important to know whether patients can interpret the data that these systems provide to generate information and knowledge that they can use to self-manage. This implies a need to acknowledge the interplay between at least two elements, both of which are in a state of flux—the system and the patients' paradigm of care. If only the ICT is changed, then this can be treated merely as another medical intervention, such as a new drug, that will be evaluated through the conventional measurement prism of clinical outcomes. However, if there is also a shift in focus regarding the role of patients in their own care, then evaluation measurements need to encompass not just clinical outcomes but also the perspectives, attitudes, insights, and experiences of individual patients. Significantly, this implies taking seriously patients' critical decision-making processes that may run counter to the decisions of a clinician. For example, a clinician's decision on treatment (often based upon the construct of an "average patient") may be countermanded by an individual patient for whom pain of treatment may be rejected in favour of higher quality, but shorter life.

While these sorts of decisions are commonplace in palliative care, they are rare in other types of care. Chronic illness currently accounts for over 70% of the burden of disease in Australia as measured in terms of disability-adjusted life years (Jordan & Osborne, 2007). This is expected to increase to 80% by 2020 (National Health Priority Action Council, 2006). In a recent publication by the Milken Institute called "An Unhealthy America: The Economic Burden of Chronic disease," it is reported that chronic health conditions cost the U.S. economy over $1 trillion a year, and this cost is likely to rise significantly in the future (DeVol, Bedroussian, Charuworn, Chatterjee, Kim, Kim, et al., 2007). As a result, the need to consider patients' perspectives is likely to increase, not because many "Internet-empowered" patients' are beginning to demand it.

While arguing for a patient-centred approach is easy, taking it seriously presents some very real challenges for those engaged in practical health projects across different patient cohorts. In approaching these challenges, this chapter is presented in two major parts. Part one examines a number of key challenges related to the emerging discourses on "empowering patients" and "e-health." These challenges underpin conventional approaches to healthcare for the chronically ill and must be understood and addressed in the development of any patient-centred e-health approach. Part two explores the implications of these challenges in a case study. The case study examines the development of a patient-centred approach aimed to assist people with chronic respiratory conditions, to achieve increased levels of self-efficacy for self-management through interactions with case mentors (community health nurses), and the adoption and use of Web and mobile information systems.

PART ONE: CONSIDERATIONS FOR A PATIENT-CENTRED APPROACH

Evidence-based medicine (EBM) proponents have developed an "hierarchy of evidence," which considers randomized controlled trials (RCT) and meta-analyses of RCTs to provide the most reliable evidence concerning the efficacy of medical interventions (Borgerson, 2005). Denny (1999) identifies EBM as reinforcing the scientific nature of medicine. Inadvertently, it also can be considered a means of fortifying the medical profession's authority. EBM tends to separate the treatment of disease from the social and environmental factors that contribute to the disease process. EBM also tends not to take into account the social situation of medicine nor patient individuality, values, experiences, and goals. It has the strong potential to obstruct patients' right to choice and their influence on decision making, thus imposing a biomedical model of medicine (Frankford, 1994) in place of patient empowerment. Simultaneously, however, EBM can be viewed as an approach that actually limits the autonomy of the medical profession, both clinically and economically, leading to increased external control by the state (Coburn, Rappolt, & Bourgeault, 1997; Rappolt, 1997). These paradoxes are underpinned by the reality that despite widespread conviction in the value of EBM, most diseases and treatments continue to lack a strong evidence base.

This is not to suggest that use of EBM is inappropriate or detrimental, rather it is to highlight that EBM is rarely well defined in theory or in practice, particularly in relation to chronic illness. EBM can be employed within a humanistic approach to provide critical information regarding scientific evidence to aid patients and practitioners in weighing the risks and benefits of treatment options (Frankford, 1994). Indeed, there is a positive trend in most developed countries towards EBM and the equalisation of relationships between health professionals and lay people (Eysenbach, 2000). The merits of this trend point towards a desire to decrease the cost of healthcare by encouraging patients to become coparticipants in their own care and to engage in self-management on the basis of being better informed. This trend has coincided with increased use of the Internet and other technologies in healthcare and the rise of the "Internet empowered" patient.

Unfortunately, most health systems have evolved to be responsive to acute conditions, but struggle to address the increasing prevalence of chronic and complex health conditions (Wagner, Austin, Davis, Hindmarsh, Schaefer, & Bonomi, 2001). Chronic conditions require treatment at a number of different levels (e.g., psychological, social, economic, and lifestyle changes, as well as the physical and treatment regimens themselves). People with chronic illness are often their own principal care-givers, and as a result, self-management and education has been recognised to be of critical importance. But this situation requires recognition of the how to facilitate a changing role for health professionals in supporting and facilitating patients as co-participants in care. This new role should be to ensure that patients with chronic illnesses "have the confidence and skills to manage their condition; the most appropriate treatments to assure optimal disease control and prevention of complications; a mutually understood care plan; and careful, continuous follow-up" (Wagner et al., 2001, pp. 66). However, in reality, if patients are involved in capturing information about their current health condition, they still do require the assistance of health professionals to interpret and provide a holistic review of their situations (Bodenheimer, Lorig, Holman, & Grumbach, 2002).

Related to issues surrounding the changing roles of health professionals and patients is recognition of how this impacts on conventional doctor-patient relationships where the doctor acts as the sole source of expertise and decision-making authority (Charles, Gafni, & Whelan, 1997). "Too often, a patient's treatments are performed 'by the book' rather than being tailored to the patient's specific needs. Others consider the care that today's patients receive is 'medicine by numbers,' which is best suited for that mythical abstraction, the 'statistically average patient.'" (Schneider & Lane, 2005, pp. iv)

Pincus (2004) describes this traditional biomedical model of health as one in which it is doctors, rather than patients or society, who are responsible for good health. Significantly, this model continues to be very successful in acute care, the setting of most medical education and training, but is increasingly recognised as problematic when applied to general health and chronic illness. The major limitation of the biomedical model is the underlying assumption that patients will conform to treatment. In many cases, patients do not do this. Patient awareness, capacity for self-management and social context are often as important as any action by health professionals in determining long-term health outcomes.

Alternatives to the traditional physician-patient relationship are more recent and are described using various names, such as *shared decision making* (Charles et al., 1997), *collaborative management* (Von Korff, Gruman, Schaefer, Curry, & Wagner, 1997), *the chronic care model* (Wagner et al., 2001), *the partnership model* (Holman & Lorig, 2000), and *patient empowerment* (Funnell, Anderson, Arnold, Barr, Donnelly, Johnson, Taylor-Moon, & White, 1991). Each concerns the same or similar notions that patient, physician, and family members should pool information and make choices together, whether the current health issue is an acute disease or long-term condition. Thus, when chronic care experts promote the incorporation of "self-management education" and "self-management support" into clinicians' practice, they are recommending the use of collaborative techniques (Barrett, 2005. pp. 16).

Kaplan, Greenfield, Gandek, Rogers, and Ware, (1996) suggest that informed patients who ask questions, consider treatment options, express opinions and state preferences tend to have better health outcomes. When patients feel they participate in decision-making, they are more likely to comply with treatment. This is particularly relevant to those with chronic conditions. The recognition of patients as people and the use of good communication skills are important in understanding symptoms, diagnosing, and gaining compliance.

In response to the ageing demographics of most first world countries, the work of the General-Practitioner (GP) is increasingly moving towards chronic disease management. However, in some instances GPs face the challenge of patients who are unwilling to "get better" or unmotivated to change unhealthy behaviours, such as smoking. This leads to frustration on the part of doctors who are expected to solve problems in which they lack authority. Indeed, many doctors feel disempowered in consultations because they lack the capacity to intervene medically in a meaningful way with these types of chronically ill patients.

More positively, Gruman and Von Korff (1996, pp. 1) have developed the following definition of self-management following a comprehensive review of over 400 articles. They define self-management as the person with the chronic disease "engaging in activities that protect and promote health, monitoring and managing of symptoms and signs of illness, managing the impacts of illness on functioning, emotions and interpersonal relationships and adhering to treatment regimes."

Evidence suggests that patients who display effective self-management skills are able to better use healthcare professionals' time (Barlow, Turner, & Wright, 2000; Lorig, Sobel, Stewart, Brown, Bandura, Ritter, et al., 1999). Clinical benefits for patients with conditions such as diabetes and hypertension have been demonstrated in systematic reviews of the effectiveness of many self-management programs, but this appears not to be the case for arthritis. Unfortunately, comparisons of the benefits of chronic disease self-management programmes are hampered by differences in the types of chronic illness examined, the theoretical frameworks deployed and the methods and assessment procedures utilised (Chodosh, Morton, Mojica, Maglione, Suttorp, Hilton, Rhodes, & Shekelle, 2005; Monninkhof, van der Aa, van der Valk, van der Palen, Zielhuis, Koning, & Pieterse, 2004; Monninkhof, van der Valk, van der Palen, van Herwaarden, Partidge, Walters, & Zielhuis, 2002; Newman, Steed, & Mulligan, 2004; Taylor, Candy, Bryar, Vrijhoef, Esmond, Wedzicha, et al., 2005; Warsi, LaValley, Wang, Avorn, & Solomon, 2003; Warsi et al., 2004; Zwar, Harris, Griffiths, Roland, Dennis, Powell Davies, & Hasan, 2006) Despite these difficulties, many evaluations report some benefit and all highlight the critical importance of health professionals in supporting these self-management behaviours.

McKinstry (2000, pp. 868) found that the "desire for involvement in decision making is variable. There is some correlation with age, illness type, social class and education level." In this study, patients nominated a preference for a more directive relationship than a partnership particularly with the older patients and those with acute conditions. Of course, this raises a further conceptual question regarding whether patients are just assuming the role of a "good patient" as a result of socialisation into the paternalistic model of health? Auerbach (2001) finds that patients want more information, but demonstrate a preference for either physician only or collaborative decision making rather than patient decision making control. Lower levels of education, serious illness, and increasing age have also been found to impact upon the desire for control (Auerbach, 2001).

At the same time, there is a rapid growth in consumer health informatics focused on patient empowerment. Patients increasingly exhibit a preference for tailored information rather than general health information. This may be due to *the inverse information law* (Eysenbach, 2000) and may be evident where access to appropriate information is particularly difficult for those who need it most. There is a worrying and widening information gap between those that have access and those who don't, particularly for those patients that have low education and low literacy, low income, poor health and inaccessibility to ICT (Eysenbach, 2000), and there is the danger of an e-health divide emerging along the same lines as the information haves and have-nots.

So where does this leave a developing patient-centred e-health model and, how can the heterogeneous characteristics of patients be accommodated in the delivery of healthcare information focused on the needs, sensitivities, and convenience of individual patients? Unfortunately, to date, there is little research that comprehensively examines how technology can be applied to a new paradigm of patient-centred healthcare. However, Barrett (2005) has developed a useful system for categorising self-management tools. He classifies tools to promote self-management into four classes of tools described below.

Subordinate tools are primarily supervisory or controlling technologies which allow external surveillance of patients. Patients tend to not interact with these tools, but are merely observed with them.

Typical *structured support tools* include home monitoring and messaging systems (Barrett, 2005). These rely upon the patients to carry out the monitoring, often in response to automated prompts, but are undertaken within a bounded set of rules. These support tools do not engage patients in developing problems solving skills, but report findings back to clinicians for interpretation. Thus, they are an aid to compliance, rather than developing or reinforcing independent self-management skills. "A really useful product would reinforce independent behaviour and help avoid long-term dependency" (Barrett, 2005, pp. 16).

Collaborative tools "involve patients using their own knowledge and making decisions jointly with clinicians. Such tools engage physicians and patients in shared decision-making envisioned by disease management advocates and clinical care theorists" (Barrett, 2005, pp. 4). The introduction of more collaborative tools will promote a patient centric approach to chronic disease management.

But the development and implementation of these emergent tools need to be considerate of both the patient and healthcare provider perspectives. As mentioned earlier in this paper, it is difficult and inappropriate to assume that the development of generic tool sets will solve all needs. There is a vast library of literature that has explored chronic health diseases and the use of ICT in health—however, there is a lack of substantive research that explores and understands the unique needs of diverse patient cohorts, which we believe may be handled best through collaborative healthcare partnerships with health providers.

Autonomous tools do not require regular input or participation by clinicians. These tools facilitate patients taking control of their health with minimal clinician participation. Introduction of autonomous tools will need to overcome significant sociocultural, professional and contextual barriers, a goal that that may be some time away.

We propose that a patient-centred approach to chronic disease requires tools that are a combination of collaborative and autonomous technologies. These types of tools are those best suited to empowering patients to understand their illnesses and to enable them to work in informed partnership with their healthcare providers.

PART TWO: IMPLICATIONS OF THE ISSUES EXAMINED

In order to explore the implications of these issues, we explored the insights, experiences and observations from a case study developed as a patient-centred approach to empower chronically ill respiratory patients in the community to self monitor and self manage their health condition with the remote support of healthcare professionals.

The case study examines alternative communication mechanisms through the use of a Web portal and mobile phone technology which has been specifically developed to aid chronically ill people undertake self-monitoring of their condition. This aims to improve their self-efficacy for self-management and encourage a partnership approach to their care.

Self-efficacy is the belief that one has the capabilities to undertake and complete a course of actions that are necessary to manage a given situation. The expectation that one can successfully complete a behaviour, or self-efficacy, is theorised to be an important predictor of whether one attempts the behaviour (Ajzen, 1985; Bandura, 1982). Aligned to this is the concept of self-management, which involves individual patients, in this case chronically ill patients, working in partnership with their carers and health professionals to manage their illness (Cummings & Turner, 2007).

Background to the Case Study

The Pathways Home for Respiratory Illness project is a controlled trial, randomised by domicile, which aims to assist people with chronic respiratory conditions, specifically COPD and CF, to achieve increased levels of self-management, self-efficacy for self-management and empowerment in relation to their conditions through ICT interventions and interactions with case mentors. Whilst it may appear that locating this research within a controlled trial environment conflicts with the critique of EBM presented within the previous section of the chapter, this is not the case. It is possible for a patient-centred ICT to underpin a controlled trial, and the evaluation of such a system can enhance the overall trial evaluation methodology. The authors have attempted to both develop and evaluate the ICT tool utilising the principles of patient-centred development, whilst the controlled trial is evaluated using positivist principles.

The project provides a means by which patients can monitor their conditions, both in relation to strict clinical indicators provided by the clinicians through EBM and in relation to individual indicators or triggers that the patient may have identified previously or may identify as a result of documented self-management. This approach acknowledges that patients are individuals and not merely bundles of clinical indicators. In this way the project is moving self-management away from simply another medical intervention to open up the possibility of supporting individualised care through the patient and his/her interactions with health professionals and the healthcare system. Following Muir Gray (2004) this involves the following actions:

- Inform and educate patients about self-management and about their condition;
- Encourage patients to reflect on their options and relate these to their own personalised priorities; and
- Facilitate individualised/personalised care interactions with health professionals based on an awareness of individual patient's preferences and self-expressed priorities and self-management experiences.

These considerations are essential if we are serious about encouraging patient self-management, as it must be anticipated that the experience will change patients' perceptions, expectations and decisions with regard to their chronic disease in ways that may be different from conventional clinical practice.

The development of self-management skills is twofold. First, access is provided to mentors with specific training in assisting patients in developing and promoting self-management skills. Second, this mentoring is aided through the provision of a range of self-monitoring tools to assist with identification and understanding the course of patients' individual illness patterns and promote informed decision making.

This patient-focused approach is premised on the view that, where possible, patients should play a central role in decisions about their own health. At the broadest level, this approach is underpinned by the perspective that providing evidence-based knowledge to patients will enhance their ability to participate in decisions about their own care and contribute to the development of an increasingly effective patient-centred healthcare system (Hill, 1998).

From a technology perspective, developing and deploying ICT to support self-efficacy and self-management amongst chronically ill patients presents numerous challenges. Most significantly, this cohort of patients exhibit diverse levels of physical and psychological capacities as a result of their illness, as well as a wide range of abilities, experiences, support mechanisms, and interests.

The project team was keen to avoid the possibility that any introduced ICT should end up simply replacing patient dependency on health professionals with a dependency on the technology, such that patients end up undertaking the monitoring of their symptoms without actually developing the self-efficacy and self-management skills necessary to respond to changes in their illness. As a result, the project team made considerable efforts to identify and accommodate the range of patient characteristics from amongst potential users of the system in the design, deployment, training and use of the ICT. In essence, this involved providing a variety of accessibility tools and a range of data entry methods to enable accessibility for all members of the disease cohort. These included paper, Internet and mobile devices, applications, and interfaces made available to different patients as part of the project.

From this experience it is argued that, for an ICT to be truly patient-centred, the characteristics of the end-users and their contexts must be considered along with ensuring that it is easy to use, fulfils a perceived need and presents a clear value proposition for adoption and utilisation. In this regard, information systems researchers within the team have spent a considerable amount of time and effort in understanding, interacting with and training all participants in the adoption and use of the technology.

Adopting this patient-centred approach acknowledges that the COPD patients are older persons, between the ages of 50 and 90. Many of the older patients have little or no experience with ICT and may have other conditions that make manipulation and/or visualisation of small pieces of equipment difficult such that a degree of individualisation of the ICTs is required. In contrast the patients in the CF cohort are between the ages of 16 and 45. These patients are more experienced with technology and many have their own computers at home or at work. Software components must be capable of being used on multiple platforms to enable choice of technology by the participants.

These accommodations enable the project to work with patients to select the technologies and technology training that best suit their current situation, capabilities, and experience, yet are flexible to changes as patients develop of greater knowledge or interest during the course of the project. In addition to the various technology-supported communication modes, a complete paper-based alternative will be available with centralised data entry. We anticipate the possibility that additional technology and information solutions may be introduced during the course of the trial in response to participant needs.

In the literature, symptom-monitoring diaries are widely recommended to encourage self-management practices. Within this project this is undertaken through the subjective interpretation of symptoms. Monitoring diaries are important, as the process can aid in clarifying when, how much, and in what context the symptoms occur. However, symptom monitoring in isolation is rarely an effective method for managing symptoms (Blanchard, Appelbaum, Radnitz, Michultka, Morrill, Kirsch, Hillhouse, Evans, Guarnieri, Attanasio, Andrasik, Jaccard, & Dentinger, 1990a; Blanchard, E., Appelbaum, Radnitz, Morrill, Michultka, Kirsch, Guarnieri, Hillhouse, Evans, Jaccard, & Barron, 1990b; Greene & Blanchard, 1994). This project utilises symptom monitoring in conjunction with mentor assisted action planning.

Partnership between patients and clinicians is an extremely important element of self-management. As suggested by Butler, Rollnick and Stott (1996):

> *Patients and clinicians are both considered experts on the patients' problems; the consultation is, therefore, a meeting between experts in which the experiential expert (the patient) meets with the clarification expert (the physician). In this view, the object of the consultation is not to convert the patient to the physician's point of view, but to enlist the patient as a therapeutic ally and to negotiate mutually acceptable plans for enhancing the patient's wellbeing* (pp. 1358).

The ICT component of the project is critical for supporting the participants in their decision-making to support self-management. ICT provides them with easily collect, transfer, and view data in different media, including the aggregated data that they have entered over a period of time. Given that deterioration in condition is frequently the result of slow, small, cumulative alterations, this ability to track minor changes over a period of time allows participants to understand trends and promotes the ability for them to intervene earlier. However, from an information systems perspective, it is clear that ensuring a successful technology implementation relies on a detailed understanding of users, their needs and the complex interactions with health professionals, the health system and the wider environment. This more holistic, patient-centred approach arises because of an awareness that while there are numerous studies supporting claims of the positive impact of ICTs in health information management and communications, questions remain over the continued lack of strong evidence on the impact of these improvements on overall patient health outcomes. Indeed, whilst the impact of new technology on driving improvements in clinical diagnosis and treatment is undoubted, the overall result of the introduction of technology in health information management and communication remains unclear, particularly where its design or implementation fails to adequately address end-user sociocultural and change management issues.

The ICT Tool

Essentially the tool provided to the participants was a diary tool to monitor their subjective symptoms and social interactions; clinical symptoms were identified by respiratory physicians within the controlled trial. This tool was available via a Web interface for both cohorts (see Figure 1) and also via mobile phone for the CF cohort (see Figure 3A). When a diary has been submitted, it is possible for the participants to view a longitudinal record online (see Figure 2) or, if using mobile phone, to request an SMS message reporting the previous seven days' diary entries in graphical format (see Figure 3B). The online longitudinal diary feedback was colour coded for ease of interpretation. The traditional traffic light colouring, green through to red, was used where green indicates normal or better symptom recording, and red indicates much worse than normal.

Methodology

Within the project, there were 108 participants recruited with COPD and 20 with CF. These participants were randomised into control and intervention groups. The use of the ICT tools was not mandatory. Adoption and subsequent use were viewed as participant choice, and the relationships between these factors and self-efficacy will be further investigated in other research.

In an effort to examine the individual's experience with self-management and the use of the ICT tools, a qualitative evaluation methodology was adopted. This methodology suited the exploratory nature of the research. Semi-structured interviews were conducted with 12 participants after they had completed a minimum of nine months within the project. Participants were selected for interview based upon the duration of their participation. The CF participants were interviewed at the completion of six months within the project. However, these interviews have not been analysed at the time of writing, and so the following results are based upon the COPD participant interviews only.

The analysis of the interview transcripts was underpinned by an interpretivist epistemology, as this was deemed to be the most logical and

Figure 1. Online daily diary

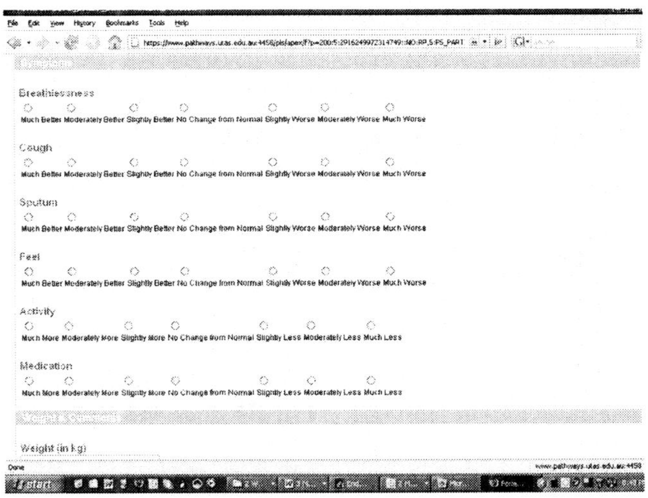

Figure 2. Online daily diary feedback

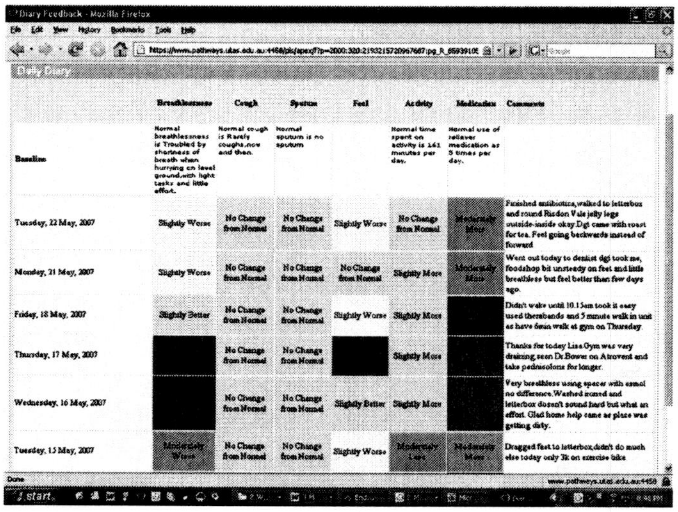

Figure 3. Mobile phone daily diary (a) and diary output (b)

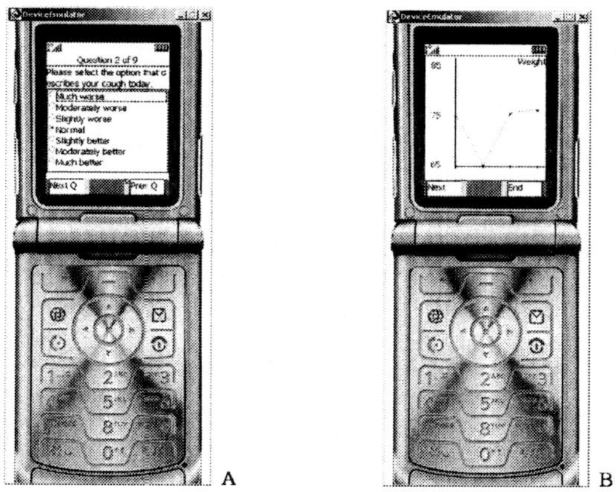

A B

appropriate approach to capture information about the perceptions and experiences of trial participants (Benbasat, Goldstein, & Mead 1987; Neuman, 2000; Zikmund, 1997).

Each interview was tape recorded and subsequently transcribed for analysis. Analysis was conducting using thematic coding drawing on the principles of grounded theory (Strauss & Corbin, 1994) starting at the sentence level to generate key concepts and themes. Following Neuman (2000), a final iteration was conducted to identify data that supported, conferred and/or showed disparity between the key themes. In presenting the analysis, the key themes that emerged are illustrated by selected quotes from interview transcripts. All data collection, analysis and interpretation were conducted in compliance with ethical research principles. All participants' details have been made anonymous, and all interview data treated in strictest confidence.

RESULTS

Initial findings from this research are presented below. Interviewees were aged between 59 and 78. Only one of the participants interviewed had any significant previous experience with using computers. Two of the interviewees had post-secondary school education levels. These people all experience moderate to severe restriction upon their daily activities, the more severe ones reported being able to walk slowly or engage in light exercise only. One participant was totally oxygen-dependent and required intranasal oxygen at rest.

The interview data have been examined in relation to the issues and challenges identified from the literature.

The Evidence-Based Approach to Chronic Illness

The disparity between the EBM approach to medical care and the requirements of those with chronic illness becomes evident when people's disease and self-management experiences are explored. These interviews reflect the issue of the depersonalised approach of EBM and demonstrate that, from the project, patients have become able to recognise the relationship between social factors and changes in their own symptoms. This is evident from many of those interviewed. For example, one female participant described effects relating to the health of her partner:

Yeah well each time the report comes back I just see the difference from week to week and I know if it is any better or any worse. Oh yeah sometimes I can see I'm alright and then sometimes I'm down and like he [partner] in the last couple of months its been because of [partner] because he has a cancer operation for it inside his face and I think that might have upset the applecart for a couple of months sort of thing but I'm just starting to come alright now but its only just every now and again I get a bit puffy (Participant 2).

The challenge of personalising care and the relationships between symptoms and other psychosocial and environmental factors is evident within the quote below. Through having access to the longitudinal record of symptoms and also the context of each diary, recorded through the use of the comments section, participants gain an understanding of the impact of life events upon their condition.

I think the comments. Looking at it overall you know because I wouldn't have, I wouldn't have taken notice of any specific thing myself..... It was written down and it caused me to have a look and think about what it was (Participant 12).

Now I wouldn't have thought through the day how much sputum I was coughing up for instance. I wouldn't have thought well on a scale of one to ten how do you feel and how's your breathlessness and stuff like this. So yes, it did force me or encourage me to look at those particular aspects whereas I wouldn't have normally done (Participant 10).

The following participant is discussing the advantage of using a computer to monitor her symptoms and the way this changes her behaviour:

I know when I look at it [the feedback] I want to do more the next day than what I did that day I put it on. And so it does push you a bit to do a bit more (Participant 4).

The Doctor-Patient Relationship

The changing doctor patient relationship and the shifting responsibilities for some decision making is evident in participant interviews, as is the need for personalised guidelines for care and the importance of coordination, collaboration and communication in a patient centric world. The increasing focus upon self-management and patient initiation of care is reflected in the quotes below:

Writing in the diary, and looking back on it and think, especially when you write something one day and you look back on it a few days later and think, 'oh my gosh, did I feel like that?' And you can sort of pick up bits and pieces of what you, sort of a pattern sometimes. You know, when I was sick, I was being sick every fortnight, and you could see a pattern on the diary – every fortnight I am sick (Participant 3).

I just get them out sometimes and just read back over, the comments I was writing when I was sick and that sort of thing (Participant 7).

I'm a bit more aware now, whereas before I wouldn't, because I know I've got to write it down, so I think, oh well (Participant 6).

For instance [the GP] said to me and I was in a bit of a dilemma with they give me the prescriptions for antibiotics and stuff and I said oh God I hate taking these. When actually do I take them 'cause he said keep them on hand in case you need them for the weekend. Then all of sudden I get a bit of a cough, I said it never occurs to me to go and get a prescription and then all of a sudden before I know where I am, I've got this horrible infection. And he said look the rule of thumb is, a change of mucus to frothy mucus, an irritating cough, he said then start thinking about getting an antibiotic because he said you can guarantee in a day or so you'll get infectious mucus he said and that's when you've got a battle. They were good guidelines for me to go on. I had the three now and since then I've been following that, I've been preparing myself and I've been able to come along quite well which to me it has kept me out of hospital for a good twelve months. I haven't been in hospital touch wood since this time last year I think it was (Participant 10).

The effect of symptom monitoring and awareness of symptoms leading to self initiation of treatment early in the course of an exacerbation is reflected in the following statement. It must be noted that it is becoming standard that people with COPD have prescriptions for antibiotics and steroids at home so that they can commence a course of treatment as soon as symptoms worsen. This reflects a change in the relationship between doctors and patients.

I wake up in the morning and I think oh God you know I feel as though a truck has run over me and I get up and go to the toilet and sometimes I can get in there and back and I think oh gee I did that without my oxygen and then other mornings I'm puffing to such a degree that I think oh no not another day like this. And you start off saying oh it has. Then I start coughing and I think well have I got any junk down there and quite often I do have and then I think right I'll go and use the puffer that [physio] gave me and this one here and I know that I do five minutes or so with that and that'll move it and that's what I have to do the rest of the day. Then I monitor the sputum and then I monitor the colour. So yes, that has given me a regular in-look sort of thing to test myself into doing it. And then at the end of the day if that doesn't work I know I'm in for another bit of a battle...so I get an antibiotic so yes, overall with the particular schedule it has made me aware and I can follow up on it (Participant 10).

The importance of the patient and doctor working as part of the team in their care is reflected in the following.

I mean years ago it was unheard of that a doctor would say to you now if this, that and something else happens you go straight and get your antibi-

otics then more or less telling you rather than go and see them and they'd tell you and they'd give you a script. They're basically putting the onus on you, which is good to a certain degree, and I've always worked in conjunction with the Pharmacist anyway so the advantage of Pathways to me has been that. It's drawn my notice and attention to how many, how often I have antibiotics which means I have to coerce with the Doctor regarding that for repeats so I might cut out the amount of times that I have to go to him (Participant 11).

[the GP said], 'well you know how you feel, he said, and if it was a different feeling you wouldn't have bothered going down for the antibiotics' (Participant 3).

Patients also need to take responsibility for maintaining a stock of prescriptions.

You must always keep one script ahead of yourself (Participant 1).

However, there is the flip side to this experience where too much responsibility is devolved to patients who are ill equipped to deal with the responsibilities inherent in a patient-centric health approach. This problem is acknowledged within the following quote from one participant where she reflects upon some of the people she has contact with through the support group she runs.

I know pretty much what I'm taking and why I'm taking it. And I prompt my doctors as to whether I need to still be on it or whether I can come off it or come down. But I would say for a lot of people especially the ones that strut to our meeting they are not ready. They can't even monitor their oxygen and I don't know I say to them 'why don't you ask your doctor? I can't tell you. You must ask your doctor.' And they say 'Well shouldn't he, wouldn't he tell me?' (Participant 10).

Collaboration and Communication with E-Health

The importance of coordination, collaboration, and communication, and the changing doctor-patient relationship is evident from the quote below. Participant 9 is a seventy-year-old man who has embraced the idea of symptom monitoring and although he chose not to use an ICT tool for this purpose he still uses the skills developed to assist in his care. He receives hard copy longitudinal data records on his diary entries by post and interprets them and also takes them to his GP to keep her informed about his progress.

So the feed back what you give me from the diaries when I've got sufficient amounts say about two months I take 'em to my Doctor.....and then she reads 'em and then I say well youse read 'em? And then she says yes I do so she knows what's going on Yeah. And she thinks it's a good thing (Participant 9).

Participants see the project and the symptom diary as being a tool to assist the doctors in coordinating their care.

Well its good. If I ever get rushed to [the hospital], I can just say I'm on the Pathways Program and hand these to the doctors down there, and then they'll have some indication of how bad I am (Participant 8).

I love it... because it's really helped me. It's brought me out a bit more and I don't feel as though I'm by myself. Before I started it I had no support. I've got support now (Participant 3).

The ultimate questions regarding the push towards the adoption of a self-management approach to care is do the individual patients want this? And are they really equipped and supported to undertake this? This requirement is reflected in the quotes below. These reflect the conflict of the changing doctor patient relationship when the patient still anticipates the doctor has more information and should dictate treatment. These participants demonstrate a lack of understanding of the purpose of the project and although they appeared to embrace all aspects it became evident that this was more an issue of compliance and an altruistic attitude towards the project rather than an understanding and embracing of the self-management approach to care.

At the moment that is useful but at the moment mine is the same colour just about. So that there is not much change in anything really. I worked that part out earlier in the piece. I could make this look real good or I could make it look bad whichever way I wanted it (Participant 5).

If I wanted to tell lies I could tell lies but no I can't see that I got anything out of it at all (Participant 1).

From what I can see that there's nothing on that computer that can improve me, and you people are not telling me anything that can. Whether you are getting anything out of it or not, I don't know but if you are, why don't you tell us? (Participant 5).

Although the formal interviews with the CF participants are yet to be analysed, the following is feedback from a young CF sufferer, who is using a mobile phone to monitor his symptoms, as described by his mentor when she asked how he felt the project had helped him.

He said that because he has to write down information for his coughing and breathing, etc. in order to text it daily, he now has a record of his symptoms and what affects them, whereas before he never took notice of how his breathing was from one day to another. I was very excited about this as you can tell. Also he has started to work again [which was his goal] but he's actually assertive with regards to his job and how it affects his CF. For example, he tells them if a task is too much physically, or if conditions exacerbate his symptoms. He noted that this is the first time that he's stood up to anyone or said no to anyone so he's pleased about that as well.

As demonstrated by the quotes above, the challenges of the use of EBM, collaboration, and communication in a patient-centric world, and the changing traditional doctor-patient relationship are key issues in the move towards the use of e-health to support a patient-centred health system.

CONCLUSION

This chapter has reflected on the learnings and experiences gained in this case study which aims to address the challenges faced by the healthcare sector supporting a patient-centred e-health paradigm. From this experience, it has been illustrated how ICT can be developed that aspires to be patient-centred. To achieve this, the chapter argues that the system's purpose, the characteristics of the end-users and their contexts all must be considered as well as ensuring that the system is easy to use, fulfils a perceived need and presents a clear value proposition for adoption and utilisation by patients. It is anticipated that this chapter has made a contribution to work aiming to support patients' becoming coparticipants in their own care. However, it is acknowledged that the challenge of changing how clinicians themselves learn to respond to this shift in the autonomy of decision-making will require further research.

ACKNOWLEDGMENT

The authors would like to acknowledge the contribution to this research of the Pathways Home for Respiratory Illness Team: Professor

Haydn Walters, Associate Professor Richard Wood Baker, Dr. David Reid, Professor Andrew Robinson, Helen Courtney-Pratt, Lyn Joseph, Helen Cameron-Tucker, Jenny Busch and Dr. Melanie Jessup.

REFERENCES

Ajzen, I. (1985). *From intentions to actions: A theory of planned behavior.* In J. Kuhl, & J. Beckmann (Eds.), *Action-control: From cognition to behavior* (pp. 11–39). Heidelberg: Springer.

Auerbach, S.M. (2001). Do patients want control over their own healthcare? A review of measures, findings, and research issues. *Journal of Health Psychology, 6*(2), 191–203.

Bandura, A. (1982). Self-efficacy mechanism in human agency. *American Psychologist, 37,* 122–147.

Barlow, J.H., Turner, A.P., & Wright, C.C. (2000). A randomized controlled study of the Arthritis Self-management Programme in the UK. *Health Education Research., 15*(6), 665–680.

Barrett, M.J. (2005). *Patient self-management tools: An overview.* Oakland, CA: California HealthCare Foundation.

Benbasat, I., Goldstein, D.K., & Mead, M. (1987). The case research strategy in studies of information systems. *MIS Quarterly, 11*(3), 369–384.

Blanchard, E., Appelbaum, K., Radnitz, C., Michultka, D., Morrill, B., Kirsch, C., Hillhouse, J., Evans, D.D., Guarnieri, P., Attanasio, V., Andrasik, F., Jaccard, J., & Dentinger, M.P. (1990). Placebo-controlled evaluation of abbreviated progressive muscle relaxation and of relaxation combined with cognitive therapy in the treatment of tension headache. *Journal of Consulting & Clinical Psychology, 58*(2), 210–215.

Blanchard, E., Appelbaum, K., Radnitz, C., Morrill, B., Michultka, D., Kirsch, C., Guarnieri, P., Hillhouse, J., Evans, D.D., Jaccard, J., & Barron, K.D. (1990). A controlled evaluation of thermal biofeedback and thermal biofeedback combined with cognitive therapy in the treatment of vascular headache. *Journal Consulting & Clinical Psychology, 58*(2), 216–224.

Bodenheimer, T., Lorig, K., Holman, H., & Grumbach, K. (2002). Patient self-management of chronic disease in primary care. *JAMA, 288*(19).

Borgerson, K. (2005). Evidence-based alternative medicine? *Perspectives in Biology and Medicine, 48*(8), 502–515.

Butler, C., Rollnick, S., & Stott, N. (1996). The practitioner, the patient and resistance to change: Recent ideas on compliance. *Canadian Medical Association Journal, 154,* 1357–1362.

Charles, C., Gafni, A., & Whelan, T. (1997). Shared decision-making in the medical encounter: What does it mean? (Or it takes at least two to tango). *Social Science & Medicine, 44*(5), 681–692.

Chodosh, J., Morton, S.C., Mojica, W., Maglione, M., Suttorp, M.J., Hilton, L., Rhodes, S., & Shekelle, P. (2005). Meta-analysis: Chronic disease self-management programs for older adults. *Annals of Internal Medicine, 143*(6), 427–438.

Coburn, D., Rappolt, S., & Bourgeault, I. (1997). Decline vs. retention of medical power through restratification: An examination of the Ontario case. *Sociology of Health and Illness, 19*(1), 1–22.

Cummings, E., & Turner, P. (2007). Considerations for deploying Web and mobile technologies to support the building of patient self-efficacy and self-management of chronic illness. In L. Al-Hakim (Ed.), *Web Mobile-Based Applications for Healthcare Management* (pp. 258–273). Hershey, PA: Idea Group, Inc.

Denny, K. (1999). Evidence-based medicine and medical authority. *Journal of Medical Humanities, 20*(4), 247–263.

DeVol, R., Bedroussian, A., Charuworn, A., Chatterjee, A., Kim, I.K., Kim, S., et al. (2007). *An unhealthy America: The economic burden of chronic disease—charting a new course to save lives and increase productivity and economic growth.* Milken Institute. Retrieved May 28, 2008, from http://www.milkeninstitute.org/publications/publications.taf

Epping-Jordan, J., Bengoa, R., Kawar, R., & Sabate, E. (2001). The challenge of chronic conditions: Who responds. *British Medical Journal, 323*(7319), 947–948.

Eysenbach, G. (2000). Recent advances: Consumer health informatics. *British Medical Journal, 320*(7251), 1713–1716.

Frankford, D. (1994). Scientism and economics in the regulation of healthcare. *Journal of Health Politics, Policy & Law, 19*(4), 773–799.

Fries, J., Friday, G., Gira, C., Cooper, P., England, M., Graves, R., Sokolov, J.J., & Wright, D. (1993). Reducing healthcare costs by reducing the need and demand for medical services. *New England Journal of Medicine, 329*, 5–9.

Funnell, M., Anderson, R., Arnold, M., Barr, P., Donnelly, M., Johnson, P., Taylor-Moon, D. & White, N.H. (1991). Empowerment an idea whose time has come in diabetes education. *The Diabetes Educator, 17*(1), 37–41.

Greene, B., & Blanchard, E. (1994). Cognitive therapy for irritable bowel syndrome. *Journal of Consulting & Clinical Psychology, 62*(3), 576–582.

Gruman, J., & Von Korff, M. (1996). *Indexed bibliography on self-management for people with chronic disease.* Washington D.C.: Centre for Advancement in Health.

Hill, S. (1998). *Using the evidence: Empowering consumers of healthcare.* Menzies Foundation. Retrieved May 28, 2008, from http://www.menziesfoundation.org.au/conferences/ebm/ebm-09hill.htm

Holman, H., & Lorig, K. (2000). Patients as partners in managing chronic disease. *British Medical Journal, 320*(7234), 526–527.

Jordan, J.E., & Osborne, R.H. (2007). Chronic disease self-management education programs: Challenges ahead. *Medical Journal of Australia, 186*(2), 84–87.

Kaplan, S., Greenfield, S., Gandek, B., Rogers, W.H., & Ware, J.E. Jr. (1996). Characteristics of physicians with participatory decision-making styles. *Annals of Internal Medicine, 124*(5), 497–504.

Lorig, K.R., Sobel, D.S., Stewart, A.L., Brown, B.W.J., Bandura, A., Ritter, P., et al. (1999). Evidence suggesting that a chronic disease self-management program can improve health status while reducing hospitalization: A randomized trial. *Medical Care, 37(*1), 5–14.

McKinstry, B. (2000). Do patients wish to be involved in decision making in the consultation? A cross sectional survey with video vignettes. *British Medical Journal, 321*(7265), 867–871.

Monninkhof, E., van der Aa, M., van der Valk, P., van der Palen, J., Zielhuis, G., Koning, K., & Pieterse, M., (2004). A qualitative evaluation of a comprehensive self-management programme for COPD patients: Effectiveness from the patients' perspective. *Patient Education and Counseling, 55*(2), 177–184.

Monninkhof, E., van der Valk, P., van der Palen, J., van Herwaarden, C., Partidge, M., Walters, E., & Zielhuis, G.A. (2002). Self-management education for chronic obstructive pulmonary disease. *Cochrane Database of Systematic Reviews: Reviews 2002*(4).

Muir Gray, J.A. (2004). Self-management in chronic illness. *The Lancet, 364*(9444), 1467–1468.

National Health Priority Action Council. (2006). *National chronic disease strategy.* Canberra: Australian Government Department of Health and Ageing. Retrieved May 28, 2008, from http://www.health.gov.au/Internet/wcms/publishing.nsf/Content/pq-ncds

Neuman, W.L. (2000). *Social research methods—qualitative and quantitative approaches (4th edition).* Needham Heights, MA: Allyn and Bacon.

Newman, S., Steed, L., & Mulligan, K. (2004). Self-management interventions for chronic illness. *The Lancet, 364*(9444), 1523–1537.

Pincus, T. (2004). Will racial and ethnic disparities in health be resolved primarily outside of standard medical care? *Annals of Internal Medicine, 141*(3), 224–225.

Rappolt, S. (1997). Clinical guidelines and the fate of medical autonomy in Ontario. *Social Science & Medicine, 44*(7), 977–987.

Schneider, S., & Lane, J. (2005). *The patient from hell: How I worked with my doctors to get the best of modern medicine and how you can too.* Cambridge, MA: Da Capo Press.

Strauss, A.L., & Corbin, J. (1994). *Grounded theory methodology: An overview.* In N.K. Denzin, & Y.S. Lincoln (Eds.), *Handbook of qualitative research* (pp. 273–285). Thousand Oaks, CA: Sage Publications.

Taylor, S., Candy, B., Bryar, R., Vrijhoef, J., Esmond, G., Wedzicha, J., et al. (2005). Effectiveness of innovations in nurse led chronic disease management for patients with chronic obstructive pulmonary disease: Systematic review of evidence. *British Medical Journal, 331*(485).

Von Korff, M., Gruman, J., Schaefer, J., Curry, S.J., & Wagner, E.H. (1997). Collaborative management of chronic illness. *Annals of Internal Medicine, 127*(12), 1097–1102.

Wagner, E.H., Austin, B.T., Davis, C., Hindmarsh, M., Schaefer, J., & Bonomi, A. (2001). Improving chronic illness care: Translating evidence into action. *Health Affairs, 20*(6), 64–78.

Warsi, A., LaValley, M.P., Wang, P.S., Avorn, J., & Solomon, D.H. (2003). Arthritis self-management education programs: A meta-analysis of the effect on pain and disability. *Arthritis & Rheumatism, 48*(8), 2207–2213.

Warsi, A., Wang, P., LaValley, M., & Avorn, J. (2004). Self-management education programs in chronic disease: A systematic review and methodological critique of the literature. *Archives of Internal Medicine, 164*(15), 1641.

Zikmund, W.G. (1997). *Business research methods (fifth edition).* Sydney, Australia: The Dryden Press.

Zwar, N., Harris, M., Griffiths, R., Roland, M., Dennis, S., Powell Davies, G., & Hasan, I. (2006). *APHCRI stream four: A systematic review of chronic disease management.* Australian National University. Retrieved May 28, 2008, from http://www.anu.edu.au/aphcri/Domain/ChronicDiseaseMgmt/Approved_25_Zwar.pdf

Chapter XIV
Incompatible Images:
Asthmatics' Non-Use of an E-Health System for Asthma Self-Management

Michel J. Sassene
Roskilde University, Denmark

Morten Hertzum
Roskilde University, Denmark

ABSTRACT

This chapter investigates asthmatics' reasons for not adopting an e-health system for asthma self-management. An understanding of these reasons is particularly relevant, because clinical evidence indicates that, if used, such systems lead to better asthma management. The investigated asthma system is, however, based on a taken-for-granted image of asthmatics as, per se, striving to be symptom-free. This image is incompatible with interviewed asthmatics' day-to-day performances of their asthma, and renders invisible (a) that their asthma performances emphasize an economy of good passages and of feeling capable, (b) that they achieve the objective of feeling capable in quite different ways, and (c) that feeling capable does not per se equal being symptom-free all the time. To attain long-term use of self-management systems and other patient-centred e-health systems, such systems must acknowledge and link into the manifold performances that comprise users' ways of living with their disease.

INTRODUCTION

Asthma, diabetes, and other chronic diseases cannot be cured. This positions these diseases at the periphery of common conceptions of diseases and their treatment. First, whereas healthcare professionals can diagnose chronic diseases and make plans for their treatment, the actual treatment, which is thus management, must to a large extent be performed by the patients themselves (Newman, Steed, & Mulligan, 2004). Second, many chronic diseases are in part caused by what can broadly be termed patients' life styles, and the management of these diseases involves as a core element comprehensive changes or restrictions in patients' habits and day-to-day lives (Butler, Rollnick, & Stott, 1996; GINA, 2005). Third, even brief failures to comply with proper management of the diseases may lead to symptoms or an irreversible worsening of the patient's condition. For many chronic diseases, patient-centred e-health systems are therefore seen as a way of supporting patients' self-management of their disease, primarily by providing information not otherwise available and by extending the communication between patients and healthcare professionals beyond infrequent, face-to-face consultations (Ball & Lillis, 2001; Safran, 2003).

This chapter analyses an e-health system for asthmatics. For reasons of anonymity, the system will be referred to as AWeb, and the company developing it as ACorp. Though asthma is a condition asthmatics have to live with, the risks of symptoms can be minimized by taking the right amount of medication. It is, however, no simple task to determine the correct amount of medication, because this depends on various risk factors, which may change dynamically and be hard to foresee. To accommodate the difficulties with dosing medication, asthmatics' self-management of their medication is considered a cornerstone in asthma treatment (Gibson, Powell, Coughlan, Wilson, Abramson, Haywood, Bauman, Hensley, & Walters, 2002; GINA, 2005). AWeb provides tools for asthmatics to manage their asthma themselves. Nevertheless, in spite of the utility of AWeb and considerable marketing by ACorp the system never attained widespread use and was discontinued after five years. To inform other initiatives toward providing e-health support for self-management of chronic diseases, we provide two accounts of the relations between asthmatics and their asthma:

- *The system's image of the user*: How does AWeb set up a way for asthmatics to think about their asthma?
- *The self-image of asthmatics*: How do asthmatics perform their asthma on a day-to-day basis?

The aim of our analysis is to elaborate and contrast these two images. We do not take asthmatics' non-use of AWeb as a rejection of self-management initiatives, but rather seek to inform future initiatives by attempting to explain why AWeb was not taken up by the targeted users.

Previous work on e-health systems for self-management of asthma has suggested several reasons for asthmatics' low uptake of such systems (Anhøj & Nielsen, 2004; Nielsen, 2005). The suggested reasons include inexperience with the Internet and computers, a latency time between starting to use a system and realizing the benefits of using it, and unpredictable interactions between the system and asthmatics' everyday lives. A limitation of this previous work is, however, that reasons for non-use have been derived from studies of asthmatics that—admittedly, to varying extents—are users of e-health systems for self-management of asthma. In the present chapter, we extend previous work by turning to non-users for input to an understanding of what "went wrong" in the AWeb project. Such an understanding is particularly relevant because a clinical test shows that, if used, Web-based asthma monitoring leads to better asthma management (in terms of symptoms suffered, lung function, and so forth) compared to monitoring by asthma specialists or general practitioners (Rasmussen, Phanareth, Nolte, & Backer, 2005).

BACKGROUND

Asthma is a chronic inflammatory disorder of the airways (GINA, 2005). This inflammatory condition causes hypersensitivity to risk factors such as stress, respiratory infections, animal fur, fungus, and smoke. The symptoms of asthma are mostly suffered as attacks, which typically involve shortness of breath, heavy coughing, troublesome and wheezing respiration, and tightness of chest. To alleviate the symptoms two types of asthma medication are currently available. *Controller medication* prevents the inflammatory condition from worsening and in the long run reduces the likelihood of attacks, but has no immediate effect. *Attack medication* is intended to immediately relieve symptoms during attacks and normally functions by temporarily enlarging the respiratory channels. Since attack medication is hard on the lungs, it is generally recommended to use it as little as possible and instead use an adequate amount of controller medication. However, it is likewise recommended not to use too much controller medication because its side effects are unclear. Hence, it is a real challenge to dose asthma medication appropriately.

In recent years, several asthma-patient education programs have advocated the use of diaries as a means of facilitating asthmatics' awareness of their asthma and commitment to effective self-management. Apart from supporting asthmatics in learning about and managing their condition, diaries are considered useful to healthcare professionals, because diaries provide them with detailed data about asthmatics' physical symptoms and use of medication (Gibson et al., 2002).

The positive experiences with the use of diaries spearheaded the design of AWeb, which was developed by ACorp in collaboration with the national Asthma and Allergy Association and an independent advisory board of asthma specialists. AWeb comprises three parts: a knowledge centre with online resources about asthma and its treatment, a discussion forum where asthmatics can submit questions to a panel of asthma experts and read answers to previously submitted questions, and a diary tool. The diary tool, which is the focus of this chapter, requires that asthmatics register as AWeb users. The intention is that asthmatics log into the diary tool every day and enter peak-flow measurements, doses of medication taken, and symptoms experienced within the last 24 hours. Based on this information AWeb advises users as to which preventive measures to take with respect to their medication, taking into consideration their asthma history and medication. In this way, the diary tool implements the step model and general self-management guidelines recommended by the Global Initiative for Asthma (GINA, 2005). The diary tool also includes graphics that show trends in peak flow and symptoms coupled with environmental data such as pollen counts; and users can write notes, for example, to elaborate on their symptoms or make notes about special circumstances. Furthermore, the diary tool is directed toward asthmatics as well as their health-care professionals, who can log in to monitor the well-being of their asthma patients and provide advice when needed. Hence, the diary tool can function both as a tool for self-management and as an extension of the patient-professional relationship.

AWeb was launched in May 2000 and attracted more than 2,000 users within the first three months. During the following year and a half, another 4,000 asthmatics registered as users. After that, new users registered at a rate of approximately 50 new users a month (Anhøj & Nielsen, 2004). However, log files show that of the initial 2,000 registered users only about 100 used the diary tool regularly and they, too, lost interest, resulting in only nine users of the diary by the end of 2000. To attract more users, ACorp initiated a marketing campaign that targeted the opinion leaders closest to asthmatics, namely general practitioners, rather than asthmatics directly. This approach was taken to counter any reluctance from asthmatics toward information and initiatives from a pharmaceutical company with vested interests. As a result, general practitioners promoted AWeb and the number of diary users reached a peak of 307 in January 2002. A year later, February 2003, the number of diary users had, however, declined to 138. Finally, in May 2005, AWeb was discontinued, primarily due to a lack of users (Anhøj & Nielsen, 2004). In explaining the low uptake of AWeb among asthmatics, the project manager we interviewed summed up:

Looking at the whole project in retrospect, the primary reason for the lack of success of [AWeb] can be attributed to the system being too complex and time consuming for the users.

While this does point to an incompatibility between AWeb and the intended users, the following analysis reveals, we will argue, that the incompatibility is more intricate and deeply rooted than a system that is too complex and time consuming for its users.

CONCEPTUAL FRAMEWORK

To analyse non-use, it is essential to avoid the pro-innovation bias, which is common in theories about diffusion of innovations (Rogers, 2003). While factors such as intrinsic motivation and perceived usefulness have been found to predict patients' behavioural intention to use e-health (Wilson & Lankton, 2004), they do not explain why some patients are unmotivated to adopt useful systems. To investigate this we turn to actor-network theory, particularly its performative approach, and to the cyborg metaphor.

Actor-network theory (Callon, 1986, 1991; Law & Singleton, 2000; Mol, 1999; Mol & Law, 2004) dissolves any inherent identity or boundary of actors by asserting that such identities and boundaries are merely ostensive and, in fact, a result of meticulous negotiations. As such, every actor is considered both a network and part of a network, and any stable identity is seen as a fact established through domination. To guide the analysis of actor networks, Callon (1986) proposes three closely coupled methodological principles: (a) *Impartiality to actors*, which implies that all actors' views are considered as is. No point of view is dismissed as inherent to the identity of the actor. (b) *Symmetry*, which implies that one general vocabulary is used to describe all involved actors, human as well as nonhuman. (c) *Free association*, which implies that the investigator should abandon a priori distinctions between actors and rather let the actors' own explanations define how they are associated with each other. To put these principles into operation, Callon (1986) suggests the use of a vocabulary of translation with four separate moments. The four moments of translation are:

- **Problematization:** How are some actors brought into motion by other actors? The meaning of the term problematization is twofold. It is both about the concrete problem to be resolved and about how some actors are defined by the way in which other actors' present the problem. In the present case study, ACorp presents AWeb as an improvement in asthma treatment.
- **Interessement:** Will the problematization incite the involved actors, such as asthmatics, to accept the identity defined for them? Interessement designates the measures taken by an actor to stabilize the identities of the other actors involved in the problematization. It comprises the means taken to incite actors to share a common goal.
- **Enrolment:** How well does the interessement succeed? Enrolment concerns how the definitions inherent in the problematization are transformed into concrete material form, such as texts and e-health systems. Through this process the problematization is negotiated and its definitions inscribed in artefacts.
- **Mobilization/displacement:** Who becomes empowered to speak on behalf of whom? Mobilization concerns the extent to which actors come to define themselves in accor-

dance with the problematization. If the actors adopt this definition their voice is displaced to the actors presenting the problematization.

By refusing to maintain absolute definitions of actors, be they asthmatics or any kind of technology, actor-network theory enables a renegotiation of their apparent identities and boundaries. As a consequence, reality becomes transitional, situated, and performed. The performative approach (Goffman, 1959; Law & Singleton, 2000; Mol, 1999; Mol & Law, 2004; Star, 1991) entails (a) that reality is not only composed of what is, but also of what is performed, and (b) that these performances could always have been done differently. Hence, to trace how asthma is actually performed, the scope of our study becomes asthmatics' concrete ways of performing their asthma. Using Moser and Law's (1999) concept of passages, the scope of our study becomes the *passages* between different ways of relating to asthma, which are provided by different ways of performing asthma.

Asthma performances are complex, and multiple experiences of asthma are often performed simultaneously and interdependently. In conceptualizing this multiplicity, we draw on the cyborg metaphor (Haraway, 1991). On a general note, the cyborg metaphor presents transgressed boundaries between categories—for example, between organism and machine. For present purposes, we will, however, focus on one characteristic—namely, the cyborg's *split vision* (Haraway, 1991). A cyborg has split vision in that it is capable of accommodating multiple, simultaneous performances that are at the same time irreducible to each other and inextricably intertwined. While a cyborg is by definition both one and many, the different identities may be more or less well-connected and the split vision may, consequently, involve boundaries at various levels of permeability between the identities. We will argue that the cyborg is a useful metaphor in understanding asthma self-management, because it is ontologically situated between categories.

METHOD

Empirical data have been collected from two target groups. To obtain data about how the AWeb project proceeded and how ACorp perceived the project and the user, two interviews were conducted with the AWeb project manager, supplemented with e-mail correspondence and published reports from the project. The authors are entirely independent of ACorp and were neither commissioned by ACorp to do the study, nor in any other way related to ACorp or AWeb. To obtain data about how asthmatics live with their asthma, four asthmatics were interviewed. All four interviewees were university students. Being young, well-educated, and technology literate, the interviewees did not span the heterogeneity of asthmatics but, on the contrary, represented the segment of asthmatics most likely to use a system like AWeb. Bearing this in mind, it is noteworthy that none of the interviewees had used AWeb. In this sense, the four interviewees are ordinary asthmatics.

All six interviews were semistructured and audio recorded. Whereas the two interviews with the project manager were explorative and clarifying, the four interviews with asthmatics were conducted as life-story interviews (Kvale, 1996). The analysis of the interviews followed a phenomenological approach in which the interviewees' statements were taken at face value and grouped into categories of related statements, each category covering a significant element of interview content. These categories were then applied to group yet more statements and produce abstractions that described patterns in the data. This process of categorization and meaning condensation was guided by our conceptual framework.

AWEB'S TRANSLATION OF ASTHMA

The development and launching of AWeb created a sociotechnical network in which "being an asthmatic" attained a specific meaning. This meaning was brought into being by the AWeb project group as an implicit consequence of the design activities, and it was embedded in AWeb as a taken-for-granted image of the user. By using the vocabulary of translation (Callon, 1986, 1991) this image of the user is revealed as created and, in turn, presented to asthmatics through the four moments of translation.

The *problematization* concerns how some actors are brought into motion by other actors. In this case we will focus on how the AWeb project group brought other actors, especially asthmatics, into motion. As the AWeb project manager remarked: "*Of course, we wanted [AWeb] to be as useful as possible to the asthmatics but we are involved in the project for commercial reasons. In the end it was a means to increase sales.*" This commercial motivation was a basic premise for ACorp to engage in the project but it should not be taken as an indication of low quality or commitment. Indeed, the project group followed recognized recommendations in their design of AWeb. The commercial motivation was, however, unlikely to incite asthmatics, and was quickly transformed by the AWeb project group into a completely different proposition: Can information technology, and indeed the Internet, support asthmatics in their self-management? This problematization enunciates several actors, including GINA, which had developed the step model that AWeb implements, general practitioners who are expected to support initiatives that are in line with recommended asthma treatment, and the asthmatics, who are seen as highly motivated, comfortable with the Internet, and eager to minimize their asthma symptoms.

In order for AWeb to be successful, the relevant actors had to become interested in the problematization. The AWeb project group applied several strategies of *interessement* to make the other actors partake in the problematization. First and most concretely, AWeb was developed. AWeb included functionality that promised to relieve many of asthmatics' symptoms and ease general practitioners' work. Second, ACorp assumed a withdrawn role and enrolled other actors to speak on behalf of the project, most notably general practitioners but also GINA and the national Asthma and Allergy Association. Third, these other actors were external to the commercial motivation for the project and represented important protectors of asthmatics' well-being. Fourth, the AWeb project group and the actors speaking on its behalf enunciated AWeb as a system that improved asthmatics' self-management and thereby reduced their symptoms.

Through the strategies of interessement the AWeb project group presented asthmatics with "a better way" of managing their asthma, available only through the use of AWeb, which at the time was the only initiative of its kind (Anhøj & Nielsen, 2004). Thus, the AWeb project group inscribed the adoption of this better way into asthmatics' decision to adopt AWeb. The number of asthmatics that adopted AWeb was however small, indicating that they approached this *enrolment* process reluctantly. Rather than engaging in regular use of AWeb, asthmatics fluctuated for some time between regular use and non-use and then reverted to non-use. In reverting to non-use the asthmatics not only discontinued their use of AWeb, they also rejected the assumptions defining AWeb as a better way to deal with asthma.

The central assumption in AWeb was that asthmatics are highly interested in their physical well-being and highly motivated toward staying symptom-free. This image of asthmatics remained unquestioned by the AWeb project group, GINA, the national Asthma and Allergy Association, and the general practitioners, but was not adopted by asthmatics to an extent that fostered regular use of AWeb. Hence, the problematization, interessement, and enrolment resulted in a very limited *mobilization* of asthmatics. While the few mobilized asthmatics that used AWeb may be considered early adopters (Rogers, 2003), they provide little basis for understanding the reluctance of most asthmatics to adopt AWeb and its image of asthmatics as, per se, striving to be symptom-free.

ASTHMATICS' PERFORMANCE OF ASTHMA

The image of asthmatics as individuals who per se prioritize being symptom-free is not restricted to the AWeb project. The same line of thinking lies beneath common categorizations of asthmatics according to their commitment to avoid symptoms, for example as either controllers or neglecters (Anhøj & Nielsen, 2004). We will argue that this is an oversimplified and somewhat misconstrued account of how asthmatics relate to their asthma. By looking at how our interviewees actually perform their asthma, we get accounts of complex asthma realities unfolding around the ways in which the interviewees handle the mundanities of their everyday life.

Four Asthma Realities

All four interviewed asthmatics use both controller and attack medication, have tried using peak-flow meters, and suffer more or less frequent asthma attacks. However, their ways of experiencing these aspects of their asthma are highly different.

Kit does not see asthma as a big problem in her day-to-day life: "*I guess many asthmatics suffer more from their asthma than I do, but again, I do have asthma, and if I am not careful I can have an attack.*" Kit previously used a peak-flow meter for training her senses by giving her a way of checking that the way her body felt was in accordance with what the peak-flow meter told her. Now, she does not use it anymore. Kit is good at taking her controller medication. Indeed, she has the controller medication under enough control that in low-risk periods, she reduces her usage of controller medication, and in certain periods, she takes no medication at all, except an occasional dose of attack medication. To Kit, it is important to try to minimize her usage of medication. In Kit's own words: "*Of course money is an issue, but to me it is more important not to feel dependent on any drugs. I would much rather try to change my way of living; do sports, keep my house clean, relax, and just listen to my body.*" Thus, Kit does not forget to take her controller medication, but at times, she deliberately omits taking it because she feels she has her asthma under control and likes the sense of being independent of medication. As such, she simply tests herself.

In contrast, John does not care much about his asthma: "*it makes no difference to me.*" In fact, John dislikes all aspects associated with asthma. When he first got diagnosed, he tried to use a peak-flow meter and a diary, but for John, these remedies were just reminders of asthma; a "thing" he felt he had quite enough of in his life as it was. He does not want to know his asthma the way a peak-flow meter makes it available to him. In general, John does not care much for understanding the effects and side effects of his medication: "*As long as it makes me breathe, I do not care about what it actually does. In fact, I often forget the brown one [the controller medication] at home. It means nothing to me.*" He goes on explaining why he often does not take his controller medication: "*Out of pure laziness, or whatever you want to call it, I sometimes do not take my [controller] medication while feeling bad; just because it feels boring to take it.*" In contrast, it is important to John to have his attack medication at hand. He often has attacks, especially at night and in the morning. His way of handling these attacks is to "*take some attack medication and go on with whatever I am doing.*" Thus, John deliberately "forgets" to take his medication because he cannot stand to be bothered with the medication, either out of what he himself terms laziness, or because he simply feels like being without it.

In Tina's view, her asthma is more or less under control. Tina has participated in clinical trials and sees this as a way of keeping her own asthma in check while at the same time contributing to the well-being of other asthmatics. And she adds: "*Besides it is only for a short period of time.*" Tina is not very good at taking her controller medication. She tells that it is probably because she cannot feel any immediate effects, which is also why she, for some time, has considered buying a peak-flow meter. She sees a peak-flow meter, which she has used during the clinical trials, as an interesting option, but she just has not gotten around buying one yet. Tina explains that she would like to take her controller medication more regularly, but mundanities repeatedly seem to get in the way:

When you take the medication you need to drink water afterward to avoid the risk of a mouth condition. And I just don't have the time for all that in the morning. But I always bring it with me to work. But when I get to work my colleagues are always late and they always do extracurricular work while on the job. And that pisses me off. So I won't do like they do. So, you see, I cannot take my medication at work.

Tina likes when someone close to her tells her to take her controller medication. Then she feels that she can legitimately spend time to take care of her asthma without seeming too preoccupied with herself. Thus, when Tina omits taking her controller medication, it is out of practical reasons, and because it seems to prevent her from seeing herself the way she wants.

Mike has taken controller medication since he was about 18 years old and says that his asthma does not cause him much trouble. He uses his controller medication on a regular basis. It keeps him virtually free of attacks and works very well for him. He therefore sees no need to test whether he could do without it. Of course, he sometimes forgets his medication, but in general he is very good at taking it. He stresses that his asthma is under control as long as he takes his controller medication. Thus, Mike practically always takes his controller medication and when he does not, it is out of accident; he never purposefully omits taking it. As the only one of the interviewees, Mike sees his general practitioner about his asthma every six months. He also has his own peak-flow meter and uses it periodically with a diary to check that everything is okay. His use of the peak-flow meter appears to be simple and problem free to Mike: "*All I have to do is blow in a tube and read a small meter. That tells me all I need to know.*" The peak-flow meter gives Mike a sense of control, and he likes the way it lets him know his asthma.

Good and Bad Passages

It is evident from the accounts above that the realities of asthma are different to the four asthmatics. In fact, each asthmatic relates to—and indeed performs—multiple asthmas depending on mood, social context, recency of his or her last attack, and other situational factors. To untangle these interwoven performances, we will draw on the theoretical notion of a passage, which refers to a performance that links other performances together (Moser & Law, 1999). Some ways of performing asthma are rendered smooth and nice to the asthmatic and thus constitute good passages. Conversely, others are rough and unpleasant and constitute bad passages. Good and bad in this connection denote what feels good and bad to the asthmatic and thereby blend physical and psychological aspects.

The four asthmatics occasionally do not take their medication, and they explain these omissions in different ways. In this respect, it is important to note that asthma medication is not only a way in which asthma is relieved, but also a way in which their lungs and their asthma are made known to asthmatics (Willems, 1998). The medication creates a new sensation of lungs and of breathing. In this sense the medication is constitutive of one performance of asthma. Omission to take medication interrupts the sensation of lungs and asthma provided by the medication and thereby constitutes yet another way of doing asthma. The four asthmatics omit to take their medication when acting upon certain specificities, specifically their present need for medication and for feeling normal and capable. While the specificities differ across asthmatics the notion of good and bad passages reveals strong similarities in the four interviewees' omissions to take controller medication. Given the choice, they all prefer to perform good passages. As such, omitting to take controller medication sometimes provides good passages.

Kit likes not to be dependent on medication all the time and performs her omissions of taking controller medication by dosing down in low-risk periods. This makes her feel capable, and thereby provides a good passage. Like Kit, John does not want to be bothered by his medication all the time. But unlike Kit, he does not plan his omissions, and consequently suffers frequent attacks. Still, being without his controller medication constitutes a good passage to him, because he experiences it as a way of avoiding an image of himself as an asthmatic. Tina cannot find the time to take her controller medication in the morning, and feels that she cannot take it at work. This tension between her self-image and her asthma seems, however, to disappear when someone close to her tells her to take her medication. Thus, she omits her medication when taking it will constitute a bad passage by interfering with the mundanities of her everyday life. Finally, Mike likes to take his medication because he finds it makes him feel well. He tries to take it consistently and feels less capable when he occasionally forgets.

Looking at the omissions of taking controller medication in terms of passages the four asthmatics seem to prefer passages that make them feel capable over being symptom-free per se. The tensions between perceiving oneself as capable and taking medication change dynamically and in making good passages they will sometimes coincide, and at other times collide. It is, for example, a better passage to take the medication in high-risk periods or when someone else creates a room for taking it without a need for performing a special relation to one's asthma self.

The asthmatics' relation to peak-flow meters provides another example of how good and bad passages are negotiated. Peak-flow meters can measure asthmatics' lung function and thereby provide a means for asthmatics to look inside their body. In the vocabulary of translation, the use of a peak-flow meter becomes a vehicle for displacing the bodily function of respiration from the respiratory system to an external device; that is, a way to excorporate asthma (Mol & Law, 2004). Hence, a peak-flow meter becomes a device for developing a new way of knowing asthma. For example, Kit previously used a peak-flow meter on a regular basis. By relating what she felt to what the peak-flow meter measured, she developed a new sensibility toward her asthma. Indeed, she developed a new asthma self. As such, the peak-flow meter not only provided objective knowledge of her asthma but also contributed to creating the way in which Kit performs her asthma. This way, the peak-flow meter was used to provide good passages. By now, Kit has, however, stopped using the peak-flow meter. It has provided her with the insight she needed to gain control of her asthma, which was her way to avoid that asthma invaded too much of her life. Now Kit has her asthma more or less under control and does not want to engage in further resource-demanding excorporations of her asthma to create a refined asthma self. For Kit, the passages provided by the peak-flow meter have changed from good to bad because the work needed to get an even better grip of her asthma does not seem worth the effort.

Applying the notion of passages to the other interviewees' relations to peak-flow meters reveals further nuances. John prefers not to adopt a peak-flow meter because it would make him more aware of his asthma by displacing the capacity of his lungs from within his body to an explicit representation outside his body. In subjectifying himself to the peak-flow meter he would have to relate to his asthma in a way that renders some of the work he does in relation to his asthma visible and thereby discords with the way he sees himself—a bad passage. Tina does not mind to use a peak-flow meter for a limited period of time in the context of a clinical trial, but she seems to resist subjectifying herself to a peak-flow meter on a regular basis. The clinical trials detach her from her performance of her own asthma by displacing it to an asthma identity that includes not only herself but also other asthmatics. This generalized asthma identity becomes available to Tina through the clinical trials' aim of benefiting asthmatics in general; and in this context—and apparently only in this context—the peak-flow meter provides good passages. Mike on the other hand has entered a symbiotic relationship with the peak-flow meter on a regular basis. The peak-flow meter provides him with a means to perform his asthma in such a way that he feels liberated from its consequences. To Mike the peak-flow meter provides good passages.

The passages relating to peak-flow meters reveal tensions between developing an experience of asthma by subjectifying to peak-flow meters and the asthmatics' image of themselves as capable. When the self-image is supported, a peak-flow meter creates good passages, which in turn can facilitate use. Conversely, when the self-image is challenged, a peak-flow meter creates bad passages and it is likely rejected.

An Economy of Passages

In relating to their medication and to peak-flow meters, the interviewees seem to perform calculations. They obviously care about how many and how severe attacks they suffer, but they seem to care at least as much about rendering their asthma smooth. For example, when Tina has an attack she thinks that maybe it is time for her to become more persistent in using controller medication. However, in the midst of all her everyday activities she finds this difficult to do and settles for less persistence: "*I guess it is because I am not that bad. Had my asthma been worse, I am sure I would have worked more with it.*" She makes an effort to tell herself and others that there are pragmatic reasons for her not taking medication and not acquiring a peak-flow meter. Hence, she does work in order not to have to do work. This work provides good passages for Tina, because it renders invisible all the efforts she puts into relating to her asthma and thus enables her to maintain an image of herself as capable.

The preference for good passages over bad passages is a persistent characteristic of the interviewees' asthma performances. Thus, their numerous specific asthma practices appear to be performed according to an overarching economy of passages, which is altogether different from the rationality of medical discourse on asthma treatment. While feeling good and capable is constitutive of the interviewees' economies of passages, they achieve this common objective in individual ways. For example, when Kit has an occasional attack all the work she has done in relation to her asthma since her last attack becomes visible to her and turns from good to bad passages; hence, in her economy of passages, it is worth her while to recap what has happened since her last attack in an effort to avoid a similar incident in the future. Conversely, Mike's economy of passages tells him that it is not worth the effort to challenge his asthma due to an occasional attack; he merely takes his attack medication. Furthermore, the interviewees dynamically adjust their ways of performing their asthma in response to practicalities and other aspects of their day-to-day lives. Sometimes being relieved of symptoms coincides with feeling capable; at other times feeling capable can imply doing things that worsen the physical condition, and as such the economy of symptoms collides with that of a capable self. Indeed, the interviewees perform not one, but a proliferation of asthmas, all of which are inextricably related through an economy of passages that emphasizes feeling capable over being symptom-free per se.

DISCUSSION

Thus far, we have approached asthma self-management from the perspective of the AWeb project with its focus on striving to be symptom-free per se and from a perspective focusing on specificities, performances, and passages in the lives of four asthmatics. These two perspectives are highly different, and our analysis points to their incompatibility as a key impediment to widespread adoption of AWeb.

A Turn to the User

Patient-centred e-health is generally seen as a potentially powerful tool for disease management because the Web offers a widely available, low cost, and flexible means of communication between patient and healthcare professional and thereby enables treatment programmes tailored to the individual patient and dynamically regulated on the basis of data entered regularly by the patient for purposes of self-management or for monitoring by a healthcare professional (Bulger & Reeves, 2000). These expectations have instigated the development of patient-centred e-health systems for diseases such as asthma, diabetes (Plougmann, Hejlesen, & Cavan, 2001), eating disorders (Carrard, Rouget, Fernández-Aranda, Volkart, Damoiseau, & Lam, 2006), and HIV/AIDS (Caceres, Gomez, Garcia, Gatell, & del Pozo, 2006). However, our analysis of AWeb reveals that even though AWeb is designed to improve asthmatics' self-management, in practice it becomes an extension of healthcare professionals' views on asthma and its treatment. Furthermore, the AWeb case demonstrates that when given the opportunity to embrace this rational medical behaviour, many asthmatics opt for a different rationale than simply striving to be free from symptoms.

This suggests that the development of self-management systems may benefit from a more thoroughly user-centred approach. While a focus on self-management may itself seem user centred, self-management systems presuppose users' active and sustained involvement and thereby become crucially dependent on being compatible with users' self-image and ways of performing their disease. Otherwise, users simply refrain from adopting such systems or cease to use them. Previous studies of asthmatics' self-management of their medication show that overuse, erratic use, and especially underuse of asthma medication are very common (Bender, Milgrom, & Rand, 1997). Reported reasons for such deviations from recommended practices include forgetfulness, denial that one is an asthmatic, inconvenience, embarrassment, and laziness (Buston & Wood, 2000). Rydström, Hartman, and Segesten (2005) find that young asthmatics' core concern is to avoid that asthma gets the upper hand over their life, and they report three strategies used by asthmatics in relating to their disease: keeping a distance to it, challenging it, and taking it into consideration. While these studies corroborate our analysis, getting to know the user can, however, be difficult because recognizing what knowledge is needed and how to obtain it may constitute major challenges. This is well illustrated in the AWeb case, where it turned out to be insufficient for ACorp to rely on asthma authorities such as GINA and the national Asthma and Allergy Association. Indeed, these authorities must be seen as part of the reason why the AWeb project came to adopt an image of the self-managing asthmatic as always striving to be symptom-free.

The present study shows how the lives of four asthmatics comprise multiple intertwined performances of asthma. Some of these asthmas are performed sequentially and others simultaneously, but all are interdependent. This way asthma can be said to be more than one and less than many in that it is neither possible to reduce the various performances of asthma to one uniform asthma performance, nor to perform the various asthmas in isolation. Rather, the asthmas constitute each other, and the resulting arrangement of irreducible practices constitutes a cyborg (Haraway, 1991). The defining characteristic of a cyborg is its ability to accommodate multiple, simultaneous performances that are at the same time irreducible to each other and inextricably intertwined. As a consequence of this split vision the cyborg is at the same time one and many, and it manages to keep itself together while being situated between categories. A cyborg has no unifying identity but several different identities, which may be more or less well-connected. The cyborg metaphor emphasizes that the individual asthmatic performs a proliferation of visible and invisible works, which are neither reducible to any one kind of work nor observable as individual works. Thus, the asthmatic cannot be adequately characterized by any one of his or her asthma performances, but only by the split vision that accommodates all the different but intrinsically intertwined performances. In this sense, getting to know the user requires attentiveness to the manifold performances that comprise users' ways of living with their disease and to the economy of passages that links the concrete performances to users' self-image.

Implications for E-Health Design

Incompatibilities between a system's image of the user and the self-image of the users constitute a major threat to adoption and use of patient-centred e-health systems. Our analysis of the self-image of asthmatics points toward three implications for the design and evaluation of systems for supporting patients' self-management:

- **Making a business case.** In most systems-development methods the decision to start a project is made on the basis of a business case that identifies a user need and argues convincingly for the viability of the envisioned solution. An understanding of good and bad passages and of the user as a cyborg will provide for the creation of business cases that more accurately reflect the viability of envisioned solutions and will, thereby, support organizations in making informed decisions about which projects to initiate—and which to avoid.
- **Designing for irreversibility.** Through the process of translation, systems bring users into motion. This is an inherent property of designing systems that aim to introduce changes to current practices, but the mobilization is merely an option presented to users. The more possibilities a system provides for linking into users' practices, the better chances it has of becoming part of some of these practices. And the more practices it becomes part of, the more it becomes ingrained in how users connect and coalesce their multiple performances of their disease. Thus, e-health systems should be designed to link into a variety of users' performances as this is how the mobilization may succeed in reaching a state where it is constitutive of users' self-image and consequently not at risk of being reverted by their day-to-day performances.
- **The performativity of evaluations.** Users are also relating to circumstances and actively performing their disease when they participate in system evaluations and clinical trials. For some users, like Tina, such evaluations provide opportunities for displacing their performance of their disease to a generalized disease identity, and thereby shifting the economy of passages toward one in which the work involved in complying with recommended practices is a good passage. For other users the circumstances of evaluations make them feel more subjected

to their disease, and this constitutes a bad passage by interfering with their image of themselves as capable. In interpreting evaluations, designers should be sensitive to these performances.

AWeb implemented state-of-the-art guidelines for asthma self-management (GINA, 2005), integrated self-management with an extended relationship between asthmatics and general practitioners, and provided personalized treatment advice at any time. Asthmatics' non-use of AWeb should not be seen as a result of dissatisfaction with these facilities, nor can system use be ensured by providing a different set of system facilities. On the contrary, the non-use of AWeb and other similar initiatives is partly explained by their narrow focus on the technology and on a medical rationality, leading to under-recognition of the myriad nontechnological, nonmedical factors involved in adopting and using e-health systems.

CONCLUSION

E-health systems for patient self-management are appearing for a number of chronic diseases including asthma. Whereas clinical trials provide evidence that such systems lead to better asthma management, practical deployment of one such system, AWeb, resulted in non-use by asthmatics. This study investigates asthmatics' reasons for not adopting AWeb by taking a performative approach and thereby keeping the practicalities of how asthmatics perform their asthma in the foreground. The analysis shows that AWeb is based on a taken-for-granted image of asthmatics as, per se, striving to be symptom-free. This image is incompatible with the four interviewed asthmatics' day-to-day performances of their asthma and renders invisible (a) that their asthma performances emphasize an economy of good passages and of feeling capable, (b) that they achieve the objective of feeling capable in quite different ways, and (c) that feeling capable does not per se equal being symptom-free all the time. The incompatibility of the system's image of the user and the self-image created and maintained by asthmatics through their asthma performances provides a basis for appreciating the manifold asthma performances such a system must incorporate in order to become and remain part of how asthmatics perform their asthma.

REFERENCES

Anhøj, J., & Nielsen, L. (2004). Quantitative and qualitative usage data of an Internet-based asthma monitoring tool. *Journal of Medical Internet Research, 6*(3), e23. Retrieved May 27, 2008, from http://www.jmir.org/2004/3/e23

Ball, M.J., & Lillis, J. (2001). E-health: Transforming the physician/patient relationship. *International Journal of Medical Informatics, 61*(1), 1-10.

Bender, B., Milgrom, H., & Rand, C. (1997). Nonadherence in asthmatic patients: Is there a solution to the problem? *Annals of Allergy, Asthma and Immunology, 79*(3), 177-186.

Bulger, D.W., & Reeves, C. (2000). Interactive Internet Web sites: A potentially powerful tool for disease management. *Disease Management & Health Outcomes, 7*(2), 67-75.

Buston, K.M., & Wood, S.F. (2000). Non-compliance amongst adolescents with asthma: Listening to what they tell us about self-management. *Family Practice, 17*(2), 134-138.

Butler, C., Rollnick, S., & Stott, N. (1996). The practitioner, the patient and resistance to change: Recent ideas on compliance. *Canadian Medical Association Journal, 154*(9), 1357-1362.

Caceres, C., Gomez, E.J., Garcia, F., Gatell, J.M., & del Pozo, F. (2006). An integral care telemedicine system for HIV/AIDS patients. *International Journal of Medical Informatics, 75*(9), 638-642.

Callon, M. (1986). Some elements of a sociology of translation: Domestication of the scallops and the fishermen of St. Brieuc Bay. In J. Law (Ed.), *Power, Action and Belief: A New Sociology of Knowledge?* (pp. 196-223). London, England: Routledge.

Callon, M. (1991). Techno-economic networks and irreversibility. In J. Law (Ed.), *A Sociology of Monsters: Essays on Power, Technology and Domination* (pp. 132-161). London, England: Routledge.

Carrard, I., Rouget, P., Fernández-Aranda, F., Volkart, A.-C., Damoiseau, M., & Lam, T. (2006). Evaluation and deployment of evidence based patient self-management support program for bulimia nervosa. *International Journal of Medical Informatics, 75*(1), 101-109.

Gibson, P.G., Powell, H., Coughlan, J., Wilson, A.J., Abramson, M., Haywood, P., Bauman, A., Hensley, M.J., & Walters, E.H. (2002). Self-management education and regular practitioner review for adults with asthma. *Cochrane Database of Systematic Reviews, Issue 3*, Art. No. CD001117. DOI: 10.1002/14651858.CD001117.

Global Initiative for Asthma (GINA). (2005). *Global strategy for asthma management and prevention.* NIH Publication No. 02-3659. Global Initiative for Asthma (GINA) workshop report. Retrieved May 27, 2008, from http://www.ginasthma.org

Goffman, E. (1959). *The presentation of self in everyday life.* Garden City, NY: Anchor Books.

Haraway, D.J. (1991). *Simians, cyborgs, and women: The reinvention of nature.* London, England: Free Association Books.

Kvale, S. (1996). *InterViews: An introduction to qualitative research interviewing.* Thousand Oaks, CA: Sage.

Law, J., & Singleton, V. (2000). Performing technology's stories: On social constructivism, performance, and performativity. *Technology and Culture, 41*(4), 765-775.

Mol, A. (1999). Ontological politics. A word and some questions. In J. Law & J. Hassard (Eds.), *Actor Network Theory and After* (pp. 74-89). Oxford, England: Blackwell.

Mol, A., & Law, J. (2004). Embodied action, enacted bodies: The example of hypoglycaemia. *Body & Society, 10*(2-3), 43-62.

Moser, I., & Law, J. (1999). Good passages, bad passages. In J. Law & J. Hassard (Eds.), *Actor Network Theory and After* (pp. 196-219). Oxford, England: Blackwell.

Newman, S., Steed, L., & Mulligan, K. (2004). Self-management interventions for chronic illness. *Lancet, 364*(9444), 1523-1537.

Nielsen, H.L. (2005). *Linking healthcare: An inquiry into the changing performances of Web-based technology for asthma monitoring.* Ph.D. thesis, Copenhagen Business School, Copenhagen, DK.

Plougmann, S., Hejlesen, O.K., & Cavan, D.A. (2001). DiasNet—A diabetes advisory system for communication and education via the Internet. *International Journal of Medical Informatics, 64*(2-3), 319-330.

Rasmussen, L.M., Phanareth, K., Nolte, H., & Backer, V. (2005). Internet-based monitoring of asthma: A long-term, randomized clinical study of 300 asthmatic subjects. *Journal of Allergy and Clinical Immunology, 115*(6), 1137-1142.

Rogers, E.M. (2003). *Diffusion of innovations (fifth edition).* New York: Free Press.

Rydström, I., Hartman, J., & Segesten, K. (2005). Not letting the disease get the upper hand over life: Strategies of teens with asthma. *Scandinavian Journal of Caring Sciences, 19*(4), 388-395.

Safran, C. (2003). The collaborative edge: Patient empowerment for vulnerable populations. *International Journal of Medical Informatics, 69*(2), 185-190.

Star, S.L. (1991). Power, technologies and the phenomenology of conventions: On being allergic to onions. In J. Law (Ed.), *A Sociology of Monsters: Essays on Power, Technology and Domination* (pp. 26-56). London, England: Routledge.

Willems, D. (1998). Inhaling drugs and making worlds: A proliferation of lungs and asthmas. In M. Berg, & A. Mol (Eds.), *Differences in Medicine: Unravelling Practices, Techniques and Bodies* (pp. 105-118). Durham, NC: Duke University Press.

Wilson, E.V, & Lankton, N.K. (2004). Modeling patients' acceptance of provider-delivered e-health. *Journal of the American Medical Informatics Association, 11*(4), 241-248.

Chapter XV
Exploring the Technology Adoption Needs of Patients Using E-Health

Linda M. Gallant
Emerson College, USA

Cynthia Irizarry
Suffolk University, USA

Gloria M. Boone
Suffolk University, USA

ABSTRACT

An extended version of the technology acceptance model (TAM) is applied to study hospital Web sites, one specific area of e-health. In a review of literature, five significant factors from TAM research are identified that are logically related to e-health sites from the user's perspective: usefulness, ease of use, trust, privacy, and personalization. All five factors emerged in the data analysis of 30 participants using a hospital Web site. We discuss the implications of this study for guiding development of effective patient-centered e-health.

INTRODUCTION

To design e-health that meets the needs and wants of users, we should consider technology adoption research and user-centered design (UCD) principles. Research in these areas can help e-health producers and providers to develop a successful UCD strategy. In general, producing high quality, functional, and usable Web sites is a goal for all businesses and services on the Internet, but particular industries and disciplines must develop Web site design strategies that encompass the specific needs and concern of their specific users. Currently, businesses are searching for successful e-commerce models (Noteberg, Christiaanse, & Wallage, 2003). In this chapter, we investigate what user-centered design strategies can be applied to develop effective e-health, using the specific example of a hospital Web site. We review the basic premises of the technology acceptance model (TAM) (Davis, 1989) and some of its extensions (e.g., Gefen, Karahanna, & Straub, 2003; Gefen & Straub, 2000; Perea y Monsuwe, Dellaert, & Ruyter, 2004; Wang, Wang, Lin, & Tang, 2003) and apply this to the research in e-health. In synthesizing these two bodies of literature, we develop an approach of experience design for e-health.

"Eighty percent of American Internet users, or some 113 million adults, have searched for information on at least one of seventeen health topics ... Most health seekers are pleased about what they find online, but some are frustrated or confused," (Fox, 2006, pp. ii). Specifically, 22% felt frustrated during their health searches, and 18% felt confused by the information they found online (Fox, 2006). Another study indicates that significant barriers to use of the Internet to find healthcare information remain for some elements of the population, such as those age 60 and older, people with 12 or fewer years of education, and residents of rural communities (Licciardone, Smith-Barbaro, & Coleridge, 2001). To increase the social and practical value of e-health, research needs to first produce answers as to what basic elements make e-health successful to its users.

What are the basic features that individuals search for on the Web? They want to find information and retrieve information easily. They want tailored health information. They want to trust the information. What is a successful e-health model? Using the technology acceptance model (TAM) as a framework, we propose to identify key factors leading to adoption of e-health. Past TAM research (Gefen et al., 2003; Gefen & Straub, 2000; Perea y Monsuwe et al., 2004; Wang, et al., 2003) gives us a starting point to shed light on the role of trust, privacy, credibility, and user perceptions of technology in the dynamic exchange between patients and provider-delivered e-health. In reviewing past research on TAM and UCD, we identified five relevant factors to explore in a case study of 30 participants using a hospital Web site. The five factors are usefulness, ease of use, trust, privacy, and personalization. These are used as sensitizing concepts in a case study to identify why potential users adopt e-health.

PRIOR RESEARCH

Using proven research approaches such as TAM and UCD to investigate patients' adoption of e-health can provide important insights. "The TAM postulates that user adoption of a new information system is determined by their intention to use the system, which in turn is determined by their beliefs about the system" (Wang, 2003, pp.335). In online technology adoption, the TAM model highlights the importance of trust, usefulness, and ease of use from the user's point of view (Gefen et al., 2003; Gefen & Straub, 2000; Perea y Monsuwe et al., 2004; Wang et al., 2003). More specifically, research using TAM in e-commerce has found that trust, privacy, and user perceptions of technology are central elements of online technology adoption (Gefen et al., 2003; Gefen & Straub, 2000; Perea y Monsuwe et al., 2004; Wang et al., 2003).

Popularity of e-health is growing. While the design and development of e-health is not well researched (Ketchum, 2005), searching the Internet for health and medical information is known to be one of the most common activities for e-health users (Akerkar & Bichile, 2004; Fox, 2006). Given that the Internet has altered the way people gain access to health information (Akerkar & Bichile, 2004; Kreps, 2003; Neuhauser & Kreps, 2003), health professionals need to understand how to design e-health using strategies that meet the needs and expectation of Internet users. In this vein, e-health has the potential to produce innovative care models in healthcare (Nash & Gremillion, 2004).

We propose that four TAM-related factors (perceived usefulness, perceived ease of use, trust, and privacy) are highly relevant to the context of e-health. An additional factor, personalization, has been found by UCD research to be a key driver of adoption and use of hospital Web sites, a form of e-health (Gallant, Irizarry, & Kreps, 2007). We review the literature relating to each of these factors in the following sections.

Usefulness

Perceived usefulness is the chief reason why people intend to use technology systems (Gefen & Straub, 2000). In TAM, usefulness is the most important source of user acceptance of new technologies (Perea y Monsuwe et al., 2004).

Perceived usefulness is defined as the extent to which a person believes that using a particular system will enhance his or her job performance, while perceived ease of use is defined as the extent to which a person believes that using a particular system will be free of effort (Wang et al., 2003, pp. 503).

Perceived usefulness is a major predictor of intended use of online technologies (Gefen et al., 2003), including e-health (Wilson & Lankton, 2004).

Ease of Use

In the sphere of the Internet, Gefen and Straub (2000) found that perceived ease of use influences individuals' intention to use an e-commerce system. Their research indicates that perceived ease of use is dependent on the tasks or types of use people expect to perform. In particular, when users perceive an intrinsic system task as easy to perform, this has a positive influence on the adoption of a technology. In the e-health context, a main task of users is searching for accurate health and medical information, which Wilson and Lankton (2004) found to be significantly correlated with patients' perceived ease of use.

Trust

Trust has been found to be a multidimensional construct invested with consumer beliefs in integrity, benevolence, ability, and predictability of the vendor (Gefen & Straub, 2004).

High levels of consumer trust encourage e-commerce, however, the appropriate conceptualization of trust has been much debated in online research, with trust levels of users being associated with personal propensity to trust (McKnight, & Chervany, 2001), perceived severity of user health problems (Fruhling, 2003; Fruhling & Lee, 2006), and Web site design factors (Shanker, Urban, & Sultan, 2005). In response, there has been a call for online trust transactions to be studied in more context and application specificity (Riegelsberger, Sasse, & McCarthy, 2005). Studying trust is important as "understanding how online trust is created and maintained can lead to improved Web sites, sales revenues, profitability, and ultimately shareholder value" (Shanker et al., 2005, pp. 326). In the context of e-health, trust is both situational and context dependent (Noteberg et al., 2003). Users provide personal information that can carry significant privacy risk (Culnan & Armstrong, 1999).

Online trust has been described as an association of networked relationships which depend on the degree of trust between the parties involved (Durkan, Durkin, & Gillen, 2003). All partners in this known network must be seen as trustworthy for members to willingly assume risk. The networking of trust extends to e-health. In the exchange between a patient and his or her healthcare provider, the provider's e-health system can provide structural assurance that the online technology environment, even with network partners, is safe and under control. This type of assurance helps to build a trusted reputation for all parties involved (Hsiao, 2003). Online interactions "include different types and levels of risk, and they are only possible if users trust each other and the systems they use to meet, communicate and transact–as well as the organizations that provide them." (Riegelsberger et al., 2005, pp. 382).

Branding is another area impacting online trust. Online trust rests in part upon the perception of a vendor's credibility. Research has shown that brand recognition can influence trust of online vendors. Durkan et al. write "Often a recognized brand name will provide a measure of credibility and thus stimulate consumer trust" (2003, pp. 99). Endorsements can also work to increase trust by decreasing uncertainty in online transaction (Noteberg et al., 2003).

Privacy

Culnan and Armstrong (1999) identify two major risks to privacy in online transactions. Once users provide personal information, they may be unable to control and protect it. Secondly, personal information could be used in other ways than were intended. Institutions must strike an appropriate balance between the personal privacy and business needs, noting that concern for privacy can be mediated by expected benefits. People will provide personal information online when an economic or social benefit can be expected (Culnan & Armstrong, 1999; Durkan et al., 2003).

Given the high sensitivity of personal health and medical information, advancement of e-health could be obstructed if users fear that their privacy is at risk. Fear of revealing personal information "to third parties without their knowledge or permission" provides a development and design challenge to e-health adoption (Wang, 2003, pp.339). Privacy is a fundamental right in most democracies (Basu, 2004), and the loss of personal privacy is a major concern of consumers in e-commerce (Noteberg et al., 2003).

Personalization

The goal of personalized care is to provide "the right information, to the right person, at the right time" (Hesse & Schneidermann, 2007, pp. 7). Hawkins, Pingree, Shaw, Gustafson, Gatzke, McDowell, and Tryon-Petith (2006) point out that the efficacy of tailored health messages has been supported across a variety of general health education domains. Other research has demonstrated that personalized or tailored information is viewed by users as more relevant and thus, more likely to be valued (Oenema, Brug & Lechner, 2001). In their study of a hospital Web site, Gallant et al. note that "users want personalized information geared to their health needs presented in a seamless and easy-to-use manner" (2007, pp. 20). While this point may seem intuitive, it is important to remember that not all e-health interfaces are designed with user goals in mind. Rigorous human-centered testing is essential for effective and useful personalization strategies.

Personalization of e-health holds much potential for preventative medicine and patient-centered care. Applying personalization strategies to e-health Web sites provides the capacity for online technologies to act in the tradition of telehealth, which has been used successfully to implement tailored healthcare management of chronic diseases, such as diabetes and asthma, and risk factors, such as high cholesterol.

METHOD

Through systematic investigation, qualitative research traditions answer questions of process, understanding, social meaning, and human action. Since we are inquiring about a process of knowledge production arising from human actions that infer meanings from product use, a qualitative research design is most appropriate. We use a case study method. Typically in qualitative case work, data is prerecorded (Stake, 2005, pp. 450). Our data was transcribed from the prerecorded usability tests and interviews. The data was analyzed for classification and pattern recognition. We conceived participant users as evaluators. From this point of view, we analyze the user data in accordance with the five sensitizing concepts described in our review of prior research. This analysis method is in accordance with an instrumental case study approach.

"...the methods of instrumental case study draw the researcher toward illustrating how the concerns of researchers and theorists are manifest in the case. Because the critical issues are more likely to be known in advance and to follow disciplinary expectations, such a design can take greater advantage of already-developed instruments and preconceived coding schemes," (Stake, 2005, pp. 450).

Participants

The 30 participants were recruited for the usability testing of a hospital Web site redesign project. Participants were paid $85.00 for up to 90 minutes of their time. Participants were selected to have a group mixed in demographics in age, gender, education, and income. See Appendix A for a breakdown of participants' demographics. All selection criteria were based on the hospital's typical patient demographic. Gender of participants was split evenly with 15 female participants, and 15 male participants. The age of participants was classified into three categories. For education, there were three categories. All participants were able to name their primary care hospital. A professional recruiting firm was hired to screen and recruit participants. The testing was done in a professional usability lab during five consecutive days of testing.

Data Collection

A high fidelity prototype of a working Web site for a Northeastern hospital was tested in a traditional usability lab. Study participants performed a task on the prototype that was accessed over the Internet from the hospital's servers. There were 34 task scenarios performed by 30 participants using a think-aloud protocol. There are three sections of the usability test designed for measuring the medical center's typical user profile. The task script was pretested on three pretest participants and minor wording changes were made. Participants had the option of reading the task along with the task being read aloud by the test facilitator.

Think-aloud protocol. This produces a verbal text of user participants' performance of task scenarios. Usability testing falls into the category of "natural techniques" in the knowledge acquisition process (Shadbolt & Milton, 1999, pp. 314). The traditional usability data collection technique of think-aloud is a process tracing method with its root in decision making research. Process tracing endeavors to let researchers observe the "natural" decision making process that participants engage in when given a task. With a think-aloud protocol, researchers gain participants' verbal utterances without interjecting any interaction that would cause a change in the participants' actions.

In-Depth Interview and Adaptive Questioning. Layering the think-aloud protocol with in-depth interviewing produces a text that provides observable and knowledge-centered data. After a participant finishes the task, the facilitator uses probing questions to elicit the user's understandings and meanings of the task, design, and overall system. As the task being performed comes to an end, the research method data collection process using interviewing becomes a codiscovery process between the participant user and test facilitator. This adaptive usability technique allows system testers the traditional behavioral measures while further providing user-centered knowledge concerning how potential customers perceive a product and its use. The latter data can be valuable to business teams across the organization.

Interviewing is a method of data collection that is well matched in the collection of information and processes "that cannot be observed effectively by other means" (Lindlof & Taylor, 2002, pp.174). Enhancing data collection with in-depth questioning at the end of tasks produces an interview procedure aimed at capturing user evaluations and knowledge of product uses and meanings. Unlike the task scenarios, the in-depth questions and probes are not predetermined. The task facilitator turns to an interviewing format that constructs a conversational environment producing questions and probes that are based on participant users' task experiences. Two trained facilitators conferred on how to approach the testing process for layering the technique of traditional think-aloud with interpretive questioning and probing, adaptive usability testing. Thus, the facilitator must adapt the post-task environment to an interviewing format. This acts as a summary of users' experiences, opinions, and evaluations of products.

Data Analysis Procedures

There were 34 task scenarios designed to measure important interaction dimensions of the Web site. The task list was developed by the lead researcher along with the hospital's marketing department team, which was responsible for the Web site development and upkeep. Tasks were divided into sections such as homepage usage, navigation, patient resources, employment, and health information. In the first part of the current investigation, a content analysis is used to measure usability problems. Measurements of the think-aloud analysis model should distinguish whether or not the usability problem was detected by observation or participant verbalization before developing a categorization of usability problems (Van Den Haak, Jong, & Schellens, 2003). The second part of the analysis seeks to learn what types of data arise from participants' responses in the post-task interviewing situation. A grounded theory approach is used. This approach is sometimes referred to as a constant-comparative method (Lindlof & Taylor, 2002, pp. 218). The analysis by the researcher is grounded in analyzing the data by aptly naming categories, making data comparisons, and overall extracting "an innovative, integrated, realistic scheme from masses of unorganized raw data" (Strauss & Corbin, 1998, pp. 13).

Traditional Analysis of Think-Aloud Data

Think-aloud protocols have been used in a variety of ways. Boren and Ramey (2000) identify that the practice of think-aloud protocols in usability testing diverge from its theoretical basis proposed by Ericsson and Simon's (1984) three-level model of verbalizations. This model in usability testing is used to identify system deficiencies (Boren & Ramey, 2000). This traditional concurrent cognitive verbalization model favors level one verbalization. Here verbalizations are not cognitively transformed before thinking aloud during a task performance (Boren & Ramey, 2000). At level two, more complex cognitive processing occurs before verbalization. Concepts such as images must be transformed into words. Level three produces the greatest amount of cognitive processing and is the least desired according to Ericsson and Simon's (1984) three-level model. Instead of simple verbalization, participants engaged in cognitive processes at level three go beyond direct task performance and verbalizing.

Analysis of Adaptive Usability and Knowledge Centered Data

At level three verbalizations, information retrieval from participants' memories is called upon to verbalize a response. Knowledge of how people perceive the usefulness of a product in their work or private life comes to bear. Knowledge management literature suggests that conversation is the key to sharing knowledge (McInerney, 2002, pp.1012). Gaining user knowledge on products is the goal of adaptive usability testing. In a qualitative interpretive methodology, talking and eliciting information can be the basis of data collection. As such, talk between the user and researcher is not a biasing factor. Using speech communication as a basis for analysis is a promising approach to usability testing.

[S]peakers cannot ignore listeners, even silent ones. Speakers expect that listeners will react to what they say, and that listeners' actions (or interactions) are reflective of that response...if we accept the view of human communication, the issue in usability testing becomes not one of disappearing from participants, but rather one of creating a highly asymmetrical speaker/listener relationship, one which maximizes the speakership of the participant and minimizes the speakership of the usability practitioner, (Boren & Ramey, 2000, pp. 268).

DATA ANALYSIS

Data used for content categories should "provide useful evidence for testing hypotheses or answering research questions," as well as "communication," an understanding of a subject (White & Marsh, 2006, pp. 27). This analysis allows participants' descriptions and opinions about hospital Web site to be communicated. It allows users' knowledge to be known.

Using five analytic constructs (usefulness, ease-of-use, trust, privacy, and personalization) drawn from TAM and UCD research, an analysis was performed on 1,800 pages of data transcripts. The five descriptive codes can also be referred to as analytic constructs. Descriptive codes "entail little interpretation" in "attributing a class of phenomena to a segment of text" (Miles & Huberman, 1994, pp. 57). Descriptive codes are more denotative in attaching face value meanings to participants' discursive text than with interpretive coding that is more connotative given a constant comparative analysis process between the developing codes and the text.

The lead author performed and initial coding analysis and developed a description of each code for hospital Web site use; participant statements that matched any category of the five codes were tagged. Appendices B through F present representative supporting quotes for each descriptive code. Based upon the set of quotes for each code set, a more precise conceptual structure for the use of hospital Web sites was defined. As a validity check, both co-authors next independently read the conceptual codes and representative quotes to compare these with the raw textual data. The coding, definition, and quotes were found to be valid and credible in transferability, dependability, and conformability.

RESULTS

The results of our analysis relating to each of the constructs we studied are reported below.

Usefulness

The usefulness of the hospital Web site as an e-health artifact centers on obtaining information about personal and family health matters, physicians, diseases, insurance plan acceptance, medical specialties, and types of medical procedures offered at the facility.

Ease of Use

Having information organized in a logical and familiar arrangement provides users a sense of flow. Especially important in this e-health context is the user's sense of timely interaction with health appointment scheduling. Participants stated the importance of having a direct sense of communicating with a medical professional instead of interacting with a nonhuman information system. Participants also emphasized the need for appropriately labeling sections and their content so that Web site users can easily find information that they need. A search function on the Web site was seen as an important user tool for finding information.

Trust

Trust was viewed as the standard of medical care associated with the reputations and specialties of physicians at the healthcare facilities. Participants wanted to view physicians' background information, including medical degrees, years of practice, and even lawsuits.

Privacy

Privacy was a concern among participants with sensitive medical conditions. Additionally, participants were more apprehensive of trusting an automated information system to properly make appointments. Participant responses suggest that as users get to know and trust a system, they feel more secure with it.

Personalization

Participants foresee an ongoing interest in acquiring tailored and up-to-date healthcare and medical information. Many participants have particular health conditions and diseases for which they are interested in obtaining targeted health information and news updates. Participants wanted to be able to access their medical records online and make appointments online.

DISCUSSION

Using an illustrative case study of a hospital Web site, we found usefulness, ease of use, trust, privacy, and personalization to hold considerable importance for participants. The finding of our case study corroborates prior research on technology adoption and suggests that these five factors should be considered when designing and building e-health systems.

Since the usefulness of new technology is a primary motivator for adoption (Perea y Monsuwe et al., 2004), people will most likely adopt e-health systems that are situationally useful in relation to illnesses, health problems, or past medical histories. This phenomenon was seen in participant quotes that show usefulness as having an easy-to-navigate hierarchy. For example, within a topology of illnesses, some users verbally distinguish aspects such as medical condition, visitor, patient, and medical professional. For others, usefulness merged with perception of ease of use. This included easy viewing and clear navigation on the Web site. Participants wanted pages that are easy to read, have large font sizes, and organize information into small segments. Factors related to navigation included a global search function, a clear primary and secondary navigation, and clear organizational principles such as alphabetical or chronological ordering. Participants wanted clear directions on how to complete forms relating to healthcare, insurance, contact information, selecting doctors, and making appointments. They wanted to be able to quickly retrieve information on financial and insurance aspects of their healthcare. Participants wondered, for example, if they could go to specific doctors with their insurance or get prescriptions filled.

While the role of trust in e-commerce has been studied by numerous researchers, proposed strategies may not be adequate to understand trust in the context of e-health (Fruhling, 2003). Yet, a mainstay of healthcare organizations' relationships with their patients and other stakeholders is trust (Hesse, Nelson, Kreps, Croyle, Arora, & Rimer, 2005). Internet users' trust of health information Web sites has also been growing (Rosenvinge, Laugerud, & Hjortdahl, 2003), with personal doctors, medical universities, and the federal government being seen as the most trusted sources of online health information (Dutta-Bergman, 2003; Kind, Wheeler, Robinson, & Cabana, 2004). This issue is prominent in our data. Participants want to search for doctors' credentials to judge whether or not the information presented and the institution owning the Web site are credible.

Online healthcare information needs to be seen as credible by users before they trust it (Rosenvinge et al., 2003). The stakes are high because use of health information can impact people's health positively or negatively (Al-Bahrani & Plusa, 2004; Luo & Najdawi, 2004; Williams, Nicholas, Huntington, McLean, 2002). A component of trust is credibility. In general, perceived credibility of an online technology attracts users (Wang et al., 2003). Our findings are in agreement with past research (Eysenbach & Kohler, 2002; & Luo & Najdawi, 2004), in that participants view e-health Web sites as more credible when source and ownership are disclosed. Trust is part of the name and reputation of the institution. Trust is also a consideration when selecting doctors as our findings suggest prospective patients want to see the biography of the doctor including specifics on education, specialties, and years of experience.

We find perceptions of online trust and privacy are contrasted to other communication methods. Participants compared the Web site functions with traditional ways of accomplishing tasks. For example, they would search to make an online appointment until they felt it was easier to fall back on the traditional communication method of making an appointment by telephone. Participants would often compare the online task to what they would do in a face-to-face interaction with a hospital employee. Thus, e-health should try to support communicative interactions people expect to have within traditional telephone and face-to-face communication with administrative and medical staff in the healthcare process. Web site users should be able to have a choice to leave the Web site to interact by telephone or in person. This would be especially helpful with users who are low in trust of general Web transactions. While some evidence in the data suggests that placing sensitive personal information on a Web site for healthcare users is an Internet privacy concern, our research design did not allow us to explore this research dimension. Future research should be undertaken to provide more insight into e-health privacy and security concerns of users.

Personalization can have impacts on issues of privacy, ease of use (usability), and usefulness. To meet the diversity needs of users, e-health Web sites can employ a personalization strategy. This process presents tailored information to users based on their personalized profile. Knowledge about a user can be used in a dynamic Web site that can specifically target information, content, and services to individual users (Adomavicius & Tuzhilin, 2005). Personalization of e-health can solve usability problems relating to user characteristics, such as disabilities and illiteracy (Denny, Ginsberg, Papp, Browne, Morgan, Kushins, & Solina, 2002). Further, the strategy of personalizing Web sites as individualized patient portals can be a useful tool for patients to gain greater access to personal health information and make better informed decisions for their health (Nguyen, Carrieri-Kohlman, Rankin, Slaughter, & Stulbarg, 2004). Personalization strategies are especially pertinent given that patients are increasingly using electronic personal health records to manage their own health (Lorbach & Detmer, 2007). Our case study data suggests that people with particular health concerns such as diabetes want to find up-to-date information on their medical conditions. People search for health information upon being diagnosed or having a family member diagnosed with a medical condition. In addition, personalization appears to enhance the expectation of usefulness. For example, personalization can allow e-health users to access RSS feeds that enable them to select useful topics, sources or information channels to access the health information.

CONCLUSION

Through analyzing several factors drawn from TAM and UCD from the user's perspective, we were able to identify a number of implications for developers of patient-centered e-health. As Hesse & Shneiderman, (2007) observed, many elegant theoretical interfaces have failed when used in real-world settings because they fail to take user needs into account. A patient-centered design focus can avoid these problems, providing e-health that is both effective for healthcare providers and empowering to patients.

REFERENCES

Adomavicius, G., & Tuzhilin, A. (2005). Personalization technologies: A process-oriented perspective. *Communications of the AMC, 48*(10), 83–90.

Akerkar, S.M., & Bichile, L.S. (2004). Health information on the Internet: Patient empowerment or patient deceit? *Indian Journal of Medical Sciences, 58*(8), 321–326.

Al-Bahrani, A., & Plusa, S.(2004). The quality of patient-orientated Internet information on colorectal cancer. *Colorectal Disease, 6,* 323–326.

Basu, S. (2004). Implementing e-commerce tax policy. *British Tax Review, (1),* 46–69.

Boren, M.T., & Ramey, J. (2000). Thinking aloud: Reconciling theory and practice. *IEEE Transactions on Professional Communication, 43*(3), 261–278.

Culnan, M.J., & Armstrong, P.K. (1999). Information privacy, Procedural fairness and impersonal trust: An empirical investigation. *Organization Science, 10*(1), 104–115.

Davis, F.D. (1989). Perceived usefulness, perceived ease of use, and user acceptance of information technology. *MIS Quarterly, 13*(3), 319–329.

Denny, J.T., Ginsberg, S., Papp, D., Browne, G., Morgan, S., Kushins, L., & Solina, A. (2002). Hospital initiatives in promoting smoking cessation: A survey of Internet and hospital-based programs target at consumers. *Chest, 122,* 692–698.

Durkan, P., Durkin, M., & Gillen, J., (2003). Exploring efforts to engender on-line trust, *Entrepreneurial Behaviour and Research, 9*(3), 93–110.

Dutta-Bergman, M. (2003). Trusted online sources of health information: Differences in demographics, health beliefs, and health-information orientation. *Journal of Medical Internet Research, 5*(3), e21. Retrieved May 27, 2008, from http://www.jmir.org/2003/3/e21/

Ericsson, K.A., & Simon, H.A. (1984). *Protocol analysis: Verbal reports as data.* Cambridge, MA: MIT Press.

Eysenbach, G., & Kohler, C. (2002) How do consumers search for and appraise health information on the world wide Web? Qualitative study using focus groups, usability tests, and in-depth interviews. *BMJ, 324,* 573–577.

Fox, S. (2006). Online health search 2006. Most Internet users start at a search engine when looking for health information online. Very few check the source and date of the information they find. *Pew Internet & American Life Project.* Retrieved

May 27, 2008, from http://www.pewInternet.org/pdfs/PIP_Online_Health_2006.pdf

Fruhling, A.L. (2003). *An empirical study of human-computer interaction: Usability factors affecting perceptions of trust of e-health consumers.* Doctoral Dissertation, University of Nebraska, 2003. Proquest, AAT3092541.

Fruhling, A.L., & Lee, S. (2006). The influence of user interface usability in rural consumers' trust of e-health services. *International Journal of Electronic Healthcare, 2*(4), 305–321.

Gallant, L., Irizarry, C., & Kreps, G.L. (2007). User centric hospital Web sites: A case for trust and personalization. *e-Service Journal, 5*(2), 5–26.

Gefen, D., Karahanna, E., & Straub, D.W. (2003). Trust and TAM in online shopping: An integrated model, *MIS Quarterly, 27*(1), 51–90.

Gefen, D., Straub, D.W. (2004). Consumer trust in B2C e-commerce and the importance

of social presence: Experiments in e-products and e-services. *Omega: The International Journal of Management Science, 32*, 407–424.

Gefen D., & Straub, D.W. (2000). The Relative importance of perceived ease-of-use in IS adoption: A study of E-commerce adoption. *Journal of the Association for Information Systems, 1*(8), 1–30.

Hawkins, R., Pingree, S., Shaw, B., Gustafson, D., Gatzke, K., McDowell, H., & Tryon-Petith, C. (2006) *Creating a dynamic, tailored, online health education and support program for women with breast cancer: A case study of the CHESS program.* Paper Presented at the Annual Meeting of the International Communication Association, Sheraton, New York. Retrieved May 27, 2008, from http://www.allacademic.com/meta/p14986_index.html

Hesse, B.W., Nelson, D.E., Kreps, G.L., Croyle, R.T., Arora, N.K., & Rimer, B.K. (2005) Trust and sources of health information. The impact of the Internet and its implications for healthcare providers: Findings from the first health information national trends survey. *Archives of Internal Medicine, 165*, 1–7.

Hesse, B.W., & Shneiderman, B. (2007). eHealth research from a user's perspective. *American Journal of Preventative Medicine, 32*(5s), 97–103.

Hsiao, R.L. (2003). Technology fears: Distrust and cultural persistence in electronic marketplace adoption. *Journal of Strategic Information Systems, 12*(3), 169–199.

Ketchum, A.M. (2005). Consumer health information Web sites: A survey of design elements found in sites developed in academic environments. *Journal of Medical Library Association, 93*(4), 496–499.

Kind, T., Wheeler, K.L., Robinson, B., & Cabana, M.D. (2004). Do the leading children's hospitals have quality Web sites? A description of children's hospital Web sites. *Journal of Medical Internet Research, 6*(2). Retrieved May 27, 2008, from http://www.jmir.org/2004/2/e20/

Kreps, G.L. (2003). E-health: Technology-mediated health communication. *Journal of Health Psychology, 8*(1), 5–6.

Licciardone, J.C., & Smith-Barbaro, P., & Coleridge, S.T. (2001). Use of the Internet as a resource for consumer health information: Results of the second osteopathic survey of healthcare in America (OSTEOSURV-II). *Journal of Medical Internet Research* 3(4):e3. Retrieved May 27, 2008, from http://www.jmir.org/2001/4/e31/

Lindlof, T.R., & Taylor, B.C. (2002). *Qualitative communication research methods (second edition).* Thousand Oaks, CA: Sage.

Lorbach, D.F., & Detmer, D.E. (2007). Research challenges for electronic health records. *Ameri-*

can Journal of Preventative Medicine, 32(5s), 104–111.

Luo, W., & Najdawi, M. (2004). Trust-building measures: A review of consumer health portals. *Communication of the ACM, 47*(1), 109–113.

McInerney, C. (2002). Knowledge management and the dynamic nature of knowledge. *Journal of the American Society for Information Systems and Technology, 53*(12), 1009–1018.

McKnight, D.H., & Chervany, N.L. (2001). What trust means in e-commerce customer relationships: An interdisciplinary conceptual typology. *International Journal of Electronic Commerce, 6(2)*, 35–59.

Miles, M.B. & Huberman, A.M. (1994). *Qualitative data analysis: An expanded sourcebook (second edition).* Thousand Oaks: Sage.

Nash, M.G., & Gremillion, C. (2004). Globalization impacts the healthcare organization of the 21st century: Demanding new ways to market product lines successfully. *Nursing Administration Quarterly, 28*(2), 86–91.

Neuhauser, L., & Kreps, G.L. (2003). The Advent of e-Health: How interactive media are transforming health communication. *Medien and Kommunikations-wissenschaft 51*(3–4), 541–556.

Nguyen, H.Q., Carrieri-Kohlman, V., Rankin, S.H., Slaughter, R., & Stulbarg, M.S. (2004). Supporting cardiac recovery through ehealth technology. *Journal of Cardiovascular Nursing, 19*(3), 200–208.

Noteberg, A., Christiaanse, E., & Wallage. (2003). Consumer trust in electronic channels: The impact of electronic commerce assurance on consumers' purchasing likelihood and risk perceptions. *e-Service Journal, 2*(2), 46–67.

Oenema, A., Brug, J., & Lechner, L. (2001). Web-based tailored nutrition education: Results of a randomized clinical trial. *Health Education Research, 16*, 647–660.

Fox, S. (2005). Health information online. Eight in ten Internet users have looked for health information online, with increased interest in diet, fitness, drug, health insurance, experimental treatments, and particular doctors and hospitals. *Pew Internet and American Life Project.* Retrieved May 27, 2008, from http://www.pewInternet.org/pdfs/PIP_Healthtopics_May05.pdf

Riegelsberger, J., Sasse, M.A., & McCarthy, J.D. (2005). The mechanics of trust: A framework for research and design. *International Journal of Human-Computer Studies. 62*, 381–422.

Rosenvinge, J.H., Laugerud, S., & Hjortdahl, P. (2003). Trust in health Web sites: A survey among Norwegian Internet users. *Journal of Telemedicine and Telecare, 9,* 161–166.

Perea y Monsuwe, T., Dellaert, B.G.C., & Ruyter, K. (2004). What drives consumers to shop online? : A literature review. *International Journal of Service Industry Management, 15*(1), 102–121.

Shadbolt, N., & Milton, N. (1999). From knowledge engineering to knowledge management. *British Journal of Management, 10,* 309–322.

Shanker, V., Urban, G.L., & Sultan, F. (2005). Online trust: A stakeholder perspective, concepts, implications, and future directions. *Journal of Strategic Information Systems, 11,* 325–344.

Sienot, M. (1997). Pretesting Web sites: A comparison between the plus-minus method and the think-aloud method for the World Wide Web. *Journal of Business and Technical Communication, 11*(4), 469–482.

Stake, R.E. (2005). *Qualitative case studies. The Sage handbook of qualitative research (third edition).* In N. Denzin, & Y. Lincoln (Eds.), (pp.443–466). Sage Publications.

Strauss, A.L., & Corbin, J. (1998). *Basics of qualitative research: Techniques and procedures for developing grounded theory (second edition).* Sage Publications.

Todd, P., & Benbasat, I. (1987). Process tracing methods in decision support systems research: Exploring the black box. *MIS Quarterly, 41*(3), 493–512.

Van Den Haak, M.J., Jong, de, M.D.T., & Schellens, P.J.(2003). Retrospective vs. concurrent think-aloud protocols: Testing the usability of an online library catalogue. *Behavior & Information Technology, 22*(5), 339–351.

Wang, Y.S. (2003). The adoption of electronic tax filing systems: an empirical study. *Government Information Quarterly, 20*(4), 333–352.

Wang, Y.S., Wang, Y.M., Lin, H.H., & Tang, T.I. (2003). Determinants of user acceptance of Internet banking: An empirical study. *International Journal of Service Industry Management, 14*(5), 501–519.

White, M.D., & Marsh, E.E. (2006). Content analysis: A flexible methodology. *Library Trends, 55*(1), 22–45.

Williams, P., Nicholas, D., Huntington, P., & McLean, F. (2002). Surfing for health: User evaluation of a health information Web site. *Health Information and Libraries Journal, 19*, 98–108.

Wilson, E.V., & Lankton, N.K. (2004). Modeling patients' acceptance of provider-delivered e-health. *Journal of the American Medical Informatics Association, 11*(4), 241–248.

APPENDIX A

Demographic	Categories	Number (percentage)
Gender		
	Male	15 (50%)
	Female	15 (50%)
Income		
	25,000 to 49,000	5 (16.6%)
	50,000 to 74,000	7 (23.3%)
	75,000 to 99,000	11 (36.6%)
	100,000 to 150,000	5 (16.6%)
	More than 150,000	2 (6.6%)
Age		
	35 to 49	13 (43.3%)
	50 to 64	13 (43.3%)
	Older than 65	4 (13.3%)
Education		
	High School Graduate	1 (3.3%)
	Some College	7 (23.3%)
	Bachelor Degree	16 (53.3%)
	Graduate Degree	6 (20%)

APPENDIX B

Usefulness
User 2: "Primary – wait a minute, primary – Finding a primary care physician. I definitely would be interested in that to see where would I go for daily checkups. And finding out the type of physician that I would want for me. And I'd probably click here to find that information out…I have a child as well and I would be interested in – especially if I'm in another healthcare, like I'm in Tufts, I'd be interested in would I have to switch doctors, especially for my son where he already has a doctor. And if I switch to [hospital name], would that same doctor be there, would be offered for me to go to that same doctor. And I would click here for that information."
User 3: "Oh, for someone like me, the most important thing would be uh – oh, let me go back to it – would be – seems like the healthcare information because this is for me, I'm trying to learn about trying to find a doctor. If I wanted to become a patient or a member, I have to – I need to know all this information. So, healthcare information."
User 7: "Maybe they would list the physicians that are affiliated with the [hospital name] and then what I would have to do is – now if my personal doctor, for example, from Watertown, I'd have to see if he's listed there. If I didn't want to bother to call his office, I'd look to see if he's affiliated with [hospital name], if I could have procedures done there, whatever. Or maybe you're looking up the names of some physicians that maybe – Maybe some information about their specialties or whatever.
User 10: "Personally? What I would use it for? I probably would – knowing me, I would probably be looking up diseases and getting information, just a general overview of it. And specifically, the type of service that's offered for that particular disease. I'm sure they don't cover everything, but I find it, what little I've moved around in it, it's very informative, so that. And I think the obvious with the patient, with the patient information, I know that with Tufts that I have a book, I don't believe there's a Web site that you can search for doctors."
User 17: "Depending on the most important to me is looking for a PCP [Primary Care Physician] that meets in my plan because if he doesn't meet your plan, I can't go to him."
User 23: "For example, my situation now, I had pain in my back, couldn't walk, my leg and so on. I want to know what was wrong, and who could treat it…So I would look for back, for example, or spinal or neurosurgery. I want to know who the doctors are, who neurosurgeons are, and how good they are. And the backgrounds they have. Their bios."

APPENDIX C

Ease of Use
User 5: "But a lot of times that's what I do. I just go to the search part of some Web sites unless it shoots out at me right away."
User 7: "Oh, I – oh, patient pharmacy. I would never think to look under there. Again I'm thinking little specialty shops. I want to get a gift. I want to get dinner. I want to get flowers or something. I would never put that together."
User 9: "This takes three days to make an appointment. If I thought it was very important, I would call up myself…This was good for – to get information. If I was going to make an appointment, I would try to do it this way if I didn't have to have it right away…I find that when I call at least the people I deal with, if they say well, can't see the doctor for two or three weeks, I'd try to speak to the doctor himself if I'm a patient of his. And tell him what my problem is and I'd tell him I need to see him sooner than three weeks. But you're on the computer, you have nobody to talk to."
User 13: "Just – it [specialty shops] could be anything. It could be a place where you just get – go buy a newspaper or you can get gifts and things like that. Flower shops or something like that. That's what I would associate it with… outpatient pharmacy, OK. Wow, I never would have looked there. Never would have looked there… Just too – not – it's more something you were going to shop for."
User 15: "You know what I'm finding, that patient service is an awfully large and important button. In fact, I would suspect that for patients or patients who are going to be referred there, that may even have to be broken out. And I can think of something here. Healthcare information divided between in-house physicians, nursing services. Something that they would like on their homepage, but for their own information. And patient related or just for newbies. People new to Lahey Clinic. The great unwashed plus patients. And I'm not saying that you have to dummy it down. But you need to make that – for example. It's nice. Medical research at Lahey, residencies and fellowships. But I'm new here. Where would I go, and it seems that oftentimes we're going through this patient service center."
User 18: "And there'd be a roster of all the physicians. And what they do and all that. After physicians, they'd do it by specialties and then the more you click on them and then get a list of the roster there. That's how I would logically go about it...And I'm sure they all link, because if you go under the disease, and then I'm sure there'll be something on the page of whatever say, kidney, that would have the physicians that would – clearly, I would think it would connect you right into the physicians, too, so there'd be a link, whether you went in one way or the other."
User 20: "OK. Specialty shops and services … I wouldn't put it with shops because as soon as shops comes into my brain, I'm seeing gift shops…And services, well, I don't know. Send a telegram. I don't know. But it doesn't say pharmacy to me."

APPENDIX D

Trust
User 2: "I'm going to scroll down to see…. Physician finder. Maybe I should look him up first before the appointment…OK, let's see. OK, so here we find him right here, residency. So I'd probably want to read a little about him."
User 6: "And then I think for – one thing that sort of provides security for patients is just seeing a little bit, like what each medical background is, like where they got their medical degree, where they've studied. You know."
User 11: "And you want to find out information like where she graduated, and her medical school, and everything … I want to know about this doctor's background…I thought it was very important when you were getting a physician finder, to be able to pull up that physician and find out – maybe that physician went to a school that you heard was really awful…I thought that was really important."
User 12: "If someone's going to [hospital name], they're going to go to [hospital name] for whatever reason, the doctors, their doctor's there, or they're good for their specific condition. No one's going to look at it [the Web site] and go oh my God what a fabulous Web site. I'm going to that hospital. Or, oh my God, this is ridiculous. I'm not going to that hell-hole."
User 20: "And I've also learned once I find that person's name, I may not be able to get it through here but, I forget now, but someone told me how to look up that person, see whether there have been lawsuits against him or things like that. It's a very helpful thing to know. I think I would definitely go to here."
User 23: "To me the most important thing is the staff, who is there, what their specialties are. Where can I get my condition treated the best. The best facilities and the best people doing it. One of the things I always look for – we're looking for a family doctor now. Our family doctor retired. We loved him and we can't find a replacement… We're looking for a family doctor, my wife and me. Internal medicine. I'm looking for somebody who is not too old, is not too young. And what I find at [hospital name], for example, is that most of the – most of the long, long lists of people in Internal Medicine, most of them got out of school in 2000, 1999, 1998. They're probably very sharp but I want somebody who said Oh, yeah, I had a case like this 12 years ago….And I like to see people who are board certified. So that page on the whatever – whatever [hospital name] is doing is very, very important to me."

APPENDIX E

Privacy
User 2: "OK at this point, honestly, at this point I'd pick up the telephone. You know? I – I use the computer a lot for information. Even when I hear some of my customers talk about – yeah, we're going on a cruise, we went through the computer to get the tickets –I go to Orbitz and (inaudible) tickets cheaper. - I'm always leery of it. I'd rather talk – after talking to all the answering machine messages, the mechanical stuff, when you finally get a hold of a human being to make an appointment, to make sure that there's no mix-up…If I was familiar with the Web site I would do that. But if I'm unfamiliar with something, I would just get on the phone and make the phone call."
User 12: "Well, I'm thinking I guess to make an appointment I've got to fill out some forms. And they're telling me about the security, that it's OK…it's not totally important to me but depending on what I'm using this for, but I could see a person that might have a problem with it, like maybe has AIDS and doesn't really need the whole world to know, or there's certain privacy issues. I always assume if it's a hospital that they have to put that here, but I am maybe naively assume that it's safe…but maybe it makes them feel good to see security but if you just saw a link I think you'd feel good knowing oh, it must be secure"
User 28: "Initially I would think to click it, to keep going, but I think it has to do with the privacy statement. So if I click on it, I think I'd probably get that click on thing…Because it's blue and it says read the privacy statement right there under it, but this made me think, keep going…But initially, that's what I want to know. You think oh, no I want to read more about the privacy statement."

APPENDIX F

Personalization
User 1: "That's what I would look for. There's very specific information about that hospital, or that organization like how to reach me, how to make an appt… If I were a regular customer with the ability to get into my records… to the extent that that's allowed, I might be able to use my SSN or some other access code to check on one big thing."
User 6: "Right, because I'm diabetic…So that's why I go online, most of the time, is to find out current news about treatments for diabetes like if there's anything new about diets, you know, for diabetics, so – you know, and not every – not every hospital or clinic treats diabetes, you know, in that sort of way, so I'd look for something. Plus I always go and look at who the doctors are, who the care – medical care givers."
User 15: "Read health information. Health information. Now that's an interesting one. Is this one the disease of the day? Can I scan, or can I search according to what I think I have, and is there information on that."
User 21: "I think it would break down into three things. An existing patient, and then what does an existing patient want to do?...Make an appointment. Check out doctors that they'd been referred to. Learn more about conditions."
User 23: "If I pop that, that's what I would expect to happen. Request an appointment – I think this would take me to some central appointment office, not to any particular doctor, and tell him who I wanted, Dr. Ollie, and I'd like an appointment for this, and that central office would somehow have available to them his free times. That's been my experience I think."
User 24: "Primarily for research, that's why I go to the other medical Web sites that I do, just for my own edification or just out of curiosity if there's something in the news, I'll just check different Web sites and plug into just, like, the general search and see what articles come up."
User 25: "I guess more articles. Articles, articles. You know, articles regarding health…Yeah, health topics….will I see news here. Sometimes – I guess…Sometimes if you're – I don't think I'd design anything – other Web sites, anyway, but – I'm just saying, sometimes, if you're in a Web site, then it'd be pretty good if it had news, you know, up-to-date news."
User 28: "Yes, see this is what – this isn't really going to help me get an appointment. I'd have to call and talk with someone. So up until this point, it's like good to use the Web site, to get the information but there's no appointment schedule that I see right away, so I would just get the phone."

Chapter XVI
Predicting Patients' Use of Provider-Delivered E-Health: The Role of Facilitating Conditions

E. Vance Wilson
Arizona State University, USA

Nancy K. Lankton
Michigan State University, USA

ABSTRACT

This chapter presents a new rational-objective (R-O) model of e-health use that accounts for effects of facilitating conditions as well as patients' behavioral intention. An online questionnaire measured patients' behavioral intention to use a new e-health application as well as proxy measures of facilitating conditions that assess prior use of and structural need for health services. A second questionnaire administered three months later collected patients' self-reported use of e-health during the intervening period. The new model increased predictions of patients' e-health use (measured in R^2) by more than 300% over predictions based upon behavioral intention alone, and all measured factors contributed significantly to prediction of use during the three-month assessment period.

INTRODUCTION

Increasingly, healthcare provider organizations offer provider-delivered e-health[1] to supply patients with health information and advanced capabilities, such as appointment scheduling, prescription refilling, and online communication with physicians and clinical staff (Hsu, Huang, Kinsman, Fireman, Miller, Selby, & Ortiz, 2005; Wilson & Lankton, 2004). Because designing, developing, and deploying e-health represents a substantial investment by providers, it is important that these applications are actually used by patients. If providers can predict levels of patient e-health use at early stages in the design process, this will help them to be more effective in allocating resources and managing risks associated with e-health delivery.

In this chapter, we propose and test a predictive model of e-health use that accounts for both situational factors (facilitating conditions) that are typically outside patients' direct control and behavioral intention that patients form toward using e-health. In the following sections, we review the background literature that motivates and supports this study, present the research model, and develop hypotheses to test relationships within the model.

BACKGROUND

Wilson and Lankton (2004) studied factors that contribute to initial acceptance of e-health among new registrants to a prototype e-health application. That study found patients' behavioral intention (BI) toward e-health use is predicted well by three prominent models of IT acceptance: the technology acceptance model (TAM) (Davis, Bagozzi, & Warshaw, 1989), the motivational model (Davis, Bagozzi, & Warshaw, 1992), and the integrated model (Venkatesh, Speier, & Morris, 2002). All are examples of *rational* models (Ajzen, 2002; Kim & Malhotra, 2005), so named because predictions are based upon individuals' beliefs regarding such factors as ease of use and usefulness of the IT. Within these models, effects of beliefs upon IT use behaviors are theorized to be fully mediated by BI that individuals form through rational processes. Wilson and Lankton (2004) also report that belief factors in the models are significantly predicted by three patient characteristics that are developed prior to use of e-health: satisfaction with the provider, information-seeking preference, and Internet dependence. This finding is important, as it implies that patients' BI toward e-health use can be predicted early in design stages of application development.

Rational models of behavior have performed well in predicting individual behaviors across a wide range of research domains. In the preponderance of published studies, a positive association is reported between BI and behavior (see reviews by Ouellette & Wood, 1998; Sheppard, Hartwick, & Warshaw, 1988). Based on this substantial literature most IT acceptance studies do not

Table 1. Review of associations between BI and self-reported IT use

Reference	IT Type	Variance in IT Use Explained by BI
Davis et al. (1989)	Word processor	12-40 %
Dishaw & Strong (1999)	Software maintenance tool	36%, including direct effect of perceived usefulness
Hartwick & Barki (1994)	Business IS application	35-74%
Horton, Buck, Waterson, & Clegg (2001)	Intranet	11%
Lai (2004)	Short message services	15%
Limayem & Hirt (2003)	Communication application	47%, including direct effects of habit and facilitating conditions
Moon & Kim (2001)	World wide Web	38%
Morris & Dillon (1997)	Netscape Web browser	19%
Shih & Fang (2004)	Internet banking	24%
Stoel & Lee (2003)	Web-based courseware	4%
Suh & Han (2002, 2003)	Internet banking	3%
Szajna (1996)	E-mail	6-32%

assess actual use, under the assumption that IT use is normatively predicted by BI (Lee, Kozar, & Larsen, 2003). Indeed, a recent review of 277 published IT acceptance studies conducted by one of the authors finds just 13 that evaluate effects of BI on self-reported IT use. Results from these 13 studies are summarized in Table 1.

As calculated from the sample sizes and correlations (actual or estimated), the weighted average correlation between BI and IT use in the studies shown in Table 1 is 36% ($R^2 = .13$), with the 95% confidence interval for correlation ranging from 25-46% and for R^2 ranging from .06-.21. At the higher end of this range BI is quite predictive of actual IT use, but predictions at the lower end of the range clearly are of limited value. In the case of the Wilson and Lankton (2004) study, a low association between BI and e-health use would essentially negate the possibility that antecedent factors mediated by BI are significantly related to e-health use.

Research to date has not reported the level of association between BI and use of e-health, but certain characteristics of the e-health context could diminish the size of this association. Patients' access to e-health often is initiated by situational factors that are outside the individual's personal control, including illness, injury, and other medical concerns. Such factors act as *facilitating conditions* which are theorized to influence individual behaviors outside the framework of beliefs and intentions that underlies rational models (Triandis, 1977, 1980). Triandis writes:

"[A]t any level of habit or behavioral intention, the absence or presence of facilitating conditions will affect the likelihood of a behavior. In an extreme case, the person's habits and behavioral intentions have no relevance if the situation does not permit him or her to behave (Triandis, 1977, pp. 206-207).

Facilitating conditions are difficult to incorporate directly into models of behavior, because of the wide range of distinct events that can promote or obstruct any specific action. For this reason, IT researchers have applied proxy measures for the presence or absence of facilitating conditions. For example, Thompson, Higgins, and Howell (1991) applied *perceived availability of guidance in selecting computer hardware and software* as a proxy measure for a facilitating condition related to the number of products that are available for an individual to select from.

Although a number of studies have applied proxy measures of facilitating conditions to model IT use, results are mixed. Some studies find significant predictions of IT use from proxy measures, including subjects' age and experience (Venkatesh, Morris, Davis, & Davis, 2003), but other studies fail to find significant effects (Thompson et al., 1991; Limayem & Hirt, 2003).

Because e-health is frequently used to respond to an unusual medical situation, facilitating conditions may be more important to e-health than to other IT. As illustrated in Table 1, typical studies address forms of IT in which incentives for use are frequent and consistent, e.g., word processing software used by MBA students (Davis et al., 1989), and in which external obstacles to use have been removed (e.g., campus computer labs provided to support student access to course communication software) (Limayem & Hirt, 2003).

Motivational and obstructive effects of facilitating conditions are especially important in the healthcare context, as patients who are willing to use health services will not necessarily have an immediate medical need (Cantor & Fallon, 1997). Although a patient may intend to use e-health in the future for accessing health information or scheduling an appointment for a medical examination, it remains unlikely that he or she will take action unless prompted by some facilitating condition, such as onset of pain. Actual use of e-health at a given moment depends upon its *microrelevance* (i.e., "the degree to which IT-use helps to solve the here-and-now problem of the user in his working process" (Spil, Schuring, & Michel-Verkerke, 2004, pp. 39)), which is predicated to a large degree upon the presence or absence of facilitating conditions. These observations suggest it is important to account for effects of facilitating conditions when modeling e-health use. However, this will require a research perspective that transcends the boundaries of rational models of IT acceptance.

RESEARCH MODEL AND HYPOTHESES

The present study tests a new research model in which the rational factor BI is augmented with objective factors representing patients' prior use of and need for healthcare services. The theoretical justification for this *rational-objective* (R-O) model is grounded in Triandis' (1977, 1980) definition of facilitating conditions as objective factors capable of directly affecting individuals' behaviors, regardless of the state of rational factors, including BI. The behavior of seeking healthcare services clearly reacts to certain facilitating conditions, such as illness or injury. For this reason, it may be anticipated that an individual's prior use of and need for healthcare services will be positively associated with presence of facilitating conditions and that these factors can provide proxy measures representative of facilitating conditions that exist in the prior context. To the extent that facilitating conditions persist across time, prior use of and need for healthcare services can further proxy for contemporaneous measurement of facilitating conditions during a subsequent period. This theorized assessment of proxy factors in predicting e-health use is illustrated in Figure 1.

The R-O research model (shown in Figure 2) posits that prediction of e-health use will be improved by augmenting BI with *offline service utilization, frequency of medical office visits,* and *structural need for medical services,* factors we propose to be associated with presence of facilitating conditions. In the following sections, hypotheses regarding relationships depicted in the research model are presented.

BI Toward Use

As discussed previously, a positive association between BI and behavior is found in a substantial prior literature, both in studies of general behavior

Figure 1. The role of proxy factors in measurement of facilitating conditions

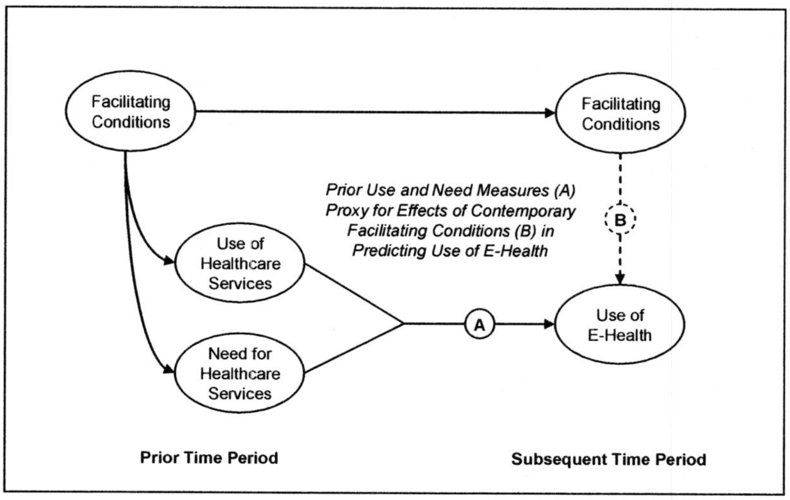

Figure 2. Rational-objective (R-O) research model

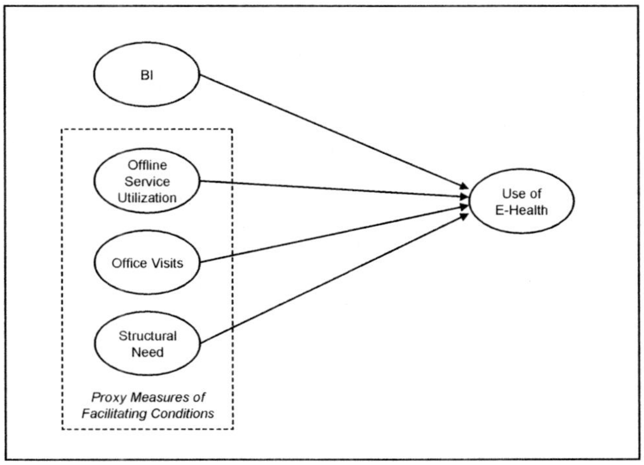

(Ouellette & Wood, 1998; Sheppard et al., 1988) and in studies directed toward IT use (Lee et al., 2003). In recognition of this precedent, a similar association is hypothesized between BI and e-health use.

H1: *BI Toward E-Health Use will Predict Use of E-Health.*

Prior Use of Offline Services

Where a certain IT has been used previously, the level of prior use can be more important than BI in predicting subsequent use (Cheung & Limayem, 2005); in some cases, prior IT use can completely subordinate effects of BI (Kim & Malhotra, 2005; Wilson, Mao, & Lankton, 2005). In the present study, participants will not have used e-health previously. However, they will have had the opportunity as patients to use health services at the provider's offline facilities that parallel the services offered via e-health. For example, filling out a prescription refill request form in the e-health application would have many similarities to requesting a prescription refill by phone or in person. Researchers find that prior utilization of an organization's service predicts future service utilization (Naessens, Baird, Jouten, Vanness, & Campbell, 2005). This suggests that e-health use will be influenced by prior use of similar offline health services.

H2: *Prior use of offline health services will predict use of e-health.*

A second way of conceptualizing prior use of health services is to assess overall utilization of provider services beyond the similar services that are offered via e-health. Frequency of office visits exemplifies this type of overall measure, based upon the rationale that patients who visit clinic offices frequently will be externally motivated to use e-health to supplement or replace their visits.

H3: *Prior number of office visits will predict use of e-health.*

Structural Need

Individual need for healthcare is associated with higher rates of healthcare use in general (Ford, Trestman, Steinberg, Tennen, & Alen, 2004; Naessens et al., 2005) and with higher rates of e-health use (Hsu et al., 2005). These observations suggest that use of e-health will increase where need for health services is *structural*, defined herein as need that is statistically associated with observable characteristics of participants. Because the association is statistical across a demographic population, we consider structural need to be a proxy measure of facilitating conditions rather than a direct measure.

H4: *Structural need for health services will predict use of e-health.*

Structural need has not been studied previously as a contributor to IT use (Lee et al., 2003). However, two factors that fit the criteria presented above are age and presence of a chronic health condition, such as diabetes. Both factors are statistically associated with increased need for health services (CDC, 2005, 2007), and Hypotheses 5a and 5b test the individual effects of these factors as contributors to structural need.

H5a: *Age will predict structural need for health services.*

H5b: *Chronic health condition will predict structural need for health services.*

Model Predictiveness

The final hypothesis tests the potency of the full R-O research model in predicting e-health use. This hypothesis contrasts the full model to the rational model—in other words, BI only, and to each alternative nested R-O model (i.e., any model that comprises BI plus a subset of objective factors contained within the full model). In order to assess trade-offs between model predictiveness and parsimony, hypothesis testing will control for differences in the number of factors between models.

H6: *The full research model will be more predictive of e-health use than alternative rational or R-O nested models.*

The following sections describe the research method and present results of hypothesis testing. The chapter concludes with a discussion of implications for practice and research.

RESEARCH METHOD

This research is conducted among patients who registered for access to an e-health application called *MyHealth* (a pseudonym), which was developed by a large Midwest U.S. provider. MyHealth presents encyclopedic health content with both browse and search access, e-mail-style connectivity with the clinic office, prescription refill ordering, and appointment scheduling. Access for patients is unrestricted, but they must first register online and thereafter login using a self-assigned ID and password. The developer of MyHealth is a provider managing approximately 100 clinics. At the time of the study, access to MyHealth was being offered to patients in four of these clinics as a pilot project. Prior to data collection, the research design was reviewed and approved by the lead researcher's Institutional Review Board.

Procedure

An invitation to volunteer for participation was sent to the e-mail addresses of 1,750 individuals who had registered for access to MyHealth following announcement of the Web site in a promotional mailing to clinic patients. On average, registrants received the e-mail invitations approximately two weeks after registration, which provided a short introductory period for them to investigate the site. 163 (9%) of the invitees responded to the invitation and 135 (8%) completed the entire initial online questionnaire. The provider declined to allow the researchers to send follow-up requests to participate. The initial questionnaire measured BI as well as demographic factors and aspects of prior offline health service utilization and need.

Three months later, a second questionnaire was administered to assess use of MyHealth during the intervening period. A request to complete the follow-up questionnaire was e-mailed to the original 135 respondents, and a second request was e-mailed two weeks later to those who had not completed the questionnaire by that time. In total, 83 of the original respondents (61%) completed the follow-up questionnaire. A one-way ANOVA conducted between early and late responders to the follow-up questionnaire showed no significant differences on measures between these groups, suggesting that participants are generally representative of the original respondents.

Responses from the initial questionnaire and the follow-up questionnaire were matched based on the participant's e-mail address. Average age of participants is 52, with a minimum age of 25, and a maximum age of 80, and 75% are women. Following registration, participants accessed MyHealth an average of 1.9 times (s.d. = 3.1 accesses).

RESULTS

Hypothesis testing was conducted using the partial least squares (PLS) approach to structural equation modeling (SEM). PLS simultaneously apportions variance across a structural model and is capable of assessing both reflective and formative latent variables (Chin, 1998; Wold, 1985, 1989), two important capabilities in operationalizing the research model used in this study.

The structural model encompasses four independent variables. BI was measured as a reflective latent variable with two indicator items. Offline service utilization was measured as the total of self-reported offline accesses to five health services, and office visits was measured as the total of self-reported visits to healthcare facilities made during the six months prior to completing the first questionnaire. Structural need was measured as a formative latent variable with two indicator items: age and presence of a chronic health condition, measured as a dichotomous variable. The dependent variable in the model, e-health use, was measured as the total of self-reported accesses to five health services offered by MyHealth during the three-month period following completion of the first questionnaire.

Construct Validation

To assess construct reliability and validity, a confirmatory factor analysis (CFA) was conducted using weighted data generated by PLS-Graph as input and modeling the items as reflective indicators of their corresponding constructs following guidelines presented by Gefen and Straub (2005). Results of the CFA analyses are presented in Table 2.

Table 2. Confirmatory factor analysis

Item \ Factor	BI	OSU	SN	OV	Use
BI: I intend to use MyHealth	**0.979**	0.104	0.134	0.032	0.229
BI: I predict I will use MyHealth	**0.985**	0.104	0.113	0.035	0.267
OSU: Offline Service Utilization	0.106	**1.000**	-0.177	0.340	0.417
SN: Structural need: Age	0.045	0.051	**0.492**	0.030	-0.153
SN: Structural need: Chronic Condition	0.115	0.171	**0.840**	-0.154	-0.260
OV: Office Visits	0.034	0.340	-0.118	**1.000**	-0.030
Use: E-Health Use	0.254	0.417	-0.310	-0.030	**1.000**

Convergent validity and discriminant validity were assessed using criteria developed by Fornell and Larcker (1981). Convergent validity is not assessed for single-item measures or formative latent variables, such as structural need. It is established for reflective latent variables when (1) all indicator loadings are significant and all loadings are above .70, (2) composite construct reliability for each factor is in excess of .80, and (3) average variance extracted (AVE) for each factor is above .50. For the BI reflective latent variable, all indicator items are above .70, composite construct reliability is .982, and AVE is .964, indicated that convergent validity is present in this factor.

Discriminant validity is established when between-construct correlations are less than the square root of AVE for each construct, which is calculated as .982 for BI and .688 for structural need. The between-construct correlations are substantially lower than the AVE figures for all factors, indicating that discriminant validity is present in both multi-item factors.

Hypothesis Tests

All hypotheses are supported. E-health use is predicted by BI (path coeff. = .254, $p < .001$), utilization of offline services (path coeff. = .410, $p < .01$), frequency of prior office visits (path coeff. = .213, $p < .05$), and presence of structural need (path coeff. = .294, $p < .001$). Structural need is predicted as a formative latent variable by age (path coeff. = .562, $p < .01$) and by chronic health condition (path coeff. = .864, $p < .001$). Finally, the full research model (shown in column 8 of Table 2) provides significantly better predictions of e-health use than any nested model ($p < .05$). Significance of R^2 differences was calculated using F-tests that control for differing number of variables in each model, as presented by Subramani (2004). Modeling of e-health use based only upon BI (shown as column 1 of Table 2) is significantly worse than other models except model 2 (BI plus office visits).

DISCUSSION AND CONCLUSION

The findings demonstrate that predictiveness of rational models of IT acceptance, such as TAM, is limited in the context of e-health. Yet these predictions can be dramatically improved by incorporating objective measures that proxy for facilitating conditions, as we did using offline service utilization, prior office visits, and structural need. These are factors that can be assessed at early stages of e-health application development to identify patient populations who are most likely to use e-health and to guide design of e-health to support targeted needs. For example, the findings regarding chronic disease suggest affected patients are disproportionately motivated to try

Table 3. Full and nested models arranged in order of increasing explained variance (R^2)

Relationship / Model	1	2	3	4	5	6	7	8
BI → E-Health Use	$.254^3$	$.255^3$	$.297^3$	$.301^3$	$.212^2$	$.212^2$	$.253^3$	$.254^3$
Offline Service Utilization → E-Health Use					$.395^2$	$.460^2$	$.341^2$	$.410^2$
Office Visits → E-Health Use		.038		.082		$.193^1$		$.213^1$
Structural need → E-Health Use			$.347^3$	$.357^3$			$.281^3$	$.294^3$
E-Health Use Model R^2	.065	.066	.183	.190	.219	.252	.294	.333

$^1 p < .05$ $^2 p < .01$ $^3 p < .001$ (one-tailed t-tests)

out e-health and are well-positioned to benefit from targeted services, such as online support for disease management.

The findings also have important implications for research. Although a number of studies have reported that prior IT use is predictive of subsequent use outside the framework of rational models (e.g., Cheung & Limayem, 2005; Kim & Malhotra, 2005; Kim, Malhotra, & Narasimhan, 2006, Limayem & Hirt, 2003), the results here indicate that prior use of offline services has similar effects on subsequent IT use. This finding suggests researchers need to reconsider the mechanisms that influence use of e-health and related IT.

Two mechanisms for explaining the effects of prior IT use are prominent in the current literature. The first mechanism proposes that prior experiences drive development of reasoned beliefs, culminating in the formation of BI toward use (Ajzen, 2002). But in the present study offline service utilization, prior office visits, and structural need factors each show significant direct effects on e-health use beyond any mediating effects of BI. The second mechanism proposes that effects of prior IT use on subsequent use occurs through formation of habits (Kim et al., 2006). However, habits are developed through repetitive action (Ouellette & Wood, 1998), and the opportunity for repetitive use of MyHealth by participants was virtually non-existent prior to administration of the first questionnaire in our study.

Thus, neither mechanism offers a satisfactory explanation of findings in the present study. However, the findings are consistent with the proposition that e-health use is predominantly determined by facilitating conditions that are essentially outside the control of individual patients. As discussed previously, past research finds facilitating conditions to be only equivocal predictors of IT use, however, most of this research has been directed toward IT in which effects of facilitating conditions are limited by the structure of the research domain, such as where external obstacles have been removed. Findings of the present study suggest that there is a class of IT, including e-health, in which facilitating conditions are exceptionally salient. It will be important for future researchers to determine what characteristics these IT share and to consider the potential effects of facilitating conditions when designing research. One idea that has been proposed is that e-health is one example of an emerging class of IT designed to support sporadic uses, and the sporadic nature of the activity reduces the importance of BI in predicting future IT use (Wilson et al., 2005).

FUTURE RESEARCH DIRECTIONS

It is interesting that contrasts among full and nested models reveal that each of the proxy factors for facilitating conditions is a significant predictor of e-health use. This finding affirms both the choice of factors in the study and the practice of implementing multiple measures, yet it also raises questions that may provide direction for future research. First, the findings show that both specific and general service utilization are predictive of use, but there is need for theory development to explain why. We need to understand which aspects of service utilization are key to motivating use of online services and whether these differ between e-health and other IT. Second, the results linking structural need to e-health use deserve additional exploration. The findings that factors of age and chronic health condition contribute to a formative latent factor suggest that e-health is well-received by populations who may benefit the most from services that e-health can readily offer, such as healthcare information and online support communities. It will be important for future researchers to study which services are most beneficial to populations with specific patterns of structural need (e.g., elderly diabetics), and to investigate other factors that may contribute to structural need. Finally, it will be equally important for researchers to study alternative proxy measures of facilitating conditions in order to identify an optimal trade-off between accuracy and parsimony.

CONCLUSION

This study of e-health use builds upon a prior study of initial acceptance (Wilson & Lankton, 2004). The combined research models tested in these two studies give providers a foundational framework for making early predictions about patients' acceptance and use of e-health applications. Joint findings of the two studies also provide researchers with a greater understanding of specific ways in which patients' interactions with e-health vary from other types of IT and demonstrate the importance of considering effects of facilitating conditions when designing e-health research.

REFERENCES

Ajzen, I. (2002). Residual effects of past on later behavior: Habituation and reasoned action perspectives. *Personality and Social Psychology Review, 6*(2), 107-122.

Cantor, C., & Fallon, B. (1997). *Phantom illness: Recognizing, understanding, and overcoming hypochondria.* Boston, MA: Houghton Mifflin.

Center of Disease Control (CDC). (2005). Annual rate of visits per person to physician offices, by patient age group—United States, 2003. *Center for Disease Control QuickStats, 54*(48), 1238. Retrieved May 27, 2008, from http://www.cdc.gov/mmwr/preview/mmwrhtml/mm5448a9.htm

Center of Disease Control (CDC). (2007). Costs of chronic disease. *Center for Disease Control Chronic Disease Overview.* Retrieved May 27, 2008, from http://www.cdc.gov/nccdphp/overview.htm#2

Cheung, C.M.K., & Limayem, M. (2005). The role of habit in information systems continuance: Examining the evolving relationship between intention and usage. In D. Avison, D. Galletta, & J. DeGross (Eds.), *Proceedings of the 26th International Conference on Information Systems* (pp. 471-482). Las Vegas, NV, USA, University of Minnesota.

Chin, W. (1998). The partial least squares approach to structural equation modeling. In G.A. Marcoulides (Ed.), *Modern Methods for Business Research* (pp. 295-336). Mahwah, NJ: Lawrence Erlbaum Associates.

Davis, F.D. (1989). Perceived usefulness, perceived ease of use, and user acceptance of information technology. *MIS Quarterly, 13,* 319-329.

Davis, F.D., Bagozzi, R.P., & Warshaw, P.R. (1989). User acceptance of computer technology: A comparison of two theoretical models. *Management Science, 35,* 982-1002.

Davis, F.D., Bagozzi, R.P., & Warshaw, P.R. (1992). Extrinsic and intrinsic motivation to use computers in the workplace. *Journal of Applied Social Psychology, 22,* 1111-1132.

Dishaw, M.T., & Strong, D.M. (1999). Extending the technology acceptance model with task-technology fit constructs. *Information & Management, 36,* 9-21.

Fishbein, M., & Ajzen, I (1975). *Belief, attitude, intention and behavior: An introduction to theory and research.* Reading, MA: Addison-Wesley.

Ford, C.A., Bearman, P.S., & Moody, J. (1999). Foregone healthcare among adolescents. *Journal of the American Medical Association, 282,* 2227-2234.

Ford, J.D., Trestman, R.L., Steinberg, K., Tennen, H., & Allen, S. (2004). Prospective association of anxiety, depressive, and addictive disorders with high utilization of primary, specialty and emergency medical care. *Social Science & Medicine, 58*(11), 2145-2148.

Fornell, C.R., & Larcker, D.F. (1981). Structural equation models with unobservable variables and measurement error: Algebra and statistics. *Journal of Marketing Research, 18*(3), 382-388.

Forrest, C.B., & Starfield, B. (1998). Entry into primary care and continuity: The effects of access. *American Journal of Public Health, 8*(9), 1330-1337.

Gefen, D., & Straub, D.W. (2005). A practical guide to factorial validity using PLS-Graph: Tutorial and annotated example. *Communications of the Association for Information Systems, 16,* Article 24, 91-109.

Harris, K.D., Donaldson, J.F., & Campbell, J.D. (2001). Introducing computer-based telemedicine in three rural Missouri counties. *Journal of End User Computing, 13*(4), 26-35.

Hartwick, J., & Barki, H. (1994). Explaining the role of user participation in information system use. *Management Science, 40*(4), 440-465.

Hong, W., Thong, J.Y.L., Wong, W.M., & Tam, K.Y. (2001). Determinants of user acceptance of digital libraries: An empirical examination of individual differences and system characteristics. *Journal of Management Information Systems, 18*(3), 97-124.

Horton, R.P., Buck, T., Waterson, P.E., & Clegg, C.W. (2001). Explaining Intranet use with the technology acceptance model. *Journal of Information Technology, 16,* 237-249.

Hsu, J., Huang, J., Kinsman, J., -Fireman, B., Miller, R., Selby, J., & Ortiz, E. (2005). Use of e-health services between 1999 and 2002: A growing digital divide. *Journal of the American Medical Informatics Association, 12,* 164-171.

Igbaria, M., Guimaraes, T., & Davis, G.B. (1995). Testing the determinants of microcomputer usage via a structural equation model. *Journal of Management Information Systems, 11*(4), 87-114.

Keil, M., Beranek, P.M., & Konsynski, B.R. (1995). Usefulness and ease of use: Field study evidence regarding task considerations. *Decision Support Systems, 13*(1), 75-91.

Kim, S.S., Malhotra, N.K., & Narasimhan, S. (2006). Two competing perspectives on automatic use: A theoretical and empirical comparison. *Information Systems Research, 14*(2), 418-435.

Kim, S.S., & Malhotra, N.K. (2005). A longitudinal model of continued IS use: An integrative view of four mechanisms underlying postadoption phenomena. *Management Science, 51*(5), 741-755.

Lai, T.L. (2004). Service quality and perceived value's impact on satisfaction, intention and usage of short message service (SMS). *Information Systems Frontiers, 6*(4), 353-368.

Lazarus, I.R. (2001). Separating myth from reality in e-health initiatives. *Managed Healthcare Executive, June*, 33-36.

Lee, Y., Kozar, K.A., & Larsen, K.R.T. (2003). The technology acceptance model: Past, present, and future. *Communications of the Association for Information Systems, 12,* Article 50, 752-780.

Leisen, B., & Hyman, M.R. (2004). Antecedents and consequences of trust in a service provider: The case of primary care physicians. *Journal of Business Research, 57*(9), 990-999.

Limayem, M., & Hirt, S.G. (2003). Force of habit and information systems usage: Theory and initial validation. *Journal of the Association for Information Systems, 4,* 65-97.

McKillen, D. (2001). E-health traffic—slow but steady growth. *Marketing and Media, 36*(9), 10-12.

Moon, J., & Kim, Y. (2001). Extending the TAM for a World-Wide-Web context. *Information & Management, 38,* 217-230.

Morris, M.G., & Dillon, A. (1997). How user perceptions influence software use. *IEEE Software, 4,* 58-65.

Naessens, J.M., Baird, M.A., Jouten, H.K.V., Vanness, D.J., & Campbell, C.R. (2005). Predicting persistently high primary care use. *Annals of Family Medicine, 3*(4), 324-330.

Ouellette, J.A., & Wood, W. (1998). Habit and intention in everyday life: The multiple processes by which past behavior predicts future behavior. *Psychological Bulletin, 12,* 54-74.

Payton, F.C., & Brennan, P.F. (1999). How a community health information network is really used. *Communications of the ACM, 42,* 85-89.

Sheppard, B.H., Hartwick, J., & Warshaw, P.R. (1988). The theory of reasoned action: A meta-analysis of past research with recommendations for modifications and future research. *Journal of Consumer Research, 15,* 325-343.

Shih, Y., & Fang, K. (2004). The use of a decomposed theory of planned behavior to study Internet banking in Taiwan. *Internet Research, 14*(3), 213-223.

Spill, T. A.M., Schuring, R.W., & Michel-Verkerke, M.B. (2004). Electronic prescription system: Do the professionals USE IT? *International Journal of Healthcare Technology Management, 6*(1), 32-55.

Stoel, L., & Lee, K.H. (2003). Modeling the effect of experience on student acceptance of Web-based courseware. *Internet Research, 13*(5), 364-374.

Subramani, M. (2004). How do suppliers benefit from information technology use in supply chain relationships? *MIS Quarterly, 28*(1), 45-74.

Suh, B., & Han, I. (2002). Effect of trust on customer acceptance of Internet banking. *Electronic Commerce Research and Applications, 1,* 247-263.

Suh, B., & Han, I. (2003). The impact of customer trust and perception of security control on the acceptance of electronic commerce. *International Journal of Electronic Commerce, 7*(3), 135-161.

Szajna, B. (1996). Empirical evaluation of the revised technology acceptance model. *Management Science, 42*(1), 85-92.

Thompson, R.L., Higgins, C.A., and Howell, J.M. (1991). Personal computing: Toward a conceptual model of utilization. *MIS Quarterly, 15*(1), 125-143.

Triandis, H.C. (1977). *Interpersonal behavior.* Brooks/Cole Publishing, Monterey, CA.

Triandis, H.C. (1980). Values, attitudes, and interpersonal behavior. In H.E. Howe & M. M. Page (Eds.), *Nebraska Symposium on Motivation 1979* (pp. 195-259). Lincoln, NE: University of Nebraska Press.

Venkatesh, V., Morris, M.G., Davis, G.B., & Davis, F.D. (2003). User acceptance of information technology: Toward a unified view. *MIS Quarterly, 27*(3), 425-478.

Venkatesh, V., Speier, C., & Morris, M.G. (2002). User acceptance enablers in individual decision making about technology: Toward an integrated model. *Decision Science, 22,* 297-316.

Wilson, E.V., & Lankton, N.K. (2004). Modeling patients' acceptance of provider-delivered e-health. *Journal of the American Medical Informatics Association, 11*(4), 241-248

Wilson, E.V., Mao, E., & Lankton, N.K. (2005). Predicting continuing acceptance of IT in conditions of sporadic use. In N.C. Romano, Jr. (Ed.), *Proceedings of the Eleventh Americas Conference on Information Systems.* Omaha, NE, USA.

Wold, H. (1989). Introduction to the second generation of multivariate analysis. In H. Wold (Ed.),

Theoretical Empiricism (pp. vii-xi). New York: Paragon House.

Wold, H. (1998). Partial least squares. In S. Kotz, & N.L. Johnson (Eds.), *Encyclopedia of Statistical Sciences* (Vol. 6, pp. 581-591). New York: Wiley.

ENDNOTE

[1] For brevity, we refer to "provider-delivered e-health" simply as *e-health* and "health-care provider organizations" as *providers* throughout the remainder of the chapter.

Compilation of References

Adler, K.G. (2006). Web portals in primary care: An evaluation of patient readiness and willingness to pay for online services. *Journal of Medical Internet Research, 8*(4), e26.

Adomavicius, G., & Tuzhilin, A. (2005). Personalization technologies: A process-oriented perspective. *Communications of the AMC, 48*(10), 83–90.

Agarwal, R., & Venkatesh, V. (2002). Assessing a firm's Web presence: A heuristic evaluation procedure for the measurement of usability. *Information Systems Research, 13*(2), 168-186.

Agency for Healthcare Research and Quality (AHRQ). (2007). *Improving healthcare quality: A guide for patients and families*. Retrieved May 26, 2008, from http://www.ahrq.gov/consumer/qntlite/

Ahern, D.K. (2007). Challenges and opportunities of eHealth research. *American Journal of Preventive Medicine, 32*(5), 75-82.

AHIC. (2007). *Community meeting: Consumer empowerment workgroup*. Mountain View, CA: American Health Information Community.

AHIMA. (2005). The role of the personal health record in the EHR. *Journal of American Health Information Management Association, 76*(7), 64A-D.

AHIMA. (2006). The value of personal health records. A joint position statement for consumers of healthcare. *Journal of American Health Information Management Association, 77*(9), 22-24.

Ajzen, I. (1985). *From intentions to actions: A theory of planned behavior*. In J. Kuhl, & J. Beckmann (Eds.), *Action-control: From cognition to behavior* (pp. 11–39). Heidelberg: Springer.

Ajzen, I. (2002). Residual effects of past on later behavior: Habituation and reasoned action perspectives. *Personality and Social Psychology Review, 6*(2), 107-122.

Akerkar, S.M., & Bichile, L.S. (2004). Health information on the Internet: Patient empowerment or patient deceit? *Indian Journal of Medical Sciences, 58*(8), 321–326.

Al-Bahrani, A., & Plusa, S.(2004). The quality of patient-orientated Internet information on colorectal cancer. *Colorectal Disease, 6,* 323–326.

Anderson, G.F., Frogner, B.F., Johns, R.A., & Reinhardt, U.E. (2006). Healthcare spending and use of information technology in OECD countries. *Health Affairs, 25,* 819-831.

Andreassen, H. K., Trondsen, M., Kummervold, P. E., Gammon, D., & Hjortdahl, P. (2006). Patients who use e-mediated communication with their doctor: New constructions of trust in the patient-doctor relationship. *Qualitative Health Research, 16*(2), 238-248.

Andreassen, H.K., Bujnowska-Fedak, M.M., Chronaki, C.E., Dumitru, R.C., Pudule, I., Santana, S., Voss, H., & Wynn, R. (2007). European citizens' use of e-health services: A study of seven countries [Electronic version]. *BMC Public Health*. Retrieved May 13, 2008, from http://www.biomedcentral.com/1471-2458/7/53

Anhøj, J., & Nielsen, L. (2004). Quantitative and qualitative usage data of an Internet-based asthma monitoring tool. *Journal of Medical Internet Research, 6*(3), e23. Retrieved May 27, 2008, from http://www.jmir.org/2004/3/e23

Armstrong, N., Hearnshaw, H., Powell, J., & Dale, J. (2007). Stakeholder perspectives on the development of a virtual clinic for diabetes care: Qualitative study. *Journal of Medical Internet Research, 9*(3), e23. Retrieved May 26, 2008, from http://www.jmir.org/20073/e23

Armstrong, N., Powell, J., Hearnshaw, H., & Dale, J. (2007). Design of a trial of internet-based self-management for diabetes. *Journal of Telemedicine and Telecare, 13*(Supplement 1), 1-2.

Arnstein, S.R. (1969). A ladder of citizen participation in the USA. *Journal of the American Institute of Planners, 35*(4), 216-224.

Auerbach, S.M. (2001). Do patients want control over their own healthcare? A review of measures, findings, and research issues. *Journal of Health Psychology, 6*(2), 191–203.

Ba, S., & Pavlou, P.A. (2002). Evidence of the effect of trust building technology in electronic markets: Price premiums and buyer behavior. *MIS Quarterly, 26*(3), 243-268.

Baier, A. (1986). Trust and antitrust. *Ethics, 96*(2), 231-260.

Bailey, P.G. (1998). Best healthcare system in the world: Where healthcare should go in the 21st century. *Vital Speeches of the Day, 64*(8), 245.

Baker, L., Wagner, T. H., Singer, S., & Bundorf, M. K. (2003). Use of the Internet and e-mail for health care information: Results from a national survey. *JAMA, 289*(18), 2400-2406.

Ball, M., Smith, C., & Bakalar, R.S. (2007). Personal health records: Empowering consumers. *Journal of Health Information Management, 21*(1), 76-86.

Ball, M.J., & Lillis, J. (2001). E-health: Transforming the physician/patient relationship. *International Journal of Medical Informatics, 61*(1), 1-10.

Bandura, A. (1982). Self-efficacy mechanism in human agency. *American Psychologist, 37,* 122–147.

Banks, P., & Lawrence, M. (2005). Transparent or opaque? Disabled people in Scotland describe their experience of applying for disability living allowance. *Journal of Social Work, 5,* 299-317.

Barber, B. (1983). *The logic and limits of trust.* New Brunswick, NJ: Rutgers University Press.

Barlow, J.H., Turner, A.P., & Wright, C.C. (2000). A randomized controlled study of the Arthritis Self-management Programme in the UK. *Health Education Research., 15*(6), 665–680.

Barrera, M. Jr., Glasgow, R.E., McKay, H.G., Boles, S.M., & Feil, E.G. (2002). Do Internet-based support interventions change perceptions of social support? An experimental trial of approaches for supporting diabetes self-management. *American Journal of Community Psychology, 30*(5), 637-654.

Barrett, M.J. (2005). *Patient self-management tools: An overview.* Oakland, CA: California HealthCare Foundation.

Basu, S. (2004). Implementing e-commerce tax policy. *British Tax Review, (1),* 46–69.

Bates, D.W., Kuperman, G.J., Wang, S., Gandhi, T., Kittler, A.,Volk, L., Spurr, C., Khorasani, R., Tanasijevic, M., & Middleton, B. (2003). Ten commandments for effective clinical decision support: Making the practice of evidence-based medicine a realty. *Journal of the American Medical Informatics Association, 10*, 523–530.

Baucus, M. (2005). Looking at the U.S. healthcare system in the rear-view mirror. *Health Affairs, 24*, 544-545.

Baxter, L., Thorne, L., & Mitchell, A. (2001). *Small voices, big noises. Lay involvement in health research: Lessons from other fields.* Exeter, UK: Washington Singer Press.

Beauregard, T.R. (2006). *Large employer views of consumer-driven healthcare: Current interest, barriers, and potential solutions.* Manhattan Institute. Retrieved

May 26, 2008, from http://www.manhattan-institute.org/consumerdrivenhealthcare/pdfs/Beauregard.pdf

Beck, R.S., Daughtridge, R., & Sloane, P. (2002). Physician-patient communication in the primary care office: A systematic review. *Journal American Board of Family Practice, 15*, 25-38.

Beckjord, E.B., Finney Rutten, L.J., Squiers, L., Arora, N.K., Volckmann, L., Moser, R. P., & Hesse B.W. (2007). Use of the internet to communicate with healthcare providers in the United States: Estimates from the 2003 and 2005 health information national trends surveys (HINTS). *Journal of Medical Internet Research, 9*(3), e20.

Beckman, H.B., Markakis, K.M., Suchman, A.L., & Frankel, R.M. (1994). The doctor-patient relationship and malpractice. Lessons from plaintiff depositions. *Archives of Internal Medicine, 154*(12), 1365-1370.

Beckman, J.F., Fernandez, C.E., & Coulter, I.D. (1996). A systems model of healthcare: A proposal. *Journal of Manipulative and Physiological Therapeutics, 19*(3), 208-215.

Bem, D.J. (1972). Self-perception theory. In L. Berkowitz (Ed.), *Advances in experimental social psychology* (pp. 1-62). New York: Academic Press.

Benbasat, I., Goldstein, D.K., & Mead, M. (1987). The case research strategy in studies of information systems. *MIS Quarterly, 11*(3), 369–384.

Bender, B., Milgrom, H., & Rand, C. (1997). Nonadherence in asthmatic patients: Is there a solution to the problem? *Annals of Allergy, Asthma and Immunology, 79*(3), 177-186.

Benz, G., & Paddison, N.V. (2004). Developing patient-based marketing strategies. *Healthcare Executive, 19*(5), 40-42.

Bergmo, T.S., Kummervold, P.E., Gammon, D., & Dahl, L.B. (2005). Electronic patient-provider communication: Will it offset office visits and telephone consultations in primary care? *International Journal of Medical Informatics, 74*, 705-710.

Berkowitz, E.N. (2006). *Essentials of healthcare marketing.* Sudbury, MA: Jones & Bartlett.

Berners-lee, T. (2000). *Weaving the Web: The original design and ultimate destiny of the world wide Web (first edition).* New York: HarperCollins Publishers.

Bernhardt, J.M., Lariscy, R.A.W., Parrott, R.L., Silk, K.J., & Felter, E.M. (2002). Perceived barriers to internet-based health communication on human genetics. *Journal of Health Communication, 7*(4), 325-340.

Berry, L.L., Seiders, K., & Wilder, S.S. (2003). Innovations in access to care: A patient-centered approach. *Annals of Internal Medicine, 139*(7), 568-575.

Berwick, D. (2003). *Escape fire: Lessons for the future of healthcare*. New York: Commonwealth Fund.

Bethell, C. (2000). *Patient-centered care measures for the national healthcare quality report (defining patient-centered care).* Retrieved May 26, 2008, from http://www.markle.org/resources/facct/doclibFiles/documentFile_168.pdf

Beyer, H., & Holtzblatt, K. (1998). *Contextual design: Defining customer-centered systems.* San Francisco: Morgan Kaufmann.

Bhattacherjee, A. (2002). Individual trust in online firms: Scale development and initial test. *Journal of Management Information Systems, 19*(1), 211-241.

Bird, J. (2003). "I wish to speak to the despisers of the body." The Internet, physicality, and psychoanalysis. *Journal for the Psychoanalysis of Culture & Society, 8*(1), 121-126.

Blanchard, E., Appelbaum, K., Radnitz, C., Michultka, D., Morrill, B., Kirsch, C., Hillhouse, J., Evans, D.D., Guarnieri, P., Attanasio, V., Andrasik, F., Jaccard, J., & Dentinger, M.P. (1990). Placebo-controlled evaluation of abbreviated progressive muscle relaxation and of relaxation combined with cognitive therapy in the treatment of tension headache. *Journal of Consulting & Clinical Psychology, 58*(2), 210–215.

Blanchard, E., Appelbaum, K., Radnitz, C., Morrill, B., Michultka, D., Kirsch, C., Guarnieri, P., Hillhouse, J.,

Evans, D.D., Jaccard, J., & Barron, K.D. (1990). A controlled evaluation of thermal biofeedback and thermal biofeedback combined with cognitive therapy in the treatment of vascular headache. *Journal Consulting & Clinical Psychology, 58*(2), 216–224.

Bodenheimer, T., Lorig, K., Holman, H., & Grumbach, K. (2002). Patient self-management of chronic disease in primary care. *JAMA, 288*(19).

Boren, M.T., & Ramey, J. (2000). Thinking aloud: Reconciling theory and practice. *IEEE Transactions on Professional Communication, 43*(3), 261–278.

Borgerson, K. (2005). Evidence-based alternative medicine? *Perspectives in Biology and Medicine, 48*(8), 502–515.

Boulos, M.N., Maramba, I., & Wheeler, S. (2006). Wikis, blogs and podcasts: A new generation of Web-based tools for virtual collaborative clinical practice and education. *BMC Medical Education, 6*, 41.

Bowers, M.R., & Kiefe, C.I. (2002). Measuring healthcare quality: Comparing and contrasting the medical and the marketing approaches. *American Journal of Medical Quality, 17*(4), 136-143.

Brailer, D.J. (2004). *The decade of health information technology: Delivering consumer-centric and information-rich healthcare*. National Coordinator for Health Information Technology. Retrieved May 26, 2008, from, from http://www.hhs.gov/healthit/documents/hitframework.pdf

Brailer, D.J. (2005) *Is there a doctor in the mouse?: Using information technology to improve healthcare.* Testimony before the U.S. House of Representatives, Committee on Government Reform, Subcommittee on Federal Workforce and Agency Organization. Retrieved May 14, 2008, from http://www.hhs.gov/healthit/t050727.html

Brailer, D.J. (2005). Interoperability: The key to the future healthcare system. *Health Affairs, Web Exclusive, W5-19-W5-21.*

Brewer, M.B., & Silver, M. (1978). Ingroup bias a function of task characteristics. *European Journal of Social Psychology, 8*(3), 393-400.

Brooks, R.G., M.D. (2006). Physicians' use of e-mail with patients: Factors influencing electronic communication and adherence to best practices. *Journal of Medical Internet Research, 8*(1), e2.

Brug, J., Campbell, M., & van Assema, P. (1999). The application and impact of computer-generated personalized nutrition education: A review of the literature. *Patient Education and Counseling, 36*(2), 145-156.

Bulger, D.W., & Reeves, C. (2000). Interactive Internet Web sites: A potentially powerful tool for disease management. *Disease Management & Health Outcomes, 7*(2), 67-75.

Burkhauser, R.V., & Houtenville, A.J. (2006). A guide to disability statistics from the current population survey. *Annual Social and Economic Supplement (March CPS).* Rehabilitation Research and Training Center on Disability Demographics and Statistics, Cornell University, Ithaca, NY. Retrieved May 21, 2008, from http://digitalcommons.ilr.cornell.edu/edicollect/1233/

Bush, G.W. (2004). *Executive order: Incentives for the use of health information technology and establishing the position of the national health information technology coordinator.* Washington D.C.: The White House.

Buston, K.M., & Wood, S.F. (2000). Non-compliance amongst adolescents with asthma: Listening to what they tell us about self-management. *Family Practice, 17*(2), 134-138.

Butler, C., Rollnick, S., & Stott, N. (1996). The practitioner, the patient and resistance to change: Recent ideas on compliance. *Canadian Medical Association Journal, 154*(9), 1357-1362.

Caceres, C., Gomez, E.J., Garcia, F., Gatell, J.M., & del Pozo, F. (2006). An integral care telemedicine system for HIV/AIDS patients. *International Journal of Medical Informatics, 75*(9), 638-642.

Callon, M. (1986). Some elements of a sociology of translation: Domestication of the scallops and the fishermen of St. Brieuc Bay. In J. Law (Ed.), *Power, Action and Belief: A New Sociology of Knowledge?* (pp. 196-223). London, England: Routledge.

Callon, M. (1991). Techno-economic networks and irreversibility. In J. Law (Ed.), *A Sociology of Monsters: Essays on Power, Technology and Domination* (pp. 132-161). London, England: Routledge.

Calongne, C.M. (2001). Designing for Web site usability. *Journal of Computing in Small Colleges, 16*(3), 39-45.

Cameron, L.D., & Nicholls, G. (1998). Expression of stressful experiences through writing: Effects of a self-regulation manipulation for pessimists and optimists. *Health Psychology, 17*(1), 84-92.

Campbell, R.S., & Pennebaker, J.W. (2003). The secret life of pronouns: Flexibility in writing style and physical health. *Psychological Science, 14*(1), 60-65.

Campion, P.D., Butler, N.M., & Cox, A.D. (1992). Principle agendas of doctors and patients in general practice consultations. *Family Practice, 9*(2), 181-190.

Cantor, C., & Fallon, B. (1997). *Phantom illness: Recognizing, understanding, and overcoming hypochondria.* Boston, MA: Houghton Mifflin.

Carrard, I., Rouget, P., Fernández-Aranda, F., Volkart, A.-C., Damoiseau, M., & Lam, T. (2006). Evaluation and deployment of evidence based patient self-management support program for bulimia nervosa. *International Journal of Medical Informatics*, *75*(1), 101-109.

Carrigan, M. (1993). The future of healthcare information systems. *Hospital Material Management Quarterly, 15*(1), 1-13.

Carroll, C., Marsden, P., Soden, P., Naylor, E., New, J., & Dornan, T. (2002). Involving users in the design and usability evaluation of a clinical decision support system. *Computer Methods and Programs in Biomedicine, 69*(2), 123-135.

Cech, C.G., & Condon, S.L. (1998). Message size constraints on discourse planning in synchronous computer-mediated communication. *Behavior Research Methods, Instruments, & Computers, 30*(2), 255-263.

Center of Disease Control (CDC). (2005). Annual rate of visits per person to physician offices, by patient age group—United States, 2003. *Center for Disease Control QuickStats, 54*(48), 1238. Retrieved May 27, 2008, from http://www.cdc.gov/mmwr/preview/mmwrhtml/mm5448a9.htm

Center of Disease Control (CDC). (2007). Costs of chronic disease. *Center for Disease Control Chronic Disease Overview.* Retrieved May 27, 2008, from http://www.cdc.gov/nccdphp/overview.htm#2

Charles, C., Gafni, A., & Whelan, T. (1997). Shared decision-making in the medical encounter: What does it mean? (Or it takes at least two to tango). *Social Science & Medicine, 44*(5), 681–692.

Cheng, S.-H., Wei, Y.-J., & Chang, H.-J. (2006). Quality competition among hospitals: The effects of perceived quality and perceived expensiveness on healthcare patients. *American Journal of Medical Quality, 21* (1), 68-75.

Cherry, C., & Anderson, S. (2002). *Refreshing the national listening exercise: Report of the findings.* London, UK: National Co-ordinating Centre for NHS Service Delivery and Organisation.

Cheung, C.M.K., & Lee, M.K.O. (2001). Trust in Internet shopping: Instrument development and validation through classical and modern approaches. *Journal of Global Information Management, 9*(3), 23-35.

Cheung, C.M.K., & Limayem, M. (2005). The role of habit in information systems continuance: Examining the evolving relationship between intention and usage. In D. Avison, D. Galletta, & J. DeGross (Eds.), *Proceedings of the 26th International Conference on Information Systems* (pp. 471-482). Las Vegas, NV, USA, University of Minnesota.

Chin, J. P., Diehl, V. A., & Norman, L. K. (1988). *Development of an instrument measuring user satisfaction of the human-computer interface*. New York: ACM Press

Chin, W. (1998). The partial least squares approach to structural equation modeling. In G.A. Marcoulides (Ed.), *Modern Methods for Business Research* (pp. 295-336). Mahwah, NJ: Lawrence Erlbaum Associates.

Chodosh, J., Morton, S.C., Mojica, W., Maglione, M., Suttorp, M.J., Hilton, L., Rhodes, S., & Shekelle, P. (2005). Meta-analysis: Chronic disease self-management programs for older adults. *Annals of Internal Medicine, 143*(6), 427–438.

Choy, A., Hudson, Z., Pritts, J., & Goldman, J. (2001). Exposed online: Why the new federal health privacy regulation doesn't offer much protection to Internet users. *Pew Internet & American Life Project*. Retrieved May 24, 2008, from http://www.pewInternet.org/pdfs/PIP_HPP_HealthPriv_report.pdf

Christensen, H., Griffiths, K.M., & Jorm, A.F. (2004). Delivering interventions for depression using the internet: Randomised controlled trial. *British Medical Journal, 328*, 265.

Christiansen, J.R. (1999). Health information technology and privacy: The legal perspective. *MDComputing: Computers in Medical Practice, 16*(4), 15-16.

Clark, R., Williams, J., Clark, J., & Clark, C. (2002). Assessing Web site usability: Construction zone. *Journal of Healthcare Information Management, 17*(2), 51-55.

Clayton, A., Oakley, P., & Pratt, B. (1997). *Empowering people: A guide to participation*. Oxford, UK: INTRAC.

Coble, J.M., Karat, J., Orland, M., & Kahn, M. (1997). Iterative usability testing: Ensuring a usable clinical workstation. In *Proceedings of AMIA Annual Symposiu* (pp. 744–748).

Coburn, D., Rappolt, S., & Bourgeault, I. (1997). Decline vs. retention of medical power through restratification: An examination of the Ontario case. *Sociology of Health and Illness, 19*(1), 1–22.

Cohn, J. (2007). *Sick: The untold story of America's healthcare crisis---and the people who pay the price*. NY: Harper Collins.

Cohn, S.P. (2006, February). *Personal health records and personal health record systems*. Chairman National Committee on Vital and Health Statistics. Retrieved May 26, 2008, from, from http://www.ncvhs.hhs.gov/0602nhiirpt.pdf

Conhaim, W.W., & Page, L. (2003). Is the doctor online? *Information Today, 20*(2), 29-31.

Conn, J. (2006). Personal and (maybe) confidential. *Modern Healthcare, 36*, 28-31.

Connecting for Health. (2003). *The personal health working group final report*. Markle Foundation. Retrieved May 14, 2008, from http://www.markle.org/downloadable_assets/final_phwg_report1.pdf

Connecting for Health. (2004). *Connecting Americans to their healthcare: Final report*. Markle Foundation. Retrieved May 14, 2008, from http://www.connectingforhealth.org/resources/wg_eis_final_report_0704.pdf

Coulter, A. (1997). Partnerships with patients: the pros and cons of shared clinical decision-making. *Journal of Health Services Research & Policy, 2*(2), 112-121.

Coulter, A. (2002). *The autonomous patient: Ending paternalism in medical care*. London, UK: The Stationery Office.

Coulter, A. (2005). What do patients and the public want from primary care? *British Medical Journal, 331*(7526), 1199-1201.

Culnan, M.J., & Armstrong, P.K. (1999). Information privacy, Procedural fairness and impersonal trust: An empirical investigation. *Organization Science, 10*(1), 104–115.

Culver, C., Moor, J., Duerfeldt, W., Kapp, M., & Sullivan, M. (1994). Privacy. *Professional Ethics 3*(3-4), 3-25.

Cummings, E., & Turner, P. (2007). Considerations for deploying Web and mobile technologies to support the building of patient self-efficacy and self-management of chronic illness. In L. Al-Hakim (Ed.), *Web Mobile-Based Applications for Healthcare Management* (pp. 258–273). Hershey, PA: Idea Group, Inc.

Currall, S.C., & Judge, T.A. (1995). Measuring trust between organizational boundary role persons. *Orga-*

nizational Behavior and Human Decision Processes, 64(2), 151-170.

Currie, W.L., & Guah, M.W. (2006). IT-enabled healthcare delivery: The U.K. National Health Service. *Information Management, 23*(2), 7-22.

Curtis, A. (2000). *Through the WEB and what Alice found there: The impact of the Internet on the therapeutic alliance.* Paper presented at the 35th Annual Australian Psychological Society Conference, Canberra.

Daft, R.L., & Lengel, R.H. (1986). Organizational information requirements, media richness and structural design. *Management Science, 32*(5), 554-571.

Danis, C., & Boies, S. (2000). Using a technique from graphic designers to develop innovative system design. In *Proceedings of DIS 2000* (pp. 20–26).

Davis, F.D. (1989). Perceived usefulness, perceived ease of use, and user acceptance of information technology. *MIS Quarterly, 13*(3), 319–329.

Davis, F.D., Bagozzi, R.P., & Warshaw, P.R. (1989). User acceptance of computer technology: A comparison of two theoretical models. *Management Science, 35,* 982-1002.

Davis, F.D., Bagozzi, R.P., & Warshaw, P.R. (1992). Extrinsic and intrinsic motivation to use computers in the workplace. *Journal of Applied Social Psychology, 22,* 1111-1132.

Davis, K., Collins, K.S., Schoen, C., & Morris, C. (1995). Choice matters: Enrollees' views of their health plans. *Health Affairs, 14*(2), 99-112.

Davis, K., Schoenbaum, S.C., & Audet, A. (2005). A 2020 vision of patient-centered care. *Journal of General Internal Medicine, 20,* 953-957.

Davison, K.P., Pennebaker, J.W., & Dickerson, S.S. (2000). Who talks? The social psychology of illness support groups. *American Psychologist, 55*(2), 205-217.

DeCew, J.W. (1997). *In pursuit privacy: Law, ethics, and the rise of technology.* Ithica, NY: Cornell University Press.

Deci, E.L., & Ryan, R.M. (1985). *Intrinsic motivation and self-determination in human behavior.* New York: Plenum.

DeNavas-Walt, C., Proctor, B.D., & Lee, C.H. (2006). U.S. census bureau, current population reports, P60-231, *Income, poverty, and health insurance coverage in the United States: 2005.* Washington D.C.: U.S. Government Printing Office.

Dennis, A.R., & Valacich, J.S. (1999). *Rethinking media richness: Towards a theory of media synchronicity.* Paper presented at the 32nd Hawaii International Conference on System Sciences, Hawaii.

Denny, J.T., Ginsberg, S., Papp, D., Browne, G., Morgan, S., Kushins, L., & Solina, A. (2002). Hospital initiatives in promoting smoking cessation: A survey of Internet and hospital-based programs target at consumers. *Chest, 122,* 692–698.

Denny, K. (1999). Evidence-based medicine and medical authority. *Journal of Medical Humanities, 20*(4), 247–263.

Denton, I.C. (2001). Will patients use electronic personal health records? Responses from a real-life experience. *Journal of Healthcare Information Management, 15*(3), 251-259.

Deutsch, M. (1958). Trust and suspicion. *Journal of Conflict Resolution, 2*(4), 265-279.

Devaraj, S., & Kohli, R. (2003). Performance impacts of information technology: Is actual usage the missing link? *Management Science, 49*(3), 273-289.

DeVol, R., Bedroussian, A., Charuworn, A., Chatterjee, A., Kim, I.K., Kim, S., et al. (2007). *An unhealthy America: The economic burden of chronic disease—charting a new course to save lives and increase productivity and economic growth.* Milken Institute. Retrieved May 28, 2008, from http://www.milkeninstitute.org/publications/publications.taf

Dishaw, M.T., & Strong, D.M. (1999). Extending the technology acceptance model with task-technology fit constructs. *Information & Management, 36,* 9-21.

Dixon, P. (2007). *World privacy forum comments about the ethical, legal, and social implications of using genetic healthcare data in electronic health records.* U.S. Department of Health and Human Services (Ed.). Washington, D.C.: World Privacy Forum.

Doney, P.M., & Cannon, J.P. (1997). An examination of the nature of trust in buyer-seller relationships. *Journal of Marketing, 61*(2), 35-51.

Dumas, J.S., & Redish J.C. (1999) *A practical guide to usability testing.* Portland, OR: Intellect Books.

Durkan, P., Durkin, M., & Gillen, J., (2003). Exploring efforts to engender on-line trust, *Entrepreneurial Behaviour and Research, 9*(3), 93–110.

Dutta-Bergman, M. (2003). Trusted online sources of health information: Differences in demographics, health beliefs, and health-information orientation. *Journal of Medical Internet Research, 5*(3), e21. Retrieved May 27, 2008, from http://www.jmir.org/2003/3/e21/

Edlin, M. (2002). Embracing e-health simplifies transactions, improves patient relations. *Managed Healthcare Executive, 12*(8), 30–32.

Eng, T.R. (2001). *The eHealth landscape: A terrain map of emerging information and communication technologies in health and healthcare.* Princeton, NJ: The Robert Wood Johnson Foundation.

Epping-Jordan, J., Bengoa, R., Kawar, R., & Sabate, E. (2001). The challenge of chronic conditions: Who responds. *British Medical Journal, 323*(7319), 947–948.

Ericsson, K.A., & Simon, H.A. (1984). *Protocol analysis: Verbal reports as data.* Cambridge, MA: The MIT Press.

Ericsson, K.A., & Simon, H.A. (1984). *Protocol analysis: Verbal reports as data.* Cambridge, MA: MIT Press.

Esquivel, A., Meric-Bernstam, F., & Bernstam, E.V. (2006). Accuracy and self correction of information received from an internet breast cancer list: Content analysis. *British Medical Journal, 332*(7547), 939-942.

Etter, J.F. (2006). Internet-based smoking cessation programs. *International Journal of Medical Informatics, 75*(1), 110-116.

Eudes, J.A. (2006). Gateway to the Web. *Marketing Health Services, 25*(4), 38-39.

Ewing, T., & Cusick, D. (2004). Knowing what to measure. *Healthcare Financial Management, 58*(6), 60-63.

Eysenbach, G. (2000). Recent advances: Consumer health informatics. *British Medical Journal, 320*(7251), 1713–1716.

Eysenbach, G., & Kohler, C. (2002) How do consumers search for and appraise health information on the world wide Web? Qualitative study using focus groups, usability tests, and in-depth interviews. *BMJ, 324,* 573–577.

Eysenbach, G., & Kohler, C. (2002). How do consumers search for and appraise health information on the world wide Web? Qualitative study using focus groups, usability tests, and in-depth interviews. *British Medical Journal, 324*(7337), 573-577.

Eysenbach, G., & Kohler, C. (2003). What is the prevalence of health-related searches on the world wide web? Qualitative and quantitative analysis of search engine queries on the internet. *2003 AMIA Annual Symposium Proceedings,* 225-229.

Faulkner, A. (2005). *Service user involvement in the UK Mental Health Research Network. Guidance for good practice.* London, UK: UK Mental Health Research Network Service User Research Group England (SURGE).

Federal Trade Commission (FTC). (1973). *The code of fair information practices.* U.S. Department of Health, Education and Welfare, Secretary's Advisory Committee on Automated Personal Data Systems, Records, Computers, and the Rights of Citizens, viii. Retrieved May 24, 2008, from http://www.epic.org/privacy/consumer

Federal Trade Commission. (1998). *Privacy online: A report to congress.* Federal Trade Commission. Retrieved May 24, 2008, from http//www.ftc.gov/reports/privacy3/

Federal Trade Commission. (2000). *Privacy online: Fair information practices in the electronic marketplace.* A report to congress. Federal Trade Commission. Retrieved May 24, 2008, from http://www.ftc.gov/reports/privacy2000/privacy2000.pdf

Ferrin, D.L., Dirks, K.T., & Shah, P.P. (2006). Direct and indirect effects of third-party relationships on interpersonal trust. *Journal of Applied Psychology, 91*(4), 870-883.

Ferriter, M. (1993). Computer aided interviewing and the psychiatric social history. *Social Work and Social Sciences Review, 4*, 255-263.

Fishbein, M., & Ajzen, I (1975). *Belief, attitude, intention and behavior: An introduction to theory and research.* Reading, MA: Addison-Wesley.

Fiske, S.T., & Taylor, S.E. (1991). *Social cognition (second edition).* New York: McGraw-Hill, Inc.

Fogg, B.J. (2002). *Persuasive technology: Using computers to change what we think and do.* San Francisco, CA: Morgan Kaufmann.

Fogg, B.J. (2003). *Persuasive technology: Using computers to change what we think and do.* San Francisco: Morgan Kaufmann Publishers.

Ford, C.A., Bearman, P.S., & Moody, J. (1999). Foregone healthcare among adolescents. *Journal of the American Medical Association, 282*, 2227-2234.

Ford, J.D., Trestman, R.L., Steinberg, K., Tennen, H., & Allen, S. (2004). Prospective association of anxiety, depressive, and addictive disorders with high utilization of primary, specialty and emergency medical care. *Social Science & Medicine, 58*(11), 2145-2148.

Fornell, C.R., & Larcker, D.F. (1981). Structural equation models with unobservable variables and measurement error: Algebra and statistics. *Journal of Marketing Research, 18*(3), 382-388.

Forrest, C.B., & Starfield, B. (1998). Entry into primary care and continuity: The effects of access. *American Journal of Public Health, 8*(9), 1330-1337.

Foucault, M. (1982). *Technologies of the self.* Retrieved May 13, 2008, from http://scholar.google.com/scholar?hl=en&lr=&q=cache:ZaTVbZuQ6xEJ:www.sp.uconn.edu/~en109vc/Old/S2002/Technologies.pdf+Foucault+Birth+of+the+clinic

Fowles, J.B., Kind, A.C., Craft, C., Kind, E.A., Mandel, J.L., & Adlis, S. (2004). Patients' interest in reading their medical record: Relation with clinical and sociodemographic characteristics and patients' approach to healthcare. *Archives of Internal Medicine, 164*(7), 793-800.

Fox, S. (2005). Health information online. Eight in ten Internet users have looked for health information online, with increased interest in diet, fitness, drug, health insurance, experimental treatments, and particular doctors and hospitals. *Pew Internet and American Life Project.* Retrieved May 27, 2008, from http://www.pewInternet.org/pdfs/PIP_Healthtopics_May05.pdf

Fox, S. (2006). Online health search 2006. Most Internet users start at a search engine when looking for health information online. Very few check the source and date of the information they find. *Pew Internet & American Life Project.* Retrieved May 27, 2008, from http://www.pewInternet.org/pdfs/PIP_Online_Health_2006.pdf

Fox, S. (2006). *Can the health informatician help seniors cross the digital divide?* Paper presented at the meeting of the American Medical Informatics Association, Washington, D.C.

Fox, S. (2007). MyHealth, circa 2007. *Pew Internet & American Life Project Presentation.* Retrieved May 22, 2008, from http://www.pewinternet.org/PPF/r/87/presentation_display.asp

Fox, S., & Fallows, D. (2003). Internet health resources. *Pew Internet & American Life Project.* Retrieved May 24, 2008, from

Fox, S., & Rainie, L. (2000) The online healthcare revolution: How the Web helps Americans take better care of themselves. *Pew Internet & American Life Project.* Retrieved May 24, 2008, from http://www.pewInternet.org/reports/toc.asp?Report=26

Fox, S., Rainie, L., Horrigan, J., Lenhart, A., Spooner, T., & Carter, C. (2000). Trust and privacy online: Why Americans want to rewrite the rules. *Pew Internet & American Life Project*. Retrieved May 24, 2008, from http://www.pewInternet.org/reports/toc.asp?Report=19

Frankford, D. (1994). Scientism and economics in the regulation of healthcare. *Journal of Health Politics, Policy & Law, 19*(4), 773–799.

Fried, C. (1970). Privacy: A rational context. Chap. IX in anatomy of values. New York: Cambridge University Press. (Reprinted from *Computers, Ethics, and* Society, pp. 51-63, M.D. Ermann, M.B. Williams, & C. Gutierrez, Eds., 1990, New York: Oxford University Press.

Fried, C. (1984). Privacy. In F.D. Schoeman (Ed.), *Philosophical dimensions of privacy: An anthology* (pp. 203-222). New York: Cambridge University Press.

Friedman, C. P., & Wyatt, J. (2006). *Evaluation methods in medical informatics* (

Fries, J., Friday, G., Gira, C., Cooper, P., England, M., Graves, R., Sokolov, J.J., & Wright, D. (1993). Reducing healthcare costs by reducing the need and demand for medical services. *New England Journal of Medicine, 329*, 5–9.

Fruhling, A., & Lee, S. (2006). The influence of user interface usability on rural consumers' trust of e-health services. *International Journal of Electronic Healthcare, 2*(4), 305–321.

Fruhling, A.L. (2003). *An empirical study of human-computer interaction: Usability factors affecting perceptions of trust of e-health consumers.* Doctoral Dissertation, University of Nebraska, 2003. Proquest, AAT3092541.

Fulda, J. (1997). From data to knowledge: Implications of data mining. *Computers of Society, 27*(4), 28.

Fung, R., & Lee, M. (1999). EC-trust (trust in electronic commerce): Exploring the antecedent factors. In W. Haseman & D. Nazareth (Eds.), *Proceedings of the Americas Conference on Information Systems* (pp. 517-519). Charlotte, NC: Association for Information Systems.

Funnell, M., Anderson, R., Arnold, M., Barr, P., Donnelly, M., Johnson, P., Taylor-Moon, D. & White, N.H. (1991). Empowerment an idea whose time has come in diabetes education. *The Diabetes Educator, 17*(1), 37–41.

Gallant, L., Irizarry, C., & Kreps, G.L. (2007). User centric hospital Web sites: A case for trust and personalization. *e-Service Journal, 5*(2), 5–26.

Gammon, D., & Rosenvinge, J. (2000). Can Internet aid persons with serious mental disorders? *Journal of the Norwegian Medical Association, 120*, 1890-1892.

Ganesan, S. (1994). Determinants of long-term orientation in buyer-seller relationships. *Journal of Marketing 58*(2), 1-19.

Garets, D., & Davis, M. (2006). Electronic medical records vs. electronic health records: Yes, there is a difference. *HIMSS Analytics.* Retrieved May 14, 2008, from http://www.himssanalytics.org/docs/WP_EMR_EHR.pdf

Garfinkel, H. (1963). A conception of, and experiments with, "trust" as a condition of stable concerted actions. In O.J. Harvey (Ed.), *Motivation and social interaction: Cognitive determinants* (pp. 187-238). New York: The Ronald Press Company.

Gefen D., & Straub, D.W. (2000). The Relative importance of perceived ease-of-use in IS adoption: A study of E-commerce adoption. *Journal of the Association for Information Systems, 1*(8), 1–30.

Gefen, D., & Straub, D.W. (2005). A practical guide to factorial validity using PLS-Graph: Tutorial and annotated example. *Communications of the Association for Information Systems, 16*, Article 24, 91-109.

Gefen, D., Karahanna, E., & Straub, D.W. (2003). Trust and TAM in online shopping: An integrated model. *MIS Quarterly, 27*(1), 51-91.

Gefen, D., Straub, D.W. (2004). Consumer trust in B2C e-commerce and the importance

Gerber, B.S., & Eiser, A.R. (2001). The patient physician relationship in the Internet age: Future prospects and the research agenda. *Journal of Medical Internet Research, 3*(2), E15.

Gibson, P.G., Powell, H., Coughlan, J., Wilson, A.J., Abramson, M., Haywood, P., Bauman, A., Hensley, M.J., & Walters, E.H. (2002). Self-management education and regular practitioner review for adults with asthma. *Cochrane Database of Systematic Reviews, Issue 3*, Art. No. CD001117. DOI: 10.1002/14651858.CD001117.

Global Initiative for Asthma (GINA). (2005). *Global strategy for asthma management and prevention.* NIH Publication No. 02-3659. Global Initiative for Asthma (GINA) workshop report. Retrieved May 27, 2008, from http://www.ginasthma.org

Goedert, J. (2005, July 1). Kaiser readies new Web portal tools. Health Data Management. Retrieved May 26, 2008, from http://www.healthdatamanagement.com/

Goffman, E. (1959). *The presentation of self in everyday life*. Garden City, NY: Anchor Books.

Goldberg, M.C. (1995). If we're lucky, the patient will complain. *American Journal of Nursing, 95*(2), 52-53.

Gotlieb, C.C. (1995). Privacy: A concept whose time has come and gone. In D. Lyon & E. Zureik (Eds.), *Surveillance, Computers and Privacy* (pp. 156-171). Minneapolis: University of Minnesota Press.

Grady, P.A. (2005). *Fiscal year 2006 budget request.* Witness appearing before the House Subcommittee on Labor-HHS-Education Appropriations. Retrieved May 26, 2008, from http://www.ninr.nih.gov/NR/rdonlyres/BF2F5680-88F0-4CBF-B86D-E12AE6101246/0/FY-2006BudgetRequest.pdf

Gray, J.A.M. (2002). *The resourceful patient.* Oxford, UK: eRosetta Press.

Greenberg, J. (2006, July 18). *Will consumer driven healthcare put the brakes on rising costs?* New Hampshire Public Radio. Retrieved May 26, 2008, from http://www.nhpr.org/node/11210

Greenberg, L., D'Andrea, G., & Lorence, D.P. (2004). Setting the public agenda for online health search: A white paper and action agenda. *Journal of Medical Internet Research, 6*(2), 1-10.

Greenberg, M.A., Wortman, C.B., & Stone, A.A. (1996). Emotional expression and physical health: Revising traumatic memories or fostering self-regulation? *Journal of Personality and Social Psychology, 71*(3), 588-602.

Greene, B., & Blanchard, E. (1994). Cognitive therapy for irritable bowel syndrome. *Journal of Consulting & Clinical Psychology, 62*(3), 576–582.

Greist, J.H., Klein, M.H., & VanCura, L. (1973). A computer interview by psychiatric patient target symptoms. *Archives of General Psychiatry, 29*, 247-253.

Griffin, S.J., Kinmonth, A.-L., Veltman, M.W.M., Gillard, S., Grant, J., & Stewart, M. (2004). Effect on health-related outcomes of interventions to alter the interaction between patients and practitioners: A systematic review of trials. *Annals of Family Medicine, 2*(6), 595-608.

Griffiths, K.M., Christensen, H., Jorm, A.F., Evans, K., & Groves, C. (2004). Effect of Web-based depression literacy and cognitive-behavioral therapy interventions on stigmatising attitudes to depression. *British Journal of Psychiatry, 185*, 342-349.

Gronroos, C.A. (1984). A service quality model and its marketing implications. *Europe Journal of Marketing, 18*, 36-44.

Gruman, J., & Von Korff, M. (1996). *Indexed bibliography on self-management for people with chronic disease.* Washington D.C.: Centre for Advancement in Health.

Guastella, A.J., & Dadds, M.R. (2006). Cognitive-behavioral models of emotional writing: A validation study. *Cognitive Therapy and Research, 30*, 397-414.

Gurbaxani, V., & Whang, S. (1991). The impact of information systems on organizations and markets. *Communications of the Association for Computing Machinery, 34*(1), 59-73.

Hadley, J. (2007). Insurance coverage, medical care use, and short-term health changes following an unintentional injury or the onset of a chronic condition. *Journal of the American Medical Association (JAMA), 297*, 1073-1084.

Haire, T. (2007). Search marketing comes into its own. *Response Magazine, 15*(7), 48-52.

Halamka, J., Aranow, M., Ascenzo, C., Bates, D., Debor, G., Glaser, J., Goroll, A., Stowe, J., Tripathi, M., & Vineyard, G. (2005). Healthcare IT collaboration in Massachusetts: The experience of regional connectivity. *Journal of American Medical International Association (JAMIA), 12,* 596-601.

Hammond, W.E. (2005). The making and adoption of health data standards. *Health Affairs, 24*(5), 1205-1213.

Hanley, B., Bradburn, J., Barnes, M., Evans, C., Goodare, H., Kelson, M., Kent, A., Oliver, S., Thomas, S. & Wallcraft, J. (2004). *Involving the public in NHS, public health, and social care research: Briefing notes for researchers (second edition).* Hampshire, UK: INVOLVE.

Hanson, K.W., Neuman, P., Dutwin, D., & Kasper, J.D. (2003). Uncovering the health challenges facing people with disabilities: The role of health insurance. *Health Affairs, Web Exclusive, W3-552-565.*

Haraway, D.J. (1991). *Simians, cyborgs, and women: The reinvention of nature*. London, England: Free Association Books.

Hardey, M. (2001). E-health: The Internet and transformation of patients into consumers and producers of health knowledge. *Information, Communication and Society, 4*(3), 388-405.

Harkness, J. (2005). *What is patient-centred healthcare? A review of definitions and principles.* London: International Alliance of Patients' Organisations.

Harris, K.D., Donaldson, J.F., & Campbell, J.D. (2001). Introducing computer-based telemedicine in three rural Missouri counties. *Journal of End User Computing, 13*(4), 26-35.

Hartman, M.J. (2006). Personal health records and electronic health records: Navigating the intersections. *Health Policy Newsletter, 19*, 1.

Hartwick, J., & Barki, H. (1994). Explaining the role of user participation in information system use. *Management Science, 40*(4), 440-465.

Hassol, A., Walker, J. M., Kidder, D., Rokita, K., Young, D., Pierdon, S., Deitz, D., Kuck, S., & Ortiz, E. (2004). Patient experiences and attitudes about access to a patient electronic healthcare record and linked Web messaging. *Journal of the American Medical Informatics Association, 11*(6), 505-513.

Havenstein, H. (2007). Aetna clients to get access to online health data. *Computerworld.* Retrieved May 14, 2008, from http://www.computerworld.com/action/article.do?command=viewArticleBasicandarticleId=278859

Hawkins, R., Pingree, S., Shaw, B., Gustafson, D., Gatzke, K., McDowell, H., & Tryon-Petith, C. (2006) *Creating a dynamic, tailored, online health education and support program for women with breast cancer: A case study of the CHESS program.* Paper Presented at the Annual Meeting of the International Communication Association, Sheraton, New York. Retrieved May 27, 2008, from http://www.allacademic.com/meta/p14986_index.html

Häyry, M., & Takala, T. (2001). Genetic information, rights, and autonomy. *Theoretical Medicine 22*, 403-414.

Health and Human Services (HHS). (2007). *Value-driven healthcare—transparency: Better care lower cost.* Retrieved May 26, 2008, from http://www.hhs.gov/transparency/

Health Level Seven. (2007). *HL7's EHR technical committee opens public comment on personal health record system (PHR-S) functional model.* Retrieved May 14, 2008, from http://www.hl7.org/documentcenter/public/pressreleases/HL7_PRESS_20070827.pdf

Healy, D. (2006). The latest mania: Selling bipolar disorder. *PLoS Medicine, 3*(4), e185.

Henwood, F., Wyatt, S., Hart, A., & Smith, J. (2003). Ignorance is bliss sometimes: Constraints on the emergence of the 'informed patient' in the changing landscapes of health information. *Sociology of Health and Illness, 25*(6), 589-607.

Herxheimer, A., & Goodare, H. (1999). Who are you, and who are we? Looking through some key words. *Health Expectations, 2*(1), 3-6.

Hesse, B.W., & Shneiderman, B. (2007). eHealth research from a user's perspective. *American Journal of Preventative Medicine, 32*(5s), 97–103.

Hesse, B.W., Nelson, D.E., Kreps, G.L., Croyle, R.T., Arora, N.K., & Rimer, B.K. (2005) Trust and sources of health information. The impact of the Internet and its implications for healthcare providers: Findings from the first health information national trends survey. *Archives of Internal Medicine, 165*, 1–7.

Heubusch, K. (2007). Piecing together the PHR. *Journal of American Health Information Management Association, 78*(4), 28-32.

Hill, S. (1998). *Using the evidence: Empowering consumers of healthcare*. Menzies Foundation. Retrieved May 28, 2008, from http://www.menziesfoundation.org.au/conferences/ebm/ebm09hill.htm

Hines, L. (2007). Healthcare targets paper trail. *Press Enterprise*. Retrieved May 14, 2008, from http://www.pe.com/localnews/inland/stories/PE_News_Local_D_medicalrecords31.27afdf2.html

HIPAA. (1996). *Health insurance portability and accountability act of 1996 (public law 104-191)*. Retrieved May 14, 2008, from http://aspe.hhs.gov/admnsimp/pl104191.htm

HIPAA. (1996). *Public law no. 104-191, section 1173, U.S.C. 201 C.F.R.* Health Insurance Portability and Accountability Act.

Hofstede, G. (1980). Motivation, leadership, and organization: Do American theories apply abroad? *Organizational Dynamics, 9*(1), 42-63.

Holman, H., & Lorig, K. (2000). Patients as partners in managing chronic disease. *British Medical Journal, 320*(7234), 526–527.

Hom, J. (1996). *The usability methods toolbox*. from http://jthom.best.vwh.net/usability

Hong, W., Thong, J.Y.L., Wong, W.M., & Tam, K.Y. (2001). Determinants of user acceptance of digital libraries: An empirical examination of individual differences and system characteristics. *Journal of Management Information Systems, 18*(3), 97-124.

Horton, R.P., Buck, T., Waterson, P.E., & Clegg, C.W. (2001). Explaining Intranet use with the technology acceptance model. *Journal of Information Technology, 16*, 237-249.

Houston, T.K., Sands, D.Z., Jenckes, M.W., & Ford, D.E. (2004). Experiences of patients who were early adopters of electronic communication with their physician: Satisfaction, benefits, and concerns. *The American Journal of Managed Care, 10*(9), 601-608.

Houtenville, A.J., Erickson, W.A., & Lee, C.G. (2005). *Disability statistics from the current population survey (CPS)*. Cornell University Rehabilitation Research and Training Center on Disability Demographics and Statistics, Ithaca, NY (StatsRRTC). Retrieved May 21, 2008, from www.disabilitystatistics.org

Howley, K. (2006, April). "I can't afford to get sick"—Think your insurance has you covered? Just wait till you need it most. *Reader's Digest*. Retrieved May 26, 2008, from http://www.rd.com/content/the-cost-of-health-care-in-america/

Hsiao, R.L. (2003). Technology fears: Distrust and cultural persistence in electronic marketplace adoption. *Journal of Strategic Information Systems, 12*(3), 169–199.

Hsu, J., Huang, J., Kinsman, J., -Fireman, B., Miller, R., Selby, J., & Ortiz, E. (2005). Use of e-health services between 1999 and 2002: A growing digital divide. *Journal of the American Medical Informatics Association, 12*, 164-171.

Hsu, J., Schmittdiel, J., Krupat, E., Stein, T., Thom, D., Fireman, B., & Selby, J. (2003). Patient choice. A randomized controlled trial of provider selection. *Journal of General Internal Medicine, 18*(5), 319-325.

Hwang, K.O., Farheen, K., Johnson, C.W., Thomas, E.J., Barnes, A.S., & Bernstam, E.V. (2007). Quality of weight loss advice on internet forums. *The American Journal of Medicine, 120*(7), 604-609.

Igbaria, M., Guimaraes, T., & Davis, G.B. (1995). Testing the determinants of microcomputer usage via a structural equation model. *Journal of Management Information Systems, 11*(4), 87-114.

Inguanzo, J.M. (1992). Taking a serious look at patient expectations. *Hospitals, 66*(17), 68.

Institute of Medicine (IOM). (1991). In R.S. Dick & E.B. Steen (Eds.), *The computer-based patient record: An essential technology for healthcare*. Washington D.C.: National Academy Press.

Institute of Medicine. (2000). *To err is human: Building a safer health system*. In L.T. Kohn, J.M. Corrigan, & M.S. Donaldson (Eds.). Washington D.C.: National Academy Press.

Institute of Medicine. (2001). Crossing the quality chasm: A new health system for the 21st century. *Committee on Quality of Healthcare in America*. Washington D.C.: National Academy.

Institute of Medicine. (2003). *Key capabilities of an electronic health record system*. Committee on Data Standards for Patient Safety. Washington D.C.: National Academy Press.

Institute of Medicine. (2006). *From cancer patient to cancer survivor. Lost in transition*. In M. Hewitt, S. Greenfield, & E. Stovall (Eds.). Washington D.C.: National Academy Press.

Institute of Medicine. (2007). *Preventing medication errors*. In P. Aspden, J. Wolcott, J.L. Bootman, & L.R. Cronenwett (Eds.). Washington D.C.: National Academy Press.

IOM. (1999). *To err is human: Building a safer health system*. Washington, DC: Institute of Medicine, National Academies Press.

Isaacs, E., Whittaker, S., Frohlich, D., & O'Conaill, B. (1994). Informal communication re-examined: New functions for video in supporting opportunistic encounters. In K.E. Finn, A.J. Sellen, & S.B. Wilbur (Eds.). *Video-Mediated Communication* (pp. 459-485). Mahwah, NJ: Lawrence Erlbaum.

Isensee, S., & Rudd, J. (1996). *The art of rapid prototyping*. MA: International Thompson Computer Press.

Jacobson, P. (2007). Empowering the physician-patient relationship: The effect of the Internet. *Partnership: The Canadian Journal of Library and Information Practice and Research, 2*(1). Retrieved May 14, 2008, from http://journal.lib.uoguelph.ca/index.php/perj/issue/view/31

Jarvenpaa, S.L., & Tractinsky, N. (1999). Consumer trust in an internet store: A cross cultural validation. *Journal of Computer-Mediated Communication, 5*(2), 1-33.

Jarvenpaa, S.L., Tractinsky, N., & Vitale, M. (2000). Consumer trust in an Internet store. *Information Technology and Management 1*, 45-71.

Järvinen, O.P.(2005). *Privacy management of e-health. Content analysis of 39 U.S. health providers' privacy policies*. PhD Thesis. Turku School of Economics, Turku, Finland. Retrieved May 24, 2008, from http://www.tukkk.fi/tutkimus/Vaitokset/default.asp

Jaspers, M.W., Steen, T., van den Bos, C., & Geenen, M. (2004). The think-aloud method: A guide to user interface design. *International Journal of Medical Informatics, 73*(11-12) 781–795.

Johnsen, J.-A.K. (2007). Constraints on message size in quasi-synchronous computer mediated communication: Effect on self-concept accessibility. *Computers in Human Behavior, 23*, 2269-2284.

Johnsen, J.-A.K., Rosenvinge, J.H., & Gammon, D. (2002). Online group interaction and mental health: An analysis of three online discussion forums. *Scandinavian Journal of Psychology, 43*, 445-449.

Johnsen, J.-A.K., Steinsvik, O.O., & Gammon, D. (2004). Health-care professionals' participation in an online discussion forum: The impact on structure, content, and interaction. *Journal of Technology in Human Services, 22*, 31-44.

Johnson, C. M., Johnson, T., & Zhang, J. (2000). Increasing productivity and reducing errors through usability analysis: A case study and recommendations. *2001 AMIA Symposium Proceedings*, 394-398.

Johnson, C.M. & Johnson, T.R. (2006). The significance of cognitive modelling in building healthcare interfaces. *International Journal of Medical Informatics, 75*(2) 163–172.

Johnson, C.M., Johnson, T.R., & Zhang, J. (2005). A user-centered framework for redesigning healthcare interfaces. *Journal of Biomedical Informatics, 38*(1) 75–87.

Johnson, D.G. (1994). *Computer ethics (second edition).* Englewood Cliffs, NJ: Prentice Hall.

Johnson-George, C., & Swap, W.C. (1982). Measurement of specific interpersonal trust: Construction and validation of a scale to assess trust in a specific other. *Journal of Personality and Social Psychology, 43*(6), 1306-1317.

Joinson, A.N. (1999). Anonymity, disinhibition and social desirability on the Internet. *Behavior Research Methods, Instruments, & Computers, 31*, 433-438.

Joinson, A.N. (2001). Knowing me, knowing you: Reciprocal self-disclosure on the Internet. *CyberPsychology & Behavior, 4*, 587-591.

Joinson, A.N. (2001). Self-disclosure in computer-mediated communication: The role of self-awareness and visual anonymity. *European Journal of Social Psychology, 31*, 177-192.

Joinson, A.N. (2004). Self-esteem, interpersonal risk, and preference for e-mail to face-to-face communication. *CyberPsychology & Behavior, 7*(4), 472-478.

Joinson, A.N., McKenna, K.Y.A., Postmes, T., & Reips, U.-D. (Eds.). (2007). *The Oxford handbook of Internet psychology.* Oxford: Oxford University Press.

Jordan, B., & Henderson, A. (1995). Interaction analysis: Foundations and practice. *Journal of the Learning Sciences, 4*(1), 39-103.

Jordan, J.E., & Osborne, R.H. (2007). Chronic disease self-management education programs: Challenges ahead. *Medical Journal of Australia, 186*(2), 84–87.

Kam, L.E., & Chismar, W.G. (2003). *A self-disclosure model for personal health information.* Paper presented at the 36th Hawaii International Conference on System Sciences, Hawaii.

Kaplan, B. (2003). Deriving design recommendations through discount usability engineering: Ethnographic observation and thinking-aloud protocol in usability testing for computer-based teaching cases. *2003 AMIA Annual Symposium Proceedings,* 346-350.

Kaplan, S., Greenfield, S., Gandek, B., Rogers, W.H., & Ware, J.E. Jr. (1996). Characteristics of physicians with participatory decision-making styles. *Annals of Internal Medicine, 124*(5), 497–504.

Kaplan, W.A. (2006). Can the ubiquitous power of mobile phones be used to improve health outcomes in developing countries? [Electronic version]. *Globalization and Health.* Retrieved May 13, 2008, from http://www.globalizationandhealth.com/content/2/1/9

Karahanna, E., Agarwal, R., & Angst, C.M. (2006). Reconceptualizing compatibility beliefs in technology acceptance research. *MIS Quarterly, 30*(4), 781-804.

Katz-Haas, R. (1998). Ten guidelines for user-centered web design. *Usability Interface, 5*(1).

Kaufman, D. R., Patel, V. L., Hilliman, C., Morin, P. C., Pevzner, J., Weinstock, R. S., et al. (2003). Usability in the real world: Assessing medical information technologies in patients' homes. *Journal of Biomedical Informatics, 36*(1-2), 45-60.

Kaushal, R., Blumenthal, D., Poon, E.G., Jha, A.K., Franz, C., Middleton, B., Glaser, J., Kuperman, G., Christino, M., Fernandopulle, R., Newhouse, J.P., Bates, D.W., & the Cost of National Health Information Working Group. (2005).The costs of a National Health Information Network. *Annals of Internal Medicine, 143*, 165-173.

Keil, M., Beranek, P.M., & Konsynski, B.R. (1995). Usefulness and ease of use: Field study evidence regarding task considerations. *Decision Support Systems, 13*(1), 75-91.

Kelly, E.P., & Unsal, F. (2002). Health Information privacy and e-healthcare. *International Journal of Healthcare Technology and Management, 4*(1/2), 41-52.

Kerwin, K.E., & Madison, J. (2002). The role of the Internet in improving healthcare quality. *Journal of Healthcare Management, 47*(4), 225-236.

Ketchum, A.M. (2005). Consumer health information Web sites: A survey of design elements found in sites developed in academic environments. *Journal of Medical Library Association, 93*(4), 496–499.

Kim, M.I., & Johnson, K.B. (2004). Patient entry of information: Evaluation of user interfaces. *Journal of Medical Internet Research, 6*(2), e13.

Kim, S.S., & Malhotra, N.K. (2005). A longitudinal model of continued IS use: An integrative view of four mechanisms underlying postadoption phenomena. *Management Science, 51*(5), 741-755.

Kim, S.S., Malhotra, N.K., & Narasimhan, S. (2006). Two competing perspectives on automatic use: A theoretical and empirical comparison. *Information Systems Research, 14*(2), 418-435.

Kind, T., Wheeler, K.L., Robinson, B., & Cabana, M.D. (2004). Do the leading children's hospitals have quality Web sites? A description of children's hospital Web sites. *Journal of Medical Internet Research, 6*(2). Retrieved May 27, 2008, from http://www.jmir.org/2004/2/e20/

King, S.A., & Moreggi, D. (1998). Internet therapy and self-help groups—The pros and cons. In J. Gackenbach (Ed.). *The psychology of the Internet: Intrapersonal, interpersonal and transpersonal implications* (pp. 77-109). San Diego, CA: Academic Press.

Kinzie, M. B., Cohn, W. F., Julian, M. F., & Knaus, W. A. (2002). A user-centered model for web site design: Needs assessment, user interface design, and rapid prototyping. *Journal of the American Medical Informatics Association, 9*(4), 320-330.

Kizer, K.W. (2001). Establishing healthcare performance standards in an era of consumerism. *Journal of the American Medical Association, 286* (10), 1213-1217.

Klein, L.R. (1998). Evaluating the potential of interactive media through a new lens: Search versus experience goods. *Journal of Business Research, 41*(3), 195-203.

Klein, R. (2007). Internet-based patient-physician electronic communication applications: Patient acceptance and trust. *e-Service Journal, 5*(2), 27-51.

Klein, R. (2007). Patient portal acceptance: An empirical examination of individual and technology based factors. *European Journal of Information Systems, 16*(6), 751-760.

Korpman, R. (2001). Managed care and e-health. *Health Management Technology, 22*(2), 12-14.

Koska, M.T. (1990). Patient-centered care: Can your hospital afford not to have IT? *Hospitals, 64*(21), 48-54.

Kotler, P., & Keller, L. (2005). *Marketing management.* Upper Saddle River, NJ: Pearson.

Kramer, R.M. (1994). The sinister attribution error: Paranoid cognition and collective distrust in organizations. *Motivation and Emotion, 18*(3), 199-230.

Kramer, R.M., Brewer, M.B., & Hanna, B.A. (1996). Collective trust and collective actions. In R.M. Kramer & T.R. Tyler (Eds.), *Trust in organizations: Frontiers of theory and research* (pp. 357-389). Thousand Oaks, CA: Sage, Inc.

Kreps, G.L. (2003). E-health: Technology-mediated health communication. *Journal of Health Psychology, 8*(1), 5–6.

Krizner, K. (2002). Telemedicine still looks for inroad to total acceptability. *Managed Healthcare Executive, 12*(5), 44–47.

Krumholz, H.M., Rathore, S.S., Chen, J., Wang, Y., & Radford, M.J. (2002). Evaluation of a consumer-oriented internet healthcare report card: The risk of quality ratings based on mortality data. *Journal of the American Medical Association, 287*(10), 1277-1287.

Kummervold, P.E., Gammon, D., Bergvik, S., Johnsen, J.-A.K., Hasvold, T., & Rosenvinge, J.H. (2002). Social support in a wired world: Use of online discussion forums in Norway. *Nordic Journal of Psychiatry, 56*(1), 59-65.

Kushniruk, A. W. & Patel, V. L. (2004). Cognitive and usability engineering methods for the evaluation of clinical information systems. *Journal of Biomedical Informatics, 37*(1), 56-76.

Kushniruk, A. W., Kaufman, D. R., Patel, V. L., Levesque, Y., & Lottin, P. (1996). Assessment of a computerized patient record system: A cognitive approach to evaluating medical technology. *MD Computing, 13*(5), 406-415.

Kushniruk, A. W., Patel, C., Patel, V. L., & Cimino, J. J. (2001). 'Televaluation' of clinical information systems: An integrative approach to assessing Web-based systems. *International Journal of Medical Informatics, 61*(1), 45-70.

Kushniruk, A., Patel, V., Cimino, J. J., & Barrows, R. A. (1996). Cognitive evaluation of the user interface and vocabulary of an outpatient information system. *1996 AMIA Annual Symposium Proceedings*, 22-26.

Kushniruk, A.W., Patel, V.L, Cimino, J.J., & Barrows, R.A. (1996). Cognitive evaluation of the user interface and vocabulary of an outpatient information system. In *Proceedings of AMIA Annual Symposium* (pp. 22–26).

Kvale, S. (1996). *InterViews: An introduction to qualitative research interviewing.* Thousand Oaks, CA: Sage.

Lai, T.L. (2004). Service quality and perceived value's impact on satisfaction, intention and usage of short message service (SMS). *Information Systems Frontiers, 6*(4), 353-368.

Langer, E.J. (1975). The illusion of control. *Journal of Personality and Social Psychology, 32*(2), 311-328.

Lansky, D. (2002). *Information for better quality care—the patients' perspective.* Foundation for Accountability. Retrieved May 26, 2008, from http://www.markle.org/resources/facct/doclibFiles/documentFile_526.ppt

Lansky, D. (2003). *A person-centered view of consumer information in the healthcare marketplace.* Federal Trade Commission/U.S. Department of Justice Joint Hearings on Healthcare and Competition Law and Policy. Retrieved May 26, 2008, from http://www.markle.org/resources/facct/doclibFiles/documentFile_595.ppt

Laurenceau, J.-P., Barrett, L.F., & Pietromonaco, P.R. (1998). Intimacy as an interpersonal process: The importance of self-disclosure, partner disclosure, and perceived partner responsiveness in interpersonal exchanges *Journal of Personality and Social Psychology, 74*(5), 1238-1251.

Law, J., & Singleton, V. (2000). Performing technology's stories: On social constructivism, performance, and performativity. *Technology and Culture, 41*(4), 765-775.

Lazarus, I.R. (2001). Separating myth from reality in e-health initiatives. *Managed Healthcare Executive, June*, 33-36.

Lea, M., & Spears, R. (1995). Love at first byte? Building personal relationships over computer networks. In J.T. Wood & S. Duck (Eds.). *Understudied relationships: Off the beaten track* (pp. 197-233). Newbury Park, CA: Sage.

Lea, M., O'Shea, T., Fung, P., & Spears, R. (1992). "Flaming" in computer-mediated communication: Observations, explanations and implications. In M. Lea (Ed.). *Contexts of computer-mediated communication* (pp. 89-112). London: Harvester-Wheatsheaf.

Leary, M.R., Tchividjian, L.R., & Kraxberger, B.E. (1994). Self-presentation can be hazardous to your health: Impression management and health risk. *Health Psychology, 13*, 461-470.

Lee, P.V., & Hoo, E. (2006). Beyond consumer-driven healthcare: Purchasers' expectations of all plans. *Health Affairs 25*(6), w544-w548. Retrieved May 26, 2008, from http://content.healthaffairs.org/cgi/content/abstract/25/6/w544

Lee, Y., Kozar, K.A., & Larsen, K.R.T. (2003). The technology acceptance model: Past, present, and future. *Communications of the Association for Information Systems, 12,* Article 50, 752-780.

Leisen, B., & Hyman, M.R. (2004). Antecedents and consequences of trust in a service provider: The case of primary care physicians. *Journal of Business Research, 57*(9), 990-999.

Lemov, P. (2006, September). Healthcare: A dose of transparency. *Governing Magazine*. Kaiser Family Foundation. Retrieved May 26, 2008, from http://www.governing.com/articles/9hcare.htm

Lenhart, A., Horrigan, J., & Fallows, D. (2004). Content creation online. *Pew Internet & American life project.* Retrieved May 14, 2008, from http://www.pewinternet.org/pdfs/PIP_Content_Creation_Report.pdf

Levenstein, J.H., McCracken, E.C., McWhinney, I.R., Stewart, M.A., & Brown, J.B. (1986). The patient-centred clinical method, 1: A model for the doctor-patient interaction in family medicine. *Family Practice, 3*(1), 24-30.

Lewis, C., & Rieman, J. (1994). *Task-centered user interface design: A practical introduction.* Retrieved December 13,2007 from http://www.hcibib.org/tcuid/

Lexchin, J. (2006). Bigger and better: How Pfizer redefined erectile dysfunction. *PLoS Medicine, 3*(4), e132.

Liaw, T., Lawrence, M., & Rendell, J. (1996). The effect of a computer-generated patient-held medical record summary and/or a written personal health record on patients' attitudes, knowledge and behaviour concerning health promotion. *Family Practice 13*(3), 289-293.

Licciardone, J.C., & Smith-Barbaro, P., & Coleridge, S.T. (2001). Use of the Internet as a resource for consumer health information: Results of the second osteopathic survey of healthcare in America (OSTEOSURV-II). *Journal of Medical Internet Research 3*(4):e3. Retrieved May 27, 2008, from http://www.jmir.org/2001/4/e31/

Limayem, M., & Hirt, S.G. (2003). Force of habit and information systems usage: Theory and initial validation. *Journal of the Association for Information Systems, 4,* 65-97.

Lin, B., & Umoh, D. (2002). E-healthcare: A vehicle of change. *American Business Review, 20*(2), 27-32.

Lindgaard, G. (1994). *Usability testing and system evaluation: A guide for designing useful computer systems.* London: Chapman & Hall.

Lindlof, T.R., & Taylor, B.C. (2002). *Qualitative communication research methods (second edition).* Thousand Oaks, CA: Sage.

Little, P., Everitt, H., Williamson, I., Warner, G., Moore, M., Gould, C., Ferrier, K., & Payne, S. (2001). Observational study of effect of patient centredness and positive approach on outcomes of general practice consultations. *British Medical Journal, 323*(7318), 908-911.

Littrell, J. (1998). Is the re-experience of painful emotion therapeutic? *Clinical Psychology Review, 18*(1), 71-102.

Lober, W., Zierler, B., Herbaugh, A., Shinstrom, S., Stolyar, A., Kim, E. & Kim, Y. (2006). Barriers to the use of a personal health record by an elderly population. In Proceedings of *2006 AMIA Annual Symposium Proceedings* (pp. 514-518).

Lorbach, D.F., & Detmer, D.E. (2007). Research challenges for electronic health records. *American Journal of Preventative Medicine, 32*(5s), 104–111.

Lorenzi, N.M. (2003, December 16). Strategies for creating successful local health information infrastructure initiatives. *Local Health Information Infrastructure Success/Failure Report.*

Lorig, K.R., Sobel, D.S., Stewart, A.L., Brown, B.W.J., Bandura, A., Ritter, P., et al. (1999). Evidence suggesting that a chronic disease self-management program can improve health status while reducing hospitalization: A randomized trial. *Medical Care, 37*(1), 5–14.

Luce, P., Phillips, J., Benjamin, R., & Wasson, J.H. (2006). Technology to support community health alliances. *Journal of Ambulatory Care Management, 27*(3), 399-407.

Luhmann, N. (1979). *Power and trust.* New York: John Wiley.

Luo, W., & Najdawi, M. (2004). Trust-building measures: A review of consumer health portals. *Communications of the Association for Computing Machinery, 47*(1), 108-113.

MacStravic, S. (1988). The patient as a partner: A competitive strategy in healthcare marketing. *Hospital & Health Services Administration, 33*(1), 15-24.

Malterud, K. (2001). The art and science of clinical knowledge: Evidence beyond measures and numbers. *Lancet, 358*, 397-400.

Marill, J. L., Miller, N., & Kitendaugh, P. (2006). The MedlinePlus public user interface: Studies of design challenges and opportunities. *Journal of the Medical Library Association, 94*(1), 30-40.

Markle Foundation. (2004). *Connecting Americans to their healthcare, final report.* The Robert Wood Johnson Foundation. Retrieved May 26, 2008, from http://www.connectingforhealth.org/resources/wg_eis_final_report_0704.pdf

Martin Ginis, K.A., & Leary, M.R. (2004). Self-presentational processes in health-damaging behavior. *Journal of Applied Sport Psychology, 16*, 59-74.

Martin, K.A., Leary, M.R., & Rejeski, W.J. (2000). Self-presentational concerns in older adults: Implications for health and well-being. *Basic and Applied Social Psychology, 22*(3), 169-179.

Marvel, M.K., Epstein, R.M., Flowers, K., & Beckman, H.B. (1999). Soliciting the patient's agenda: Have we improved? *Journal of the American Medical Association, 281*(3), 283-287.

Mason, J.K., McCall, & Smith, R.A. (1999). *Law and medical ethics (fifth edition).* London, England: Butterworths.

Mathieu, J. (2007). Blogs, podcasts, and wikis: The new names in information dissemination. *Journal of the American Dietetic Association, 107*(4), 553-555.

Mauro, C. L. (2000). Formal definition of user-centered design (UCD). Retrieved May, 2007, from http://www.taskz.com/definitions.php

Mayer, R.C., Davis, J.H., & Schoorman, F.D. (1995). An integration model of organizational trust. *Academy of Management Review, 20*(3), 709-734.

Mayer, R.J., Davis, J.H., & Schoorman, F.D. (1995). An integrative model of organizational trust. *Academy of Management Review, 20*, 709-734.

McArthur, R.L. (2001). Reasonable expectation of privacy. *Ethics and Information Technology, 3*, 123-128.

McFall, L. (1987). Integrity. *Ethics, 9*(1), 5-20.

McGoldrick, C., & O'Dell, S. (2000). The road to e-health: Marketing implications. *Marketing Health Services, 20*(4), 32-34.

McInerney, C. (2002). Knowledge management and the dynamic nature of knowledge. *Journal of the American Society for Information Systems and Technology, 53*(12), 1009–1018.

McKenna, K.Y.A., & Bargh, J.A. (1998). Coming out in the age of the internet: Identity demarginalization through virtual group participation. *Journal of Personality and Social Psychology, 75*(3), 681-694.

McKenna, K.Y.A., & Bargh, J.A. (1999). Causes and consequences of social interaction on the Internet: A conceptual framework. *Media Psychology, 1*, 249-269.

McKenna, K.Y.A., Green, A.S., & Gleason, M.E.J. (2002). Relationship formation on the Internet: What's the big attraction? *Journal of Social Issues, 58*(1), 9-31.

McKillen, D. (2001). E-health traffic—slow but steady growth. *Marketing and Media, 36*(9), 10-12.

McKinstry, B. (2000). Do patients wish to be involved in decision making in the consultation? A cross sectional survey with video vignettes. *British Medical Journal, 321*(7265), 867–871.

McKnight, D.H., & Chervany, N.L. (2001). What trust means in e-commerce customer relationships: An interdisciplinary conceptual typology. *International Journal of Electronic Commerce, 6(2)*, 35–59.

McKnight, D.H., Choudhury, V., & Kacmar, C. (2002). Developing and validating trust measures for e-commerce: An integrative typology. *Information Systems Research, 13*(3), 334-359.

McKnight, D.H., Choudhury, V., & Kacmar, C. (2002). The impact of initial consumer trust on intentions to transact with a Web site: A trust building model. *Journal of Strategic Information Systems, 11*(3-4), 297-323.

McKnight, D.H., Cummings, L.L., & Chervany, N.L. (1998). Initial trust formation in new organizational relationships. *Academy of Management Review, 23*(3), 473-490.

McWilliams, J.M., Meara, E., Zaslavsky, A.M., & Ayanian, J.Z. (2007). Use of health services by previously uninsured Medicare beneficiaries. *New England Journal of Medicine, 357,* 143-153.

Menachemi, N., & Brooks, R.G. (2006). Reviewing the benefits of electronic health records and associated patient safety technologies. *Journal of Medical Systems, 30*(3), 159-168.

Mettler, M., & Kemper, D.W. (2005). Information therapy: The strategic role of prescribed information in disease self-management. *Studies in Health Technology and Informatics, 8*(2), 69-76.

Michelfelder, D.P. (2001). The moral value of informational privacy in cyberspace. *Ethics and Information Technology, 3*, 129-135.

Miles, M.B. & Huberman, A.M. (1994). *Qualitative data analysis: An expanded sourcebook (second edition).* Thousand Oaks: Sage.

Miller, W.L., & Crabtree, B.F. (1999). Depth interviewing. In W.L. Miller, & B.F. Crabtree (Eds.), *Doing Qualitative Research* (pp. 89-108). Thousand Oaks CA: Sage Publications.

MNT. (2006). AHIP, BCBSA issue standards for personal health records. *Medical News Today.* Retrieved May 14, 2008, from http://www.medicalnewstoday.com/articles/59052.php

Moen, A., & Brennan, P.F. (2005). Health@Home: The work of health information management in the household (HIMH): Implications for consumer health informatics (CHI) innovations. *Journal of the American Medical Informatics Association, 12*(6), 648-656.

Mol, A. (1999). Ontological politics. A word and some questions. In J. Law & J. Hassard (Eds.), *Actor Network Theory and After* (pp. 74-89). Oxford, England: Blackwell.

Mol, A., & Law, J. (2004). Embodied action, enacted bodies: The example of hypoglycaemia. *Body & Society, 10*(2-3), 43-62.

Monninkhof, E., van der Aa, M., van der Valk, P., van der Palen, J., Zielhuis, G., Koning, K., & Pieterse, M., (2004). A qualitative evaluation of a comprehensive self-management programme for COPD patients: Effectiveness from the patients' perspective. *Patient Education and Counseling, 55*(2), 177–184.

Monninkhof, E., van der Valk, P., van der Palen, J., van Herwaarden, C., Partidge, M., Walters, E., & Zielhuis, G.A. (2002). Self-management education for chronic obstructive pulmonary disease. *Cochrane Database of Systematic Reviews: Reviews 2002*(4).

Moon, J., & Kim, Y. (2001). Extending the TAM for a World-Wide-Web context. *Information & Management, 38,* 217-230.

Moor, J.H. (1997). Towards a theory of privacy in the information age. *Computers and Society, 27*(3), 27-32.

Moor, J.H. (1998). Reason, relativity, and responsibility in computer ethics. *Computers and Society, 28*(1), 14-21.

Moore, G.E. (1965). Cramming more components onto integrated circuits. *Electronics, 38*(8), 114-117.

Moore, L.G., & Wasson, J.H. (2006). An introduction to technology for patient-centered, collaborative care. *Journal of Ambulatory Care Management, 29*(3), 195-198.

Mootee, I. (2004). *High intensity marketing.* Toronto, ON: SA Press.

Morgan, R.M., & Hunt, S.D. (1994). The commitment-trust theory of relationship marketing. *Journal of Marketing, 58*(3), 20-38.

Morris, M.G., & Dillon, A. (1997). How user perceptions influence software use. *IEEE Software, 4,* 58-65.

Morrissey, J. (2005). But what does the public think? For consumers to adopt PHRs, they need reasons that hit home. *Journal of American Health Information Management Association, 76*(10), 42-44.

Moser, I., & Law, J. (1999). Good passages, bad passages. In J. Law & J. Hassard (Eds.), *Actor Network Theory and After* (pp. 196-219). Oxford, England: Blackwell.

Muir Gray, J.A. (2004). Self-management in chronic illness. *The Lancet, 364*(9444), 1467–1468.

Murdoch, M., van Ryn, M., Hodges, J., & Cowper, D. (2005). Mitigating effect of department of veterans affairs disability benefits for posttraumatic stress disorder on low income. *Military Medicine, 170*, 137-140.

Naessens, J.M., Baird, M.A., Jouten, H.K.V., Vanness, D.J., & Campbell, C.R. (2005). Predicting persistently high primary care use. *Annals of Family Medicine, 3*(4), 324-330.

Nardi, B., Whittaker, S., & Bradner, E. (2000). *Interaction and outeraction: Instant messaging in action.* Paper presented at the CSCW 2000, Philadelphia, PA, USA.

Narins, C.R., Dozier, A.M., Ling, F.S., & Zareba, W. (2005). The influence of public reporting of outcome data on medical decision making by physicians. *Archives of Internal Medicine, 165*(1), 83-87.

Nash, M.G., & Gremillion, C. (2004). Globalization impacts the healthcare organization of the 21st century: Demanding new ways to market product lines successfully. *Nursing Administration Quarterly, 28*(2), 86–91.

National Health Interview Survey. (2006). *Public use data release. NHIS survey description.* Division of Health Interview Statistics. National Center for Health Statistics Hyattsville, Maryland Centers for Disease Control and Prevention U.S. Department of Health and Human Services. Retrieved May 21, 2008, from http://www.cdc.gov/nchs/about/major/nhis/quest_data_related_1997_forward.htm

National Health Priority Action Council. (2006). *National chronic disease strategy.* Canberra: Australian Government Department of Health and Ageing. Retrieved May 28, 2008, from http://www.health.gov.au/Internet/wcms/publishing.nsf/Content/pq-ncds

NCVHS. (2001). A strategy for building the national health information infrastructure. *National Committee on Vital and Health Statistics.* Washington DC: U.S. Department of Health and Human Services.

Neuhauser, L., & Kreps, G.L. (2003). The Advent of e-Health: How interactive media are transforming health communication. *Medien and Kommunikationswissenschaft 51*(3–4), 541–556.

Neuman, W.L. (2000). *Social research methods—qualitative and quantitative approaches (4th edition).* Needham Heights, MA: Allyn and Bacon.

Newman, S., Steed, L., & Mulligan, K. (2004). Self-management interventions for chronic illness. *The Lancet, 364*(9444), 1523–1537.

Nguyen, H.Q., Carrieri-Kohlman, V., Rankin, S.H., Slaughter, R., & Stulbarg, M.S. (2004).Supporting cardiac recovery through ehealth technology. *Journal of Cardiovascular Nursing, 19*(3), 200–208.

Nielsen, H.L. (2005). *Linking healthcare: An inquiry into the changing performances of Web-based technology for asthma monitoring.* Ph.D. thesis, Copenhagen Business School, Copenhagen, DK.

Nielsen, J. (1993). *Usability engineering.* Boston: Academic Press.

Nielsen, J. (2000). *Jakob Nielsen's alertbox, March 19, 2000: Why you only need to test with 5 users.* Retrieved May 26, 2008, from http://www.useit.com/alertbox/20000319.html

Nielsen, J., & Landauer, T. K. 1993. A mathematical model of the finding of usability problems. *Proceedings ACM/IFIP INTERCHI'93 Conference* (Amsterdam, The Netherlands, April 24-29), 206-213.

Nielsen, J., & Mack, R. L. (1994). *Usability inspection methods.* New York: Wiley.

Njølstad, I., & Aaraas, I. (1992). Look at the patient, not the notes. *Lancet, 340*(8816), 413.

Norman, C.D., & Skinner, H.A. (2006). E-health literacy: Essential skills for consumer health in a networked world. *Journal of Medical Internet Research, 8*(2), e9. Retrieved May 26, 2008, from at http://www.jmir.org/2006/2/e9/

Noteberg, A., Christiaanse, E., & Wallage. (2003). Consumer trust in electronic channels: The impact of electronic commerce assurance on consumers' purchasing likelihood and risk perceptions. *e-Service Journal, 2*(2), 46–67.

O'Sullivan, P.B. (2000). What you don't know won't hurt me: Impression management functions of communication channels in relationships. *Human Communication Research, 26*(3), 403-431.

Oenema, A., Brug, J., & Lechner, L. (2001). Web-based tailored nutrition education: Results of a randomized clinical trial. *Health Education Research, 16*, 647–660.

of social presence: Experiments in e-products and e-services. *Omega: The International Journal of Management Science*, *32*, 407–424.

Office of Disease Prevention and Health Promotion (ODPHP). (2000). *Healthy people 2010: Volume 1 (Second edition).* Washington, DC: Health and Human Services Dept.

Oliver, M.I., Pearson, N., Coe, N., & Gunnell, D. (2005). Help-seeking behaviour in men and women with common mental health problems: Cross-sectional study. *British Journal of Psychiatry, 186*(4), 297-301.

Openshaw, J. (2006, October 31). Checkup lines: Americans need to learn to shop for healthcare. *Market watch.* Retrieved May 26, 2008, from http://www.marketwatch.com/News/Story/consumers-need-become-better-health-care/story.aspx?guid=%7B09F2F091-A840-4D08-AAE3-C4CDD9A8C02C%7D

Orbell, J., Dawes, R., & Schwartz-Shea, P. (1994). Trust, social categories, and individuals: The case of gender. *Motivation and Emotion, 18*(2), 109-128.

Ouellette, J.A., & Wood, W. (1998). Habit and intention in everyday life: The multiple processes by which past behavior predicts future behavior. *Psychological Bulletin, 12,* 54-74.

Page, L., Brin, S., Motwani, R., & Winograd, T. (1998). The PageRank citation ranking: Bringing order to the Web. *Stanford Digital Library Technologies Project.* Retrieved May 22, 2008, from http://dbpubs.stanford.edu:8090/pub/1999-66

Pamben, D. (2007). Spreading the message. *Cabinet Maker, 5536*, 10.

Parks, M.R., & Floyd, K. (1996). Making friends in cyberspace. *Journal of Communication, 46*(1), 80-97.

Parks, M.R., & Roberts, L.E. (1998). "Making mOOsic": The development of personal relationships on-line and a comparison to their off-line counterparts. *Journal of Social and Personal Relationships, 15*(4), 517-537.

Parsons, T. (1951). *The social system*. London: Routledge.

Patel, V. L., & Kaufman, D. R. (1998). Medical informatics and the science of cognition. *Journal of the American Medical Informatics Association, 5*(6), 493-502.

Patt, M.R., Houston, T.K., Jenckes, M.W., Sands, D.Z., & Ford, D.E. (2003). Doctors who are using e-mail with their patients: A qualitative exploration. *Journal of Medical Internet Research. 5*(2), e9.

Pavlou, P.A., & Gefen, D. (2004). Building effective online marketplaces with institution-based trust. *Information Systems Research, 15*(1), 37-59.

Payton, F.C., & Brennan, P.F. (1999). How a community health information network is really used. *Communications of the ACM, 42,* 85-89.

Pennebaker, J.W. (1997). *Opening up: The healing power of expressing emotions (second edition).* New York: The Guilford Press.

Pennebaker, J.W. (2004). Theories, therapies, and taxpayers: On the complexities of the expressive writing paradigm. *Clinical Psychology: Science and Practice, 11*, 138-142.

Pennebaker, J.W., & Beall, S.K. (1986). Confronting a traumatic event: Toward an understanding of inhibition and disease. *Journal of Abnormal Psychology, 95*, 274-281.

Pennebaker, J.W., & Francis, M.E. (1996). Cognitive, emotional and language processes in disclosure. *Cognition and Emotion, 10*, 621-626.

Pennebaker, J.W., Mayne, T.J., & Francis, M.E. (1997). Linguistic predictors of adaptive bereavement. *Journal of Personality and Social Psychology, 72*, 863-871.

Perea y Monsuwe, T., Dellaert, B.G.C., & Ruyter, K. (2004). What drives consumers to shop online? : A literature review. *International Journal of Service Industry Management, 15*(1), 102–121.

Peterson, M.C., Holbrook, J.H., Von Hales, D., Smith, N.L., & Staker, L.V. (1992). Contributions of the history, physical examination, and laboratory investigation in making medical diagnoses. *Western Journal of Medicine, 156*(2), 163-165.

Pincus, T. (2004). Will racial and ethnic disparities in health be resolved primarily outside of standard medical care? *Annals of Internal Medicine, 141*(3), 224–225.

Plazzotta, F., Otero, P., Campos, F., Pedernera, F., Navas, H., Martínez, M., et al. (2005). *Estrategias para agilizar la atención ambulatoria: integración de los sistemas de información.* Paper presented at the 8mo Simposio de Informática en Salud - 34 JAIIO, Santa Fé, Argentina.

Plougmann, S., Hejlesen, O.K., & Cavan, D.A. (2001). DiasNet—A diabetes advisory system for communication and education via the Internet. *International Journal of Medical Informatics, 64*(2-3), 319-330.

Plovnick, R. M., & Zeng, Q. T. (2004). Reformulation of consumer health queries with professional terminology: a pilot study. *J Med Internet Res, 6*(3), e27.

Pope, C., & Mays, N. (2006). *Qualitative research in health care* (Third edition). Malden, MA: Blackwell Pub./BMJ Books.

Postmes, T., & Spears, R. (1998). Deindividuation and anti-normative behavior: A meta-analysis. *Psychological Bulletin, 123*, 238-259.

Postmes, T., Spears, R., & Lea, M. (1998). Breaching or building social boundaries? SIDE effects of computer-mediated communication. *Communication Research, 25*(6), 689-715.

Postmes, T., Spears, R., & Lea, M. (2000). The formation of group norms in computer-mediated communication. *Human Communication Research, 26*(3), 341-371.

Postmes, T., Spears, R., Sakhel, K., & de Groot, D. (2001). Social influence in computer-mediated communication: The effects of anonymity on group behavior. *Personality and Social Psychology Bulletin, 27*(10), 1243-1254.

Powell, W.W. (1996). Trust-based forms of governance. In R.M. Kramer & T.R. Tyler (Eds.), *Trust in organizations: Frontiers of theory and research* (pp. 51-67). Thousand Oaks, CA: Sage, Inc.

Pransky, G.S., & Dempsey, P.G. (2004). Practical aspects of functional capacity evaluations. *Journal of Occupational Rehabilitation, 14*, 217-229.

Pratt, W., Unruh, K., Civan, A., & Skeels, M. (2006). Personal health information management. *Communications of the ACM, 49*(1), 51-55.

Preece, J., Rogers, Y., & Sharp, H. (2002). *Interaction design: Beyond human-computer interaction.* New York: John Wiley & Sons, Inc.

Rachels, J. (1975). Why is privacy important? Philosophy and public affairs, *12*(4). (Reprinted from *Computers, Ethics, & Social Values*, pp. 351-357, D.G. Johnson & H. Nissenbaum, Eds., 1995, Englewood Cliffs, NJ: Prentice Hall.

Rappolt, S. (1997). Clinical guidelines and the fate of medical autonomy in Ontario. *Social Science & Medicine, 44*(7), 977–987.

Rasmussen, L.M., Phanareth, K., Nolte, H., & Backer, V. (2005). Internet-based monitoring of asthma: A long-term, randomized clinical study of 300 asthmatic subjects. *Journal of Allergy and Clinical Immunology, 115*(6), 1137-1142.

Rea, M & Parker, R. A. (2005). *Designing and conducting survey research: A comprehensive guide* (Third edition). San Francisco: Jossey-Bass.

Regan, P. (1995). *Legislating privacy: Technology, social values, and public policy.* Chapel Hill, NC: University of North Carolina Press.

Reicher, S.D., Spears, R., & Postmes, T. (1995). A social identity model of deindividuation phenomena. In W. Stroebe & M. Hewstone (Eds.). *European Review of Social Psychology* (Vol. 6, pp. 161-198). Chichester, U.K.: Wiley.

Revere, D., & Dunbar, P.J. (2001). Review of computer-generated outpatient health behavior interventions: Clinical encounters "in absentia." *Journal of the American Medical Informatics Association, 8*(1), 62-79.

Rheingold, H. (1993). *The virtual community: Homesteading on the electronic frontier.* New York: Perseus Books.

Rickwood, D., Deane, F.P., Wilson, C.J., & Ciarrochi, J. (2005). Young people's help-seeking for mental health problems [Electronic version]. *Australian e-Journal for the Advancement of Mental Health.* Retrieved May 13, 2008, from http://www.auseinet.com/journal/vol4iss3-suppl/rickwood.pdf

Riegelsberger, J., Sasse, M.A., & McCarthy, J.D. (2005). The mechanics of trust: A framework for research and design. *International Journal of Human-Computer Studies. 62*, 381–422.

Rieh, S.Y., & Belkin, N.J. (1998). Understanding judgment of information quality and cognitive authority in the www. *Journal of the American Society for Information Science, 35*, 279-289.

Rindfleisch, T.C. (1997). Privacy, information technology, and healthcare. *Communication of the ACM, 40*(8), 92-100.

Robinson, R., & West, R. (1992). A comparison of computer and questionnaire methods of history-taking in a genito-urinary clinic. *Psychology and Health, 6*, 77-84.

Rogers, E.M. (2003). *Diffusion of innovations (fifth edition).* New York: The Free Press.

Rose, A.F., Schnipper, J.L., Park, E.R., Poon, E.G., Li, Q., & Middleton, B. (2005). Using qualitative studies to improve the usability of an EMR. *Journal of Biomedical Informatics, 38*(1), 51–60.

Rosenstein, A.H. (1986). Applications of consumer behavior in medical care. *Journal of Professional Services Marketing, 1*(4), 31-37.

Rosenvinge, J.H., Laugerud, S., & Hjortdahl, P. (2003). Trust in health Web sites: A survey among Norwegian Internet users. *Journal of Telemedicine and Telecare, 9*, 161–166.

Rousseau, P.L., & Wachtel, P. (1998). Financial intermediation and economic performance: Historical evidence from five industrialized countries. *Journal of Money, Credit and Banking, 30*(4), 657-678.

Rubin, J. (1994) *Handbook of usability testing: How to plan, design, and conduct effective tests.* New York: John Wiley and Sons.

Rydström, I., Hartman, J., & Segesten, K. (2005). Not letting the disease get the upper hand over life: Strategies of teens with asthma. *Scandinavian Journal of Caring Sciences, 19*(4), 388-395.

Safavi, K. (2006). Patient-centered pay for performance: Are we missing the target? *Journal of Healthcare Management, 51*(4), 215-218.

Safran, C. (2003). The collaborative edge: Patient empowerment for vulnerable populations. *International Journal of Medical Informatics, 69*(2), 185-190.

Sanchez, P.M. (2002). Refocusing Web site marketing: Physician-patient relationships. *Health Marketing Quarterly, 20*(1), 37.

Sandrick, K. (1998). Calculating ROI for CPRs. *Health Management Technology, 19*(6), 16-20.

Schlenker, B.R. (2003). Self-presentation. In M.R. Leary & J.P. Tangney (Eds.). *Handbook of self and identity* (pp. 492-518). New York: The Guilford Press.

Schliemann, T., Asting, T., Følstad, A., & Heim, J. (2002). *Medium preference and medium effects in person-person communication*. Paper presented at the CHI 2002, Minneapolis, MN, USA.

Schmit, J. (2006, August 28). Could walk-in retail clinics help slow rising health costs? *USA Today*. Retrieved May 26, 2008, from http://www.usatoday.com/money/industries/health/2006-08-24-walk-in-clinic-usat_x.htm

Schmitt, K.F., & Wofford, D.A. (2002). Financial analysis projects clear returns from electronic medical records. *Healthcare Financial Management, 56*(1), 52-57.

Schmittdiel, J., Selby, J.V., Grumbach, K., & Quesenberry, C.P., Jr. (1997). Choice of a personal physician and patient satisfaction in a health maintenance organization. *Journal of the American Medical Association, 278*(19), 1596-1599.

Schneider, S., & Lane, J. (2005). *The patient from hell: How I worked with my doctors to get the best of modern medicine and how you can too*. Cambridge, MA: Da Capo Press.

Schultz, A. S. H., Bottorff, J. L., & Johnson, J. L. (2006). An ethnographic study of tobacco control in hospital settings. *Tobacco Control, 15*(4), 317-322.

Second edition). New York: Springer.

Shadbolt, N., & Milton, N. (1999). From knowledge engineering to knowledge management. *British Journal of Management, 10*, 309–322.

Shanker, V., Urban, G.L., & Sultan, F. (2005). Online trust: A stakeholder perspective, concepts, implications, and future directions. *Journal of Strategic Information Systems, 11*, 325–344.

Shapiro, S.P. (1987). Policing trust. In C.D. Shearing & P.C. Stenning (Eds.), *Private policing* (pp. 194-220). Newbury Park, CA: Sage Publications, Inc.

Sharda, P., Das, A. L., Cohen, T.A., & Patel, V. (2006). Customizing clinical narratives for the electronic medical record interface using cognitive methods. *International Journal of Medical Informatics, 75*(5), 346–368.

Sheppard, B.H., Hartwick, J., & Warshaw, P.R. (1988). The theory of reasoned action: A meta-analysis of past research with recommendations for modifications and future research. *Journal of Consumer Research, 15*, 325-343.

Shih, Y., & Fang, K. (2004). The use of a decomposed theory of planned behavior to study Internet banking in Taiwan. *Internet Research, 14*(3), 213-223.

Siau, K., Southbard, P., & Hong, S. (2002). E-healthcare strategies and implementation. *International Journal of Healthcare Technology and Management, 4*(1-2), 118-131.

Siegel, D. A. (2003). The business case for user-centered design: Increasing your power of persuasion. *Interactions, 10*(3), 30-36.

Siegel, E.R., Logan, R.A., Harnsberger, R.L., Cravedi, K., Krause, J.A., Lyon, B., Hajarian, K., Uhl, J., Ruffin, A., & Lindberg, D.A. (2006). Information Rx: Evaluation of a new informatics tool for physicians, patients, and libraries. *Information Services and Use, 26*(1), 1-10.

Sienot, M. (1997). Pretesting Web sites: A comparison between the plus-minus method and the think-aloud method for the World Wide Web. *Journal of Business and Technical Communication, 11*(4), 469–482.

Sitkin, S., & Roth, N.L. (1993). Explaining the limited effectiveness of legalistic remedies for trust/distrust. *Organization Science, 4*(3), 367-392.

Sitkin, S.B. (1995). On the positive effect of legalization on trust. In R.J. Bies, B.H. Sheppard & R.J. Lewicki (Eds.), *Research on negotiation in organizations* (pp. 185-217). Greenwich, CT: JAI Press.

Smyth, J.M. (1998). Written emotional expression: Effect sizes, outcome types, and moderating variables. *Journal of Consulting and Clinical Psychology, 66*(1), 174-184.

Sneha, S., & Varshney, U. (2005, August 11-14). A wireless ECG monitoring system for healthcare. In *Proceedings of the Eleventh Americas Conference on Information Systems* (pp. 2539-2549). Omaha, NE.

Social Security Administration (SSA). (2006). *Social Security disability benefits*. SSA Publication No. 05-10029.

ICN 456000. Retrieved May 21, 2008, from http://www.ssa.gov/pubs/10029.html#part2

Social Security Administration. (2006). *Disability evaluation under social security. Blue book.* SSA Publication No. 64-039 ICN 468600. Retrieved May 21, 2008, from http://www.ssa.gov/disability/professionals/bluebook/

Social Security Administration. (2007). *Annual statistical supplement to the Social Security bulletin.* SSA Publication No. 13-11700. Social Security Administration, Office of Policy, Office of Research, Evaluation, and Statistics: Washington D.C. Retrieved May 21, 2008, from http://www.socialsecurity.gov/policy/docs/statcomps/supplement/2006/supplement06.pdf

Sofaer, S., Crofton, C., Goldstein, E., Hoy, E., & Crabb, J. (2005). What do consumers want to know about the quality of care in hospitals? *Health Services Research, 40*(6), 2030.

Somerville, A. (1999). English V. Genetic privacy: Orthodoxy or oxymoron? *Journal of Medical Ethics, 25*, 144-150.

Spears, R., Lea, M., & Postmes, T. (2001). Social psychological theories of computer-mediated communication: Social pain or social gain. In W.P. Robinson & H. Giles (Eds.). *The New Handbook of Language and Social Psychology.* Chichester, U.K.: John Wiley & Sons Ltd.

Spill, T. A.M., Schuring, R.W., & Michel-Verkerke, M.B. (2004). Electronic prescription system: Do the professionals USE IT? *International Journal of Healthcare Technology Management, 6*(1), 32-55.

Sprague, L. (2006). *Personal health records: The peoples' choice?* (Publication No. 820). Washington D.C.; National Health Policy Forum. Retrieved May 14, 2008, from http://www.nhpf.org/pdfs_ib/IB820_PHRs_11-30-06.pdf

Stake, R.E. (2005). *Qualitative case studies. The Sage handbook of qualitative research (third edition).* In N. Denzin, & Y. Lincoln (Eds.), (pp.443–466). Sage Publications.

Star, S.L. (1991). Power, technologies and the phenomenology of conventions: On being allergic to onions. In J. Law (Ed.), *A Sociology of Monsters: Essays on Power, Technology and Domination* (pp. 26-56). London, England: Routledge.

Stead, W.W., Kelly, B.J., & Kolodner, R.M. (2005). Achievable steps toward building a national health information infrastructure in the United States. *JAMIA, 12*(2), 113-120.

Stead, W.W., Kelly, B.J., & Kolodner, R.M. (2005). Achievable steps toward building a National Health Information infrastructure in the United States. *Journal of the American Medical Informatics Association, 12*(2), 113-120.

Stensland, P., & Malterud, K. (1997). New gateways to dialogue in general practice: Development of an illness diary to expand communication. *Scandinavian Journal of Primary Healthcare, 15*, 175-179.

Stewart, K.J. (2003). Trust transfer on the World Wide Web. *Organization Science, 14*(1), 5-17.

Stoel, L., & Lee, K.H. (2003). Modeling the effect of experience on student acceptance of Web-based courseware. *Internet Research, 13*(5), 364-374.

Strauss, A.L., & Corbin, J. (1994). *Grounded theory methodology: An overview.* In N.K. Denzin, & Y.S. Lincoln (Eds.), *Handbook of qualitative research* (pp. 273–285). Thousand Oaks, CA: Sage Publications.

Strauss, A.L., & Corbin, J. (1998). *Basics of qualitative research: Techniques and procedures fordeveloping grounded theory (second edition).* Sage Publications.

Street, R. L., Jr. (2003). Mediated consumer-provider communication in cancer care: The empowering potential of new technologies. *Patient Education Counseling, 50*(1), 99-104.

Subramani, M. (2004). How do suppliers benefit from information technology use in supply chain relationships? *MIS Quarterly, 28*(1), 45-74.

Suh, B., & Han, I. (2002). Effect of trust on customer acceptance of Internet banking. *Electronic Commerce Research and Applications, 1*, 247-263.

Suh, B., & Han, I. (2003). The impact of customer trust and perception of security control on the acceptance of electronic commerce. *International Journal of Electronic Commerce, 7*(3), 135-161.

Suler, J.R. (2000). Psychotherapy in cyberspace: A 5-dimensional model of online and computer-mediated psychotherapy. *CyberPsychology & Behavior, 3*(2), 151-159.

Szajna, B. (1996). Empirical evaluation of the revised technology acceptance model. *Management Science, 42*(1), 85-92.

Tang, P.C., & Lansky, D. (2005). The missing link: Bridging the patient-provider health information gap. *Health Affairs, 24*(5), 1290-1295.

Tang, P.C., & McDonald, C.J. (2001). Computer-based patient-record systems. In E.H. Shortliffe & L.E. Perreault (Eds.). *Medical informatics: Computer applications in healthcare and biomedicine* (Second edition, pp. 327-358). New York: Springer-Verlag.

Tang, P.C., Ash, J.S., Bates, D.W., Overhage, J.M., & Sands, D.Z. (2006). Personal health records: Definitions, benefits, and strategies for overcoming barriers to adoption. *Journal of the American Medical Informatics Association, 13*(2), 121-126.

Tang, P.C., Black, W., Buchanan, J., Young, C.Y., Hooper, D., Lane, S.R., et al. (2003). *PAMFOnline: Integrating EHealth with an electronic medical record system.* Paper presented at the 2003 AMIA Annual Symposium Proceedings.

Tauzin, B. (2006). Building a healthcare system. *Vital Speeches of the Day, April 1, 2006, 72*(12), 378-381.

Tavani, H.T. (1999). Informational privacy, data mining, and the Internet. *Ethics and Information Technology, 1*, 137-145.

Tavani, H.T. (1999). KDD, Data mining, and the challenge for normative privacy. *Ethics and Information Technology, 1*, 265-273.

Taylor, A.R., Cool, C., Belkin, N.J., & Amadio, W.J. (2007). Relationships between categories of relevance criteria and stage in task completion. *Information Processing & Management, 43*(4), 1071-1084.

Taylor, S., Candy, B., Bryar, R., Vrijhoef, J., Esmond, G., Wedzicha, J., et al. (2005). Effectiveness of innovations in nurse led chronic disease management for patients with chronic obstructive pulmonary disease: Systematic review of evidence. *British Medical Journal, 331*(485).

Taylor-Mendes, C. (2007). Proceed with caution: Using Wikipedia as a reference. *Neonatal Network, 26*(3), 140-141.

Teece, D.J. (1980). Economies of scope and the scope of the enterprise. *Journal of Economic Behavior and Organization, 1*(3), 223-247.

The Foundation for Accountability (FACCT). (2000). *Patients and quality: What do they know? What do they want? Results from FACCT consumer research 1996-2000.* Retrieved May 26, 2008, from http://www.markle.org/resources/facct/doclibFiles/documentFile_196.pdf

Thibaut, J.W., & Kelley, H.H. (1959). *The social psychology of groups.* New York: Wiley.

Thompson, P.B. (2001). Privacy, secrecy and security. *Ethics and Information Technology, 3*, 13-19.

Thompson, R.L., Higgins, C.A., and Howell, J.M. (1991). Personal computing: Toward a conceptual model of utilization. *MIS Quarterly, 15*(1), 125-143.

Tidwell, L.C., & Walther, J.B. (2002). Computer-mediated communication effects on disclosure, impressions, and interpersonal evaluations: Getting to know one another a bit at a time. *Human Communication Research, 28*(3), 317-348.

Tobias, R. L. (1996). Healthcare in the information age: An integrated system wide approach. *Vital Speeches of the Day, April 15, 1996, 13*, 411.

Todd, P., & Benbasat, I. (1987). Process tracing methods in decision support systems research: Exploring the black box. *MIS Quarterly, 41*(3), 493–512.

Tornatzky, L.G., & Klein, K.J. (1982). Innovation characteristics and innovation adoption-implementation: A meta-analysis of findings. *IEEE Transactions on Engineering Management, 29*(1), 28-45.

Tran, D.T., Zhang, X., Stolyar, A., & Lober, W.B. (2005) Patient-centered design for a personal health record system. In *Proceedings of AMIA Annual Symposium* (pp. 1140).

Triandis, H.C. (1977). *Interpersonal behavior.* Brooks/Cole Publishing, Monterey, CA.

Triandis, H.C. (1980). Values, attitudes, and interpersonal behavior. In H.E. Howe & M. M. Page (Eds.), *Nebraska Symposium on Motivation 1979* (pp. 195-259). Lincoln, NE: University of Nebraska Press.

Tsiknakis, M., Katehakis, D.G., & Orphanoudakis, S.C. (2002). An open, component-based information infrastructure for integrated health information networks. *International Journal of Medical Informatics 68*, 3-26.

Tulu, B., & Chatterjee, S. (2003, August 4-6). A new security framework for HIPAA-compliant health information systems. In *Proceedings of Americas Conference on Information Systems (AMCIS)* (pp. 929-938). Tampa, FL.

Turkle, S. (1995). *Life on the screen: Identity in the age of the Internet.* New York: Simon & Schuster, Inc.

Turner M., & Beresford, P. (2005). *User controlled research. Its meanings and potential. Final report.* Hampshire, UK: INVOLVE.

UsabilityNet (2006). Key principles of user-centred design. Retrieved June 2006, from http://www.usabilitynet.org/management/b_design.htm

Uslaner, E.M. (2000). *Trust, civic engagement, and the Internet.* European Consortium for Political Research. University of Grenoble, April 6-11. Retrieved May 24, 2008, from http://www.bsos.umd.edu/gvpt/uslaner/Internettrust.pdf

van den Brink, J.L., Moorman, P.W., de Boer, M.F., Pruyn, J.F.A., Verwoerd, C.D. A., & van Bemmel, J.H. (2005). Involving the patient: A prospective study on use, appreciation and effectiveness of an information system in head and neck cancer care. *International Journal of Medical Informatics, 74*, 839-849.

Van Den Haak, M.J., Jong, de, M.D.T., & Schellens, P.J.(2003). Retrospective vs. concurrent think-aloud protocols: Testing the usability of an online library catalogue. *Behavior & Information Technology, 22*(5), 339–351.

Vence, D.L. (2007). SRO SEO. *Marketing News, 41*(13), 4.

Venkatesh, V., Morris, M.G., Davis, G.B., & Davis, F.D. (2003). User acceptance of information technology: Toward a unified view. *MIS Quarterly, 27*(3), 425-478.

Venkatesh, V., Speier, C., & Morris, M.G. (2002). User acceptance enablers in individual decision making about technology: Toward an integrated model. *Decision Science, 22,* 297-316.

Von Korff, M., Gruman, J., Schaefer, J., Curry, S.J., & Wagner, E.H. (1997). Collaborative management of chronic illness. *Annals of Internal Medicine, 127*(12), 1097–1102.

von Neuman, J., & Morgenstern, O. (1944). *The theory of games and economic behavior.* Princeton, NJ: Princeton University Press.

Wagner, E.H., Austin, B.T., Davis, C., Hindmarsh, M., Schaefer, J., & Bonomi, A. (2001). Improving chronic illness care: Translating evidence into action. *Health Affairs, 20*(6), 64–78.

Waitzkin, H. (1984). Doctor-patient communication. Clinical implications of social scientific research. *Journal of the American Medical Association, 252*(17), 2441-2446.

Walker, J., Pan, E., Johnston, D., Adler-Milstein, J., Bates, D.W., & Middleton, B. (2005). The value of healthcare information exchange and interoperability. *Health Affairs Web Exclusive, W5-10-W5-18.*

Wallach, H.S., & Bar-Zvi, M. (2007). Virtual-reality-assisted treatment of flight phobia. *The Israel Journal of Psychiatry and Related Sciences, 44*(1), 29-32.

Waller, A., Franklin, V., Pagliari, C., & Greene, S. (2007) Participatory design of a text message scheduling system to support young people with diabetes. *Health Informatics Journal, 12*(4), 307–321.

Wal-Mart. (2007). *400 health clinics to open in Wal-mart stores during next three years.* Retrieved May 14, 2008, from http://www.walmartfacts.com/articles/default.aspx?id=4973

Walter, Z., & Tung, Y.A. (2002). E-healthcare system design: A consumer preference approach. *International Journal of Healthcare Technology and Management, 4*(1/2), 53-70.

Walters, B., Barnard, D., & Paris, S. (2006). Patient portals and e-visits. *Journal of Ambulatory Care Management, 29*(3), 222-224.

Walther, J.B., & Burgoon, J.K. (1992). Relational communication in computer-mediated interaction. *Human Communication Research, 19*, 50-88.

Wang, F., Helian, N., & Jayaram, N. (2002, June 6-8). A management information system for public health. *European Conference on Information Systems 2002* (pp. 1454-1464). Gdansk, Poland.

Wang, S.J., Middleton, B., Prosser, L.A., Bardon, C.G., Spurr, C.D., Carchidi, P.J., et al., (2003). A cost-benefit analysis of electronic medical records in primary care. *The American Journal of Medicine, 114*(5), 397-403.

Wang, W., & Benbasat, I. (2005). Trust in and adoption of online recommendation agents. *Journal of the Association for Information Systems, 6*(3), 72-101.

Wang, Y.S. (2003). The adoption of electronic tax filing systems: an empirical study. *Government Information Quarterly, 20*(4), 333–352.

Wang, Y.S., Wang, Y.M., Lin, H.H., & Tang, T.I. (2003). Determinants of user acceptance of Internet banking: An empirical study. *International Journal of Service Industry Management, 14*(5), 501–519.

Wangberg, S., Gammon, D., & Spitznogle, K. (2007). In the eyes of the beholder: Exploring psychologists' attitudes towards and use of eTherapy in Norway. *CyberPsychology & Behaviour, 10*(3), 418-423.

Wangberg, S.C. (2007). An Internet-based diabetes self-care intervention tailored to self-efficacy [Electronic Version]. *Health Education Research.* Retrieved May 13, 2008, from http://her.oxfordjournals.org/cgi/content/full/cym014v1

Wareham, J., & Klein, R. (2003). Intermediation structures in electronic healthcare portals. In A. Armoni (Ed.), *Effective healthcare information systems* (pp. 237-248). Hersey, PA: IRM Press.

Warren, S., & Brandeis, L.D. (1890). The right to privacy. *Harvard Law Review, 4*, 193-220.

Warsi, A., LaValley, M.P., Wang, P.S., Avorn, J., & Solomon, D.H. (2003). Arthritis self-management education programs: A meta-analysis of the effect on pain and disability. *Arthritis & Rheumatism, 48*(8), 2207–2213.

Warsi, A., Wang, P., LaValley, M., & Avorn, J. (2004). Self-management education programs in chronic disease: A systematic review and methodological critique of the literature. *Archives of Internal Medicine, 164*(15), 1641.

Wasson, J.H. (2006). When all things are not equal. *Journal of Ambulatory Care Management, 29*(3), 235-237.

White, M.D., & Marsh, E.E. (2006). Content analysis: A flexible methodology. *Library Trends, 55*(1), 22–45.

Wichowski, H.C., & Kubsch, S.M. (1997). The relationship of self-perception of illness and compliance with healthcare regimens. *Journal of Advanced Nursing, 25*, 548-553.

Wickramasinghe, N., & Goldberg, S. (2005, June 6-8). A framework for delivering M-health excellence. In *Proceedings of the 18th Bled eConference eIntegration in Action* (pp. 1-21). Bled, Slovenia.

Wickramasinghe, N., & Mills, G.L. (2001, June 27-29). Knowledge management systems: A healthcare initiative with lessons for us all. In *Proceedings of the 9th European Conference on Information Systems* (pp. 763-774). Bled, Slovenia.

Willems, D. (1998). Inhaling drugs and making worlds: A proliferation of lungs and asthmas. In M. Berg, & A. Mol (Eds.), *Differences in Medicine: Unravelling Practices, Techniques and Bodies* (pp. 105-118). Durham, NC: Duke University Press.

Williams, P., Nicholas, D., Huntington, P., & McLean, F. (2002). Surfing for health: User evaluation of a health information Web site. *Health Information and Libraries Journal, 19*, 98–108.

Williamson, C. (2001). What does involving consumers in research mean? *QJM: An International Journal of Medicine, 94*(12), 661-664.

Wilson, E.V. (2003). Asynchronous healthcare communication. *Communications of the ACM, 46*(6), 79-84.

Wilson, E.V. (2008). Creating patient-centered e-health. In N. Wickramasinghe, & E. Geisler (Eds.), *Encyclopedia of Healthcare Information Systems,* (pp. 318-324). Hershey, PA: IGI Publishing.

Wilson, E.V., & Lankton, N.K. (2004). Modeling patients' acceptance of provider-delivered e-health. *Journal of the American Medical Informatics Association, 11*(4), 241-248

Wilson, E.V., Mao, E., & Lankton, N.K. (2005). Predicting continuing acceptance of IT in conditions of sporadic use. In N.C. Romano, Jr. (Ed.), *Proceedings of the Eleventh Americas Conference on Information Systems.* Omaha, NE, USA.

Wold, H. (1989). Introduction to the second generation of multivariate analysis. In H. Wold (Ed.), *Theoretical Empiricism* (pp. vii-xi). New York: Paragon House.

Wold, H. (1998). Partial least squares. In S. Kotz, & N.L. Johnson (Eds.), *Encyclopedia of Statistical Sciences* (Vol. 6, pp. 581-591). New York: Wiley.

Woodard, T.D. (2005). Addressing variation in hospital quality: Is six sigma the answer? *Journal of Healthcare Management, 50*(4), 226-236.

Worden, J.K., & Flynn, B.S. (2001). The case for persuasive health messages. *Effective Clinical Practice, 4*(2), 73-75.

Wright, J. (2002). Online counselling: Learning from writing therapy. *British Journal of Guidance & Counselling, 30*(3), 287-298.

Wrightsman, L.S. (1991). Interpersonal trust and attitudes toward human nature. In J.P. Robinson, P.R. Shaver & L.S. Wrightsman (Eds.), *Measures of personality and social psychological attitudes: Volume 1: Measures of social psychological attitudes* (pp. 373-412). San Diego, CA: Academic Press, Inc.

Wroblewski, L. (2002). *Site-seeing: A visual approach to Web usability.* New York: Hungry Minds, Inc.

Wroblewski, L. (2006). *Where visual design meets usability.* Retrieved May 26, 2008, from http://www.lukew.com/ff/entry.asp?363

Xu, Y., & Chen, Z. (2006). Relevance judgment: What do information consumers consider beyond topicality? *Journal of the American Society for Information Science and Technology, 57*(7), 961-973.

Yasnoff, W.A., Humphreys, B.L., Overhage, J.M., Detmer, D.E., Brennan, P.F., Morris, R.W., Middleton, B., Bates, D.W., & Fanning, J.P. (2004). A consensus action agenda for achieving the national health information infrastructure. *Journal of American Medical International Association, 11*(4), 332-228.

Ydreborg, B., Ekberg, K., & Nordlund, A. (2006). Health, quality of life, social network and use of healthcare: A comparison between those granted and those not granted disability pensions. *Disability and Rehabilitation, 28*, 25-32.

Yellowlees, P.M., & Cook, J.N. (2006). Education about hallucinations using an Internet virtual reality system: A qualitative survey. *Academic Psychiatry, 30*(6), 534-539.

Zaheer, A., McEvily, B., & Perrone, V. (1998). Does trust matter: Exploring the effects of interorganizational and interpersonal trust on performance. *Organization Science, 9*(2), 141-159.

Zhang, J. (2005). Guest editorial: Human-centered computing in health information systems. *Journal of Biomedical Informatics, 38*(1), 1–3.

Zhang, J., Johnson, T.R., Patel, V.L., Paige, D.L., & Kubose, T. (2003). Using usability heuristics to evaluate patient safety of medical devices. *Journal of Biomedical Informatics, 36*(1–2), 23–30.

Zikmund, W.G. (1997). *Business research methods (fifth edition).* Sydney, Australia: The Dryden Press.

Zucker, L.G. (1986). Production of trust: Institutional sources of economic structure 1840-1920. In B.M. Straw & L.L. Cummings (Eds.), *Research in organizational behavior* (pp. 53-111). Greenwich, CT: JAI Press.

Zwar, N., Harris, M., Griffiths, R., Roland, M., Dennis, S., Powell Davies, G., & Hasan, I. (2006). *APHCRI stream four: A systematic review of chronic disease management.* Australian National University. Retrieved May 28, 2008, from http://www.anu.edu.au/aphcri/Domain/ChronicDiseaseMgmt/Approved_25_Zwar.pdf

About the Contributors

E. Vance Wilson received a PhD in information systems in 1995 from the University of Colorado at Boulder. He is currently an associate clinical professor at Arizona State University. Prof. Wilson's research focuses on organizational aspects of human-computer interaction with specific interests in e-health, computer-mediated communication, decisional guidance, and supporting technology for software development teams. He is supervising editor of the Information Systems and Healthcare Department at *Communications of the AIS*.

* * *

Natalie Armstrong currently holds a post-doctoral fellowship at the Health Sciences Research Institute, Warwick Medical School, University of Warwick, UK. Her background is in medical sociology, and her research interests lie primarily in the exploration of lay perceptions and experiences of health, illness, and healthcare, using qualitative methods and drawing on sociological theory. She has published work on women's experiences and understandings of cervical cancer screening, and on patients' and health professionals' perspectives on e-health within diabetes care. She is currently working on a programme of research exploring the use of an Internet-based self-management system for diabetes care.

Elaine A. Blechman received her PhD in social and clinical psychology from UCLA in 1971. She is a professor of psychology at University of Colorado-Boulder. Her research and policy work on resilience-promoting long-term care has been supported by the National Institute of Mental Health and the National Institute of Drug Abuse and has resulted in seven books and several hundred journal articles and chapters. Dr. Blechman is the President of Prosocial Applications, Inc., supplier of The Smart PHR™, an unbound, consumer-controlled PHR system. Embedded care plans automate delivery of known effective treatments to individuals with chronic conditions, including cancer survivors. She is active in setting standards for consumer-centered health information technology and serves as cochair of the consumer empowerment technical committee of the ANSI/HIMSS Health Information Technology Standards panel. With colleagues at several universities and medical centers, Dr. Blechman is investigating how an unbound PHR system can improve quality, access, and efficiency of long-term healthcare.

Gloria Boone is a professor of communication at Suffolk University in Boston, Massachusetts. She teaches classes in advertising, new media, usability, Web design, and rhetoric. She has published books on rhetorical communication and on business communication. Her articles deal with usability of Web sites, social media marketing, advertising, and rhetoric. She consults with businesses and healthcare organizations on advertising, usability, communication, and integrated marketing communication. As a classically trained rhetorician, she believes that the arts and the humanities inform "new" developments in Web design, technology, and communication. She holds a PhD from Ohio University. Visit Gloria's Web site at http://infoacrs.com.

Carlo Busolin graduated in industrial design at the Faculty of Art and Design IUAV in Venice and received a Master in Medical Design in Venice. He works as a designer in a company related to architecture and naval preparation fields. He has worked for the new Venice-Mestre Hospital where he contributed to create the guidance signs project. He has been involved in developing research projects on e-Health. Some of his projects were reported and published in important design competitions.

Stephen Chau is a general manager for Verdant Health. In this role, he is currently involved in a number of e-health developments, both commercial and research. He was previously a research fellow in the Smart Internet Technology CRC and undertook a number of research projects in e-health. He graduated from the University of Tasmania initially with a BEc and a Grad Dip Sci (IT). He returned to the university in 1995 to complete an honours degree in computing and later commence a PhD in the School of Information Systems. His doctoral research explored the utilisation of e-commerce amongst thirty-four SMEs from two states of Australia.

Diego Conforti received the first degree in cognitive psychology at the University of Trento, Italy. Until 2005, he had been an officer at the Health Planning and Research Unit of the Department of Health of the Autonomous Province of Trento, Italy. Since 2006, he has been the key person for e-health programs and activities at the Health Services Organization Unit of the Department of Health, Trento (Italy). His main interests are innovative e-health services for citizens and integrated health information systems.

Elizabeth Cummings commenced her PhD in 2004 and is researching the impact of ICTs on health outcomes. She has been involved in a number of research projects in this area. Elizabeth has over 25 years' experience in healthcare in Australia. Elizabeth is a registered nurse and midwife and has worked in both clinical and administrative positions in nursing. She has also worked as strategic information manager for the state-based organisation the Tasmanian General Practice Divisions. Elizabeth has been involved in developing and implementing general practice ICT initiatives, and closely involved with national e-health initiatives. In 2005, she joined the Smart Internet Technology Cooperative Research Centre.

Juanita Dawson is a doctoral student in the School of Information Systems and Technology at Claremont Graduate University. She is also a research scholar in engineering and information technology at Raytheon Corporation. She holds a BS in mathematics from Grambling State University, an MBA in computer information systems from California State University, and an MS in information systems and Technology from Claremont Graduate University. Her research is focused on privacy, security, and interoperability of information systems. Her current research projects include employer-sponsored personal health records and patient-centered e-health information systems. She is a member of the American Medical Informatics Association (AMIA), the Association of Computer Machinery (ACM), and IEEE Computer Society, and has been published in conferences including AMIA and SIGMIS.

Gonzalez Bernaldo de Quirós, MD, is vice director of strategic planning in the Hospital Italiano de Buenos Aires in Argentina. He also has academic appointments in the Internal Medicine Division, and he is head of human physiology at the School of Medicine in HIBA. He has developed research and educational programs in medical informatics, clinical management and chronic disease management, and clinical research in internal medicine. More than 20 fellows have been trained in these programs under the supervision of the Department of Research and Education at the Hospital Italiano. His research focuses on the development of electronic medical records and disease management programs

Michael Dinger is currently a doctoral student in management information systems at Clemson University. His research interests include the IT workforce, absorptive capacity, trust in online environments, and electronic commerce. Michael earned a BS in business administration at Presbyterian College.

Claudio Eccher graduated cum laude in physics in 1996 at the University of Trento, Italy. In 2006, he received the PhD degree in communication and information technology from the ICT International Doctorate School, University of Trento. He has worked as researcher at the e-Health Applied Research Unit of the Bruno Kessler Foundation since 1997. His current research field focuses on knowledge-based services aimed to healthcare professionals. In the past, he has worked on several research topics: image analysis in medicine, computer-based collaborative systems supporting the care process, and modeling languages for systems biology.

Stefano Forti received the MS degree in physics from the University of Trento, Italy, in 1987. He is head of the E-Health Applied Research Unit at Bruno Kessler Foundation, Trento, Italy. His current research interests are in the field of e-Health, and are mainly focused on consumer health informatics and user-centered design in health information systems. In the past, he worked on a variety of research topics, including integrated electronic patient records, Web-based distributed cooperative systems, clinical decision support systems, and tools for continuous monitoring of quality of clinical care.

Ann Fruhling is an assistant professor at the University of Nebraska at Omaha. Her research includes agile system development methods, human computer interaction usability, user interface design, and e-health acceptance. Dr. Fruhling is the principle investigator of an extensive research project that involves designing and implementing a public health emergency response system. She has published papers in journals such as *Journal of Management Information Systems, Communications of the AIS, Journal of Computer Information Systems, International Journal of Electronic Healthcare, International Journal of Cooperative Information Systems,* and *Journal of Electronic Commerce Research.*

Linda Gallant's teaching and research interests include the application of research methods to social computing, and the maximization of information and communication technology (ICT) to advance human communication in multiple contexts—healthcare, politics, and the workplace. She is published in *Personal and Ubiquitous Computing, Academic Exchange Quarterly, Qualitative Research Reports in Communication, First Monday,* and *e-Service Journal.* She brings a disciplinary background in communication studies to a burgeoning area of user experience design. Specifically, she investigates how New Media facilitate human communication by investigating Internet-based technologies as social artifacts. A central interest in her research and teaching is how a technology's design and development (information architecture, usability, and rhetorical strategies) impacts its social and cultural uses, whether these uses were intended or unintended by the technology's original engineers and designers.

Deede Gammon is a psychologist with nearly 20 years of experience in telemedicine and e-health research and development (R&D). She has led a number of R&D programs at Norwegian Centre for Telemedicine, along with being a part-time associate professorship at the Faculty of Medicine, University of Tromsø. Her focus has been on increasing knowledge about patients' and the public's use of information and communication technologies for health purposes as a basis understanding the implications of e-health for patients, the public, health providers, and health policy.

Morten Hertzum received his PhD from University of Copenhagen, Denmark, in 1994, and has since 2003 held a position as associate professor in computer science at Roskilde University, Denmark. Dr. Hertzum's overall research interest concerns how technologies support—and otherwise affect—human activities. This interest has led to research in the areas of human-computer interaction, computer supported cooperative work, information seeking and retrieval, and software engineering. Dr. Hertzum is currently involved in research projects on healthcare IT, effects-driven IT development, and cultural aspects of usability evaluation.

Thomas A. Horan, PhD, is director of the Kay Center for E-Health Research and associate professor at Claremont Graduate University's School of Information Systems and Technology. In this capacity, Dr. Horan is responsible for directing a wide range of research and policy studies on health information systems. He also serves in an advisory role for several private sector companies and heath agencies. Dr. Horan is a member of the American Medical Informatics Association (AMIA), the Association of Computer Machinery (ACM), and the Association of Information Systems (AIS). He has published numerous technical articles in journals such as *Communications of the ACM*, *Communications of the AIS*, and *International Journal of Healthcare Technology and Management*. Dr. Horan has his Master's and PhD degrees from Claremont Graduate University.

Cynthia A. Irizarry, PhD, is an associate professor of communication studies at Stetson University. Her areas of research include organizational and corporate communication, particularly in healthcare contexts, utilizing qualitative research design. Her research has appeared in a variety of publications, including *e-Service Journal* and *Qualitative Research Reports in Communication*. She has also worked as a consultant with governmental and private agencies exploring mediated message design in health promotion and corporate communication campaigns.

Olli Järvinen received a PhD from the Turku School of Economics, Department of Management, and a PhLic from the University of Turku, Department of Information Technology. Dr. Järvinen has worked in ICT for nearly 30 years, including 15 years as a senior system analyst in a large hospital, and has visited as a researcher at North Carolina State University on a Fulbright Scholarship. Currently, he is head of ICT for the Finnish Game and Fisheries Research Institute. Dr. Järvinen's research interests focus on organizational privacy policies and practices.

Jan-Are K. Johnsen is a psychologist and project manager at the Norwegian Centre for Telemedicine. He is currently pursuing a PhD within the fields of computer mediated communication and psychology.

His line of research focuses on how people use text-based communication to manage self-presentation, and in turn, how this knowledge can be utilized in designing systems for interpersonal communication, including e-health systems.

Richard Klein is an assistant professor of Mmanagement at Clemson University. He holds a PhD in business administration from Georgia State University; MS in technology management from Mercer University; and MA in economics from Boston University. Dr. Klein researches electronic business initiatives, intermediation, and digitally-enabled supply chain management with an emphasis on the healthcare industry. He has published in top journals including *Decision Sciences, Journal of Management Information Systems,* and *Journal of Operations Management.* Dr. Klein has presented his work at national and international conferences, including the Annual Meeting of the Academy of Management, the Americas Conference on Information Systems, the European Conference on Information Systems, and the Institute for Operations Research and the Management Sciences Annual Meeting.

Nancy Lankton received the PhD in computer information systems at Arizona State University in 2000. She is an assistant professor in the Department of Accounting and Information Systems at Michigan State University and teaches database technology and information systems controls. Prior to this, she had extensive work experience in accounting and auditing. Her research interests include technology acceptance and continuance, e-services, habit, trust, and technology investment decisions. She has published in the *Journal of the American Medical Informatics Association, Communications of the AIS, E-Service Journal,* and *International Journal of Healthcare Management & Technology.* Dr. Lankton is a member of the Association for Information Systems (AIS) and the Information Systems Auditing and Control Association (ISACA).

Cynthia LeRouge, PhD, is an assistant professor at Saint Louis University. Her current research interests relate to healthcare information systems, and in particular telemedicine. Dr. LeRouge has held various management roles in practice in the software, healthcare, public accounting, and petrochemical industries. She has over 35 publications including research articles in journals, including *Decision Support Systems, International Journal of Healthcare Technology and Management, Journal, International Journal of Human Computer Studies, Journal of Computer Information Systems, Journal of Information Technology Education, Journal of Information Systems Education,* and *Communications of the AIS,* edited chapters in research-based books, and peer-reviewed conference proceedings. Dr. LeRouge has a PhD in information systems from the University of South Florida.

Nicolò Luppino received his first degree in industrial design from the IUAV University in Venice, Italy. Here, he also received the University Master's degree in medical design and is taking the MS degree in product design. Today, he's actively collaborating with Bruno Kessler Foundation, Trento, to the realization of a personal health record system. In the recent past, he has worked on realization of a visual information system in the New Venice-Mestre Hospital. He is interested in all design aspects, from health to daily life.

Jiao Ma, PhD, is an assistant professor at Saint Louis University (SLU). Dr. Ma holds a secondary appointment at Center for Outcomes Research/Internal Medicine, SLU. Her research interests are in human factors engineering (specifically, human error investigation, user-centered design, data mining applications in aviation, and healthcare). Dr. Ma received her PhD and MS in human factors engineering from the State University of New York at Buffalo in 2005 and 2002, respectively. She produced nearly 20 journal/proceeding papers and Federal Aviation Administration technical reports. Before joining SLU, Dr. Ma worked as a senior usability consultant and led user-centered design for healthcare applications. Her clients included Metlife and Healthlink.

Giovanni Martini took a degree in sociology at the University of Trento. Until April 2007, he was the director of Health Innovation and Education Unit of the Department of Health of the Autonomous Province of Trento (Italy). Since May 2007, he has been a freelance social researcher and is involved in international projects, mainly funded by the European Union, about the development of technological infrastructures to support the daily activities of frail elderly people. His main interests have been health policy, health promotion, equity in health, health research, bioethics, health education and training, e-health, domotics, and social use of new technologies.

Alejandro Mauro, MD is a third-year resident of Medical Informatics Program at the Hospital Italiano de Buenos Aires (HIBA). He has been working as leader project in the development of HIBA's Personal Health Record System (PHRS) for the last two years, working with HMO patients and applying UCD techniques for the design and evaluation of the PHRS (see Web site at http://www.alejandro.mauro.name). His research interests center around the design, development, usability evaluation, and implementation of computer-based health information systems.

John Powell is associate clinical professor of epidemiology and public health at the Health Sciences Research Institute, Warwick Medical School, University of Warwick, UK, where he leads an e-health research group. He has degrees in Social and Political Sciences and Clinical Medicine, and trained in psychiatry before becoming an academic public health physician. His research interests are in consumer use of the Internet, particularly in the area of mental health. He is currently working on a programme of research with NHS Direct Online, the largest provider of online health information in the UK.

Barbara Purin graduated in mathematics from the University of Trento (Italy). Since 2002, she has been working at the Telemedicine and Medical Informatics Laboratory of the Centre for Scientific and Technological Research (now e-Health Applied Research Unit at the Bruno Kessler Foundation). The activities of the Research Unit cover basic and applied research in the field of consumer health informatics and user-centred design in health information systems. Her research interests focus mainly on designing and conducting usability tests of innovative PHR prototypes, and then on analysing the collected data.

Ebrahim Randeree is currently an assistant professor in the College of Information at Florida State University, USA. He has published in many journals and conferences. His research interests are related to technology adoption, outsourcing, information assurance, strategic information technology, and knowledge management with a focus on the healthcare arena. He teaches health informatics, strategic management, and information technology.

Michel Sassene is in the process of completing his master's degree in computer science and international development studies at Roskilde University, Denmark. Michel Sassene's research interests centre upon the intersections between organisations, people, and IT. These interests have thus far led to work in the healthcare sector with special attention to IT-supported self-management of chronic diseases and collaboration between the primary and secondary sectors. After October 2007, Michel Sassene will join the State Employer's Authority to work on the implementation of large-scale e-learning projects for state employees.

Joseph Tan, PhD, is editor-in-chief, *International Journal of Healthcare Information Systems and Informatics*. His professional background spans a broad spectrum of disciplines and research interests with demonstrated ability to serve in both academia and industry. He is a lead investigator in redefining the frontiers of interdisciplinary and translational business and health IT knowledge development and expansion, including active involvement in collaborative research and multidisciplinary joint-grant submissions. He has achieved recognized scholarship in teaching and learning with students' yearly nominations for teaching excellence awards and networks widely with key decision and policy makers, as well as academic scholars and practitioners at local, provincial/state, national and international levels, including private, public, and nongovernmental organizations and universities. His has taken leadership in curriculum and program accreditation, peer-reviewed journal publications and book reviews, online education and programming, planning and organization of symposiums and conferences, development of book series, special issue journals, and federal grant proposals. His last 20-year academic experience includes full-time employment in academia; private and nonprofit sector organizations, as well as consulting and executive program development activities catering to executives and foreign delegation. His overall career focus is on reshaping the landscape of IS/IT applications and promotion in e-Health informatics through cross-disciplinary thinking/project partnering with diverse practitioners, clinicians, researchers, and a variety of user communities.

Bengisu Tulu, PhD, is an assistant professor in the Department of Management at Worcester Polytechnic Institute, Massachusetts. She is also a research fellow in the Kay Center for E-Health Research at Claremont Graduate University. She holds a BS in mathematics from Middle East Technical University, Turkey and an MS and PhD in information systems and technology from Claremont Graduate University. Her research is focused on the use of information technology within healthcare. Her current research projects include user centric personal health records for people with disabilities, Internet-based telemedicine, business value of telemedicine and healthcare outsourcing. Dr. Tulu has published in respected scholarly journals and refereed conferences, including *Telemedicine & e-Health Journal, IEEE Network, IEEE Journal on Selected Areas in Communications,* and *Communications of the AIS.*

Paul Turner is an associate professor at the University of Tasmania. Since joining the university in the year 2000, Paul has been very active in conducting and coordinating research at basic, applied, and strategic levels across a range of industry sectors with a particular focus on systems approaches in e-health, forensic computing, and e-business. These research activities have led to Paul having been directly involved in raising research grants, consultancies, and scholarships to a value of more than $4.5 million. Paul has built a strong reputation for his capacity to make original and innovative contributions to information systems research, and is particularly well-known for his involvement in multidisciplinary research, most notably with the schools of medicine, pharmacy, and nursing. Since 2001, Paul has also published more than 100 peer-reviewed papers in academic journals, books, and conferences.

John A. Valenza is associate professor, Department of Diagnostic Sciences and Executive Associate Dean, the University of Texas Dental Branch at Houston. Since joining the faculty in 1987, he has served as director, General Practice Residency Program, associate dean for patient care, and interim chair, Department of Diagnostic Sciences. As Executive Associate Dean of the Dental Branch, he led the school's conversion to electronic patient records, digital radiography, clinical simulation and faculty practice, and oversees the school's educational technology. He has numerous publications on technology and patient care, and has lectured extensively on computers in dental practice.

Muhammad Walji is assistant professor in the Department of Diagnostic Sciences at the University of Texas Dental Branch focused on informatics research. He has a MS and PhD in Health Informatics and was trained as a National Library of Medicine (NLM) fellow from 2003–2006. He has published numerous papers and conducted extensive research in the area of consumer-health informatics, human-computer interaction, and persuasive technology. He is a member of the Health Information Management Systems Society, American Medical Informatics Association, the American Dental Education Association, and the International Association of Dental Researchers.

Melinda Whetstone is a doctoral student in the College of Information at Florida State University, USA. Her research interests are related to electronic health record systems, personal health records, patient empowerment, and knowledge management with a focus on healthcare.

Jiajie Zhang is the Doris L. Ross professor and the associate dean of Research at School of Health Information Sciences at University of Texas at Houston. He has done extensive research in biomedical informatics, cognitive science, human-centered computing, information visualization, decision making, and computational modeling. He is a fellow of American College of Medical Informatics.

Index

W